THE GOUT

A Medical Microcosm
in a Changing World

THE GOUT

A Medical Microcosm
in a Changing World

Dorian Haskard

World Scientific

NEW JERSEY · LONDON · SINGAPORE · BEIJING · SHANGHAI · TAIPEI · CHENNAI

Published by

World Scientific Publishing Europe Ltd.

57 Shelton Street, Covent Garden, London WC2H 9HE

Head office: 5 Toh Tuck Link, Singapore 596224

USA office: 27 Warren Street, Suite 401-402, Hackensack, NJ 07601

Library of Congress Cataloging-in-Publication Data

Names: Haskard, Dorian, author.

Title: The gout : a medical microcosm in a changing world / Dorian Haskard.

Description: New Jersey : World Scientific, [2025] | Includes bibliographical references and index. |
   Contents: Thomas Sydenham and His Associates -- Some Gout Physicians of the Eighteenth
   Century -- Pills, Powders and Other Potions -- The French Remedy -- The Discovery of
   Uric Acid -- More Pills and Potions -- Controlling Uric Acid -- Crystallising Inflammation --
   From Colchicum to Colchicine -- In the Family -- Triggers and Protectors --
   The Humanness of Gout -- Food, Gout and Global Health.

Identifiers: LCCN 2025006462 | ISBN 9781800616486 (hardcover) |
   ISBN 9781800616493 (ebook for institutions) | ISBN 9781800616509 (ebook for individuals)

Subjects: MESH: Gout--history | Gout--therapy | Gout Suppressants | Life Style--history |
   Socioeconomic Factors--history

Classification: LCC RC629 | NLM WE 11.1 | DDC 616.3/999--dc23/eng/20250212

LC record available at https://lccn.loc.gov/2025006462

British Library Cataloguing-in-Publication Data

A catalogue record for this book is available from the British Library.

Cover image by James Gillray, *Punch Cures the Gout, the Colic and the Tisick* (1799).
Courtesy of the Yale Center for British Art (Paul Mellon Collection), public domain.

First published 2025 (hardcover)
Reprinted 2025 (in paperback edition)
ISBN 978-1-80061-879-4 (pbk)

For any available supplementary material, please visit
https://www.worldscientific.com/worldscibooks/10.1142/Q0486#t=suppl

Desk Editors: Nambirajan Karuppiah/Rosie Williamson

Typeset by Stallion Press
Email: enquiries@stallionpress.com

About the Author

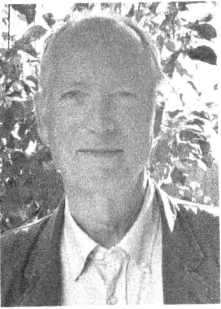

Dorian Haskard is a professor of cardiovascular medicine and rheumatology at Imperial College London. He took a winding path into medicine, with interests including geology, physiology and psychology. After undergraduate years at the University of Oxford, he trained as a doctor at the Middlesex, Royal London and Guy's Hospitals in London and spent two years studying at the University of Texas Southwestern Medical School in Dallas. Having qualified as a physician, he practised for many years as a consultant rheumatologist at the Hammersmith Hospital in London. In parallel, he has pursued an academic career researching the cell and molecular bases of heart attacks, strokes and other cardiovascular problems in rheumatic diseases. He advocates a holistic approach to health and the importance of multidisciplinary teamwork in clinical medicine and medical research. To this end, he initiated the popular Imperial College Science in Medicine School Team Prize being held for the fifth time in 2025. He is a British Heart Foundation Emeritus Professor and a fellow of the Linnean Society of London, the Royal College of Physicians and the UK Academy of Medical Sciences. His pastimes include gardening and thinking about connectivity in the environment.

Preface

G out is a legend among diseases. There can be few other topics in the history of medicine upon which so many social, scientific and medical prejudices and assumptions have been assembled. The very word is ambiguous, as 'the Gout' and 'gout' are not the same. While 'the Gout' was a loosely defined concept, linked in our minds to Georgian excess, 'gout' refers to the modern disease. This story charts how one emerged scientifically from the other and how changes in treatment, mostly commercially driven, tailgated onto the changing understanding of the condition. The book addresses whether it is fair to blame an unhealthy lifestyle, given what we now know about individual genetic variations that render some individuals particularly susceptible, all superimposed on the genetic changes during evolution that have made gout a peculiarly human condition. Although, historically, gout was a disease of the rich, no longer is this solely the case, and the story has an uncertain ending with gout now among the consequences of poor living in our deteriorating environment.

I should say from the outset that I do not suffer from gout and can only sympathise with those that have experienced its terrible torments and tortures. My interest is as a doctor rather than as a patient and dates back to long ago when I was instructed as a junior to make a presentation on a patient with gout to the Medical Staff Round at the London (now Royal London) Hospital. It was daunting, as I knew that the senior staff would be there, eager to show the clear sky between their knowledge and mine, as would my peer group, who perhaps would bear happy witness! Adding to the challenge, a dip into the textbooks quickly revealed how much there was to know about gout that I had not been taught as a medical student. I put the time into preparing the talk, and it went fine, but the sense in the room was not electric. Was it my immature delivery style, or was it that I simply did not know enough about the subject? It seemed to me to be a truly fascinating topic with a rich cultural and scientific history. So, why were they not more excited?

A week or two later, I visited my professor of rheumatology, Harry Currey (1925–1998), to get some feedback. Now fired up, I asked about opportunities for research. He coughed a bit before he spoke, as was usual, and gave me his frank and honest opinion. My presentation had been okay, but gout was yesterday's disease and was academically dead. Everyone knew it was caused by uric acid, and we have good drugs to treat acute painful attacks, and to lower uric acid levels and prevent the attacks from happening in the first place. He also mentioned that cutting back on the beer was often a solution. Anyway, there was not much gout about, and that was why I had not been taught more about it at medical school. He offered me a different project, which I snapped up and moved on.

Some 10 years later, much water had passed under the bridge. I had had some success in researching the biology of inflammation at the Southwestern Medical School in Dallas, Texas, under the guidance of the great Morris Ziff (1913–2005). When I returned to London, I was invited to set up a laboratory at the Royal Postgraduate Medical School at the Hammersmith, long since absorbed into Imperial College. In looking for a disease into which to apply some of my insights, my thoughts returned to gout. Over the next few years, my colleagues and I published a series of papers providing new cellular and molecular details on how an acute inflammatory attack of gout kick-starts and then how it spontaneously resolves. I started to give lectures on inflammation in gout and, always curious, to read about broader aspects in the long textbook chapters I had previously skimmed and then older books describing a condition ever more nebulous as I penetrated backwards in time.

So, why go to the trouble of writing a book when so much has been written already? The vast existing library on 'the Gout' and on

modern gout splits into five categories. In the first are the ancient manuscripts. Assuming one is armed with a mastery of the old languages,
one can enjoy writings on gout dating back to Greece, Rome and
the Byzantine era. For me, these worthy parchments are mostly best
left to classicists. However, many of the speculations contained therein
held a pride of place in the thinking of orthodox physicians well into
the seventeenth century. With the Enlightenment and the beginning
of modern scientific endeavour, confidence that important truths were
hidden within old manuscripts ebbed away. The poet physician Richard
Blackmore (1654–1729), writing in 1723, was scathing of the attention paid
to the classical physicians. He reserved especial derision for Hippocrates
(ca. 460–ca. 370 BCE), the Greek physician who lived on the Island of
Kos and who we still revere for providing the Oath that acts as the blue-
print for doctors' good behaviour. Blackmore considered Hippocrates's
aphorisms as:

> … so poor and vulgar, that they are not greatly superior to such
> remarks as these: If a man eats and sleeps, it is a good sign. If a
> man refuses Meat and cannot rest, it is bad. If he rejects his Med-
> icines it is ill, nor is it well if he has a violent Pain in his Side. If a
> man sprains his leg, it is ill, if he breaks it is worse: such as these
> are many of his certain Aphorisms. But his dubious ones are like
> a String of logical Topicks, or probable Doctrines in the Church
> of Rome, which are sometimes true and sometimes false, and as
> often fail as they hold good.[1]

Actually, although on the whole it is easy to agree with Blackmore on
the utility of the classic texts, Hippocrates's five aphorisms on gout have
largely stood the test of time:

VI-28: eunuchs do not take the gout, nor become bald.
VI-29: a woman does not take the gout, unless her menses be
stopped.
VI-30: a youth does not get gout before sexual intercourse.

VI-40: in gouty affections, inflammation subsides within 40 days.
XI-55: gouty affections become active in spring and autumn.

Aphorism XI-55 is somewhat enigmatic, but it was widely accepted as true by the seventeenth- and eighteenth-century physicians. Perhaps it was the seasonal foods that did it, something we no longer notice now that globalisation provides food from around the world throughout the year.

In the second category, there is a long and distinguished pedigree of books, discourses, dissertations, treatises, essays, chapters and pamphlets with which one can trace the very slow transition of 'the Gout' into modern gout, starting for my purposes with *Treatise on the Gout or Joint-Evil* by Benjamin Welles (ca. 1616–1678) (Figure P.1).[2] The challenge of writing about gout in the early days of scientific medicine was nicely captured by the physician William Gairdner (1793–1867):

> In describing this disease, we are almost irresistibly led to employ a figurative and somewhat poetical language. Its phenomena readily adapt themselves to the metaphor of a surging mass, a coction, or a wandering vapour, and authors endow its assumed matter with a kind of separate existence, describing its wanderings to and fro, up and down in the body, till it chooses its local habitation there to mature its strength, exhaust its fire, and thence be eliminated from the system.[3]

Up to the twentieth century, many of these authors, if not most, considered that they suffered from gout themselves, and their own sufferings add empathy and insight into their writing. However, interesting as they are, many of the early works cannot be taken scientifically much beyond their times. They were written in an age of nascent science, and the science has moved on. That said, many demonstrate a very high standard of writing that is often quite humbling. Others are rambling, repetitive, and dull, and often just pufferies to attract patients. Some stray on to sounding boards and expound on matters of personal interest, curiosity or importance to

Benjamin Welles (1669)	*A Treatise on the Gout or Joint-Evil*
Thomas Sydenham (1683)	*A Treatise on the Gout and Dropsy*
Thomas Willis (1685)	*The London Practice of Physick*
Clopton Havers (1691)	*Osteologia Nova*
John Colbatch (1697)	*A Treatise of the Gout*
William Musgrave (1703)	*De Arthritide Symptomatica Dissertatio*
George Cheyne (1721)	*An Essay on the Gout*
Richard Blackmore (1726)	*The Gout, a Rheumatism and the King's Evil*
William Stukeley (1734)	*Of the Gout*
William Oliver (1751)	*A Practical Essay on … Warm Bathing in Gouty Cases*
Nicholas Robinson (1755)	*An Essay on the Gout*
John Hill (G. Crine) (1758)	*The Management of the Gout*
William Cadogan (1771)	*A Dissertation on the Gout*
William Rowley (1792)	*Treatise on the Regular, Irregular, Atonic and Flying Gout*
Richard Kentish (1791)	*Advice to Gouty Persons*
Murray Forbes (1793)	*A Treatise Upon Gravel and Upon Gout*
John Latham (1796)	*On Rheumatism and Gout*
William Heberden (1802)	*Commentaries on the History and Cure of Diseases*
Richard Reece (1803)	*The Medical Guide*
Thomas Beddoes (1803)	*Observations on … the Newly Discovered Medicine in Gout*
Robert Kinglake (1804)	*Dissertation on Gout*
James Parkinson (1805)	*Observations on the Nature and Cure of Gout*
John Ring (1811)	*A Treatise on the Gout*
Charles Scudamore (1816)	*A Treatice on the Nature and Cure of Gout*
Robert Thomas (1821)	*Modern Practice of Physic*
William Robinson (1845)	*On the Nature and Treatment of Gout*
William Gairdner (1849)	*On Gout: Its History, Its Causes and Its Cure*
Alfred Garrod (1859)	*The Nature and Treatment of Gout and Rheumatic Gout*
William Fuller (1864)	*On Rheumatism, Rheumatic Gout, and Sciatica*
Dyce Duckworth (1889)	*A Treatise on Gout*
William Ewart (1896)	*Gout and Goutiness: and Their Treatment*
Arthur Luff (1898)	*Gout: Its Pathology and Treatment*
Llewellyn J. Llewellyn (1921)	*Gout*
William Copeman (1974)	*A Short History of the Gout*

Figure P.1.

A selection of medical treaties, books, essays and pamphlets written by doctors on the subject.

the author, and you may find that in places I am guilty of the same. If and when I do, the views will be my own and will not represent any of the many organisations with which I am happy to be affiliated, be it a charity, club, professional body or university.

Research reports fall into the third category. In Britain, this starts with the *Philosophical Transactions* of the Royal Society,[a] just past its 350th anniversary, but, equally, there are the proceedings of similar scientific societies, for example of France, Germany and other European countries and the United States. Most original medical and scientific research writing is now published in journals, and there is now an enormous and ever expanding 'literature' of papers presenting research data and of review articles collating them. According to the US National Library of Medicine PubMed, in the year 1981, when I gave my presentation at the Royal London, there were 190 scientific journal articles published worldwide involving gout and 440 involving uric acid. Unexpectedly, research on gout and uric acid has grown massively, with the respective numbers in 2022 being 1,325 and 2,679. The sheer number of articles being published year on year certainly argues that these are far from yesterday's topics – the academic effort continues unabated.

The fourth category contains information for patients. Books continue to emerge on a regular basis aimed at advising people how to live with the disease, and these are now supplemented by information on websites, internet posts, blogs, etc. They may be written either by medics eager to help or by well-meaning laypersons. They usually take the form of an account of the symptoms, along with various dietary and drug options. Many contain sensible advice based on science, many less so. My book does not aim to provide any direct guidance, but hopefully gout sufferers will enjoy understanding the basis of their disease.

---

[a] Much is made of the Royal Society in the following chapters. This was and remains Britain's leading scientific organisation, and fellowship of the Royal Society is a strong sign of scientific eminence.

The final category deals more with the social side of things. The outstanding example is *Gout: The Patrician Malady* by George Rousseau and the late Roy Porter (1946–2002), first published in 1988.[4] This highly readable *tour de force* deals wonderfully with the cultural history of the Gout, albeit slanted, as the title suggests, in a perhaps understandably left-wing direction. My work also has a political undertone, which, as we will see, is inseparable from the bigger picture of gout as largely a disease of civilisation.

My book does not fit neatly into any of these categories. The central axis is a history of how 'the Gout', once thought to be incurable, transformed over three hundred and fifty years into the modern correctable disease (Chapters 2, 3, 6 and 9). Upon this hang two subthemes. The first is how changing views influenced innovations in treatment and the interactions between commerce and doctors in driving the process (Chapters 4, 5, 7, 8 and 10); the second subtheme is the nature *versus* nurture controversy and focuses on the disconnect between lifestyle and the environment our species evolved genetically to live in (Chapters 11–14). The work brings together some of the forgotten past, the false starts, blind alleys and detours, placing them in the often contentious social and scientific contexts of their times.

Once I started collecting information and finding out more background, I decided to devote as much space to the people involved as to their discoveries. Science depersonalises scientists, and I felt a need to restore them to the story. Who were the people lost behind the names mentioned *en passant* in modern reviews or entirely left behind in academic *cul-de-sacs*? What were they trying to achieve? What were their scientific, medical and social backgrounds? What were their other interests and achievements? These questions always recurred, and then by delving into the various nooks and crannies where help could be found, I unearthed captivating facets to the lives of those I knew of just as names, as well as amazing personalities that I had not heard of at all. I do not dwell so much on gout's 'martyrs', who have been well covered elsewhere.[5]

Many of those who form the fabric of the story were pioneers of their fields and received a very high level of professional and public recognition during their lifetimes, with elections to fellowship of the Royal Society or the equivalent in other nations, Nobel Prizes, Lasker awards, knighthoods and so on, testifying to their outstanding calibre. Titles and honours have been omitted from the text as the use of only the first and last names simplifies the narrative, not least by sidestepping issues about when honours were bestowed in relation to achievements. To preserve the names of authors who have passed away, I have tended to refer to them directly in the text, whereas work by living authors is mostly just referenced.

I have to admit a serious proviso to emphasising 'Great Men'. This is the easiest way to approach the historical aspects, as often we simply do not know enough about actual circumstances. However, although we like to make a hero, we need to recognise that, in so doing, we are often perpetuating the myth of a single-handed genius. While in the past some scientists certainly did work as a one-man band, nowadays multidisciplinary teams are usually needed for real progress. Furthermore, a scientific field tends to move forward collectively. That said, hanging the stories upon specific individuals with what we know of their social networks and cross-cutting interests helps illustrate the wide bandwidth of enquiry of yesterday's scientists. Nowadays, academic specialisation is necessary for success but tends to sacrifice intellectual breadth for scientific depth.

I have written the book from a somewhat personal perspective, and the choices of who to include have mainly been British and Continental European up to 1900 and mainly American thereafter, reflecting a shift in the centre of gravity of medical research and development. I apologise if any glaring omission pricks some national, university or family pride, but I doubt the overall message would be much affected. Along the same lines, it has been difficult at times to know whether to refer to England, Scotland, Wales, Ireland or just Britain, and I beg forgiveness if I have transgressed heartfelt issues of regional sovereignty and independence.

Hippocrates was fully aware of the gender bias to having gout (aphorisms VI-28, -29 and -30 above). It is true that gout is rare in men before puberty and in women before menopause. VI-28 is likely to be accurate; however, it is hard to find enough eunuchs nowadays to be sure. On the discovery side, readers can hardly fail to observe that the scientists, medical practitioners and the like in the story were mostly men. That is how things were. Some strong women do get mention, including the satirical print publisher Hannah Humphrey (ca. 1745–ca. 1818), the intrepid traveller Hester Stanhope (1776–1839), the early geneticist Edith 'Becky' Saunders (1865–1945), the clinical biochemist Willey Denis (1879–1929), the uric acid physiologist and gout physician Ts'ai Fan Yu (1911–2007) and the medicinal chemist and Nobel Laureate Gertrude Elion (1918–1999). Early on in her career, Elion had struggled to find a job in a chemistry laboratory, being told a woman would be a distracting influence.[6] Thankfully, life in medical science is very different nowadays.

I have made plentiful use of quotes, sometimes extensively. I have done this not just to preserve the message but often to celebrate the language. I hope that the reader will find my choices justified, as how much or how little to cite verbatim is a matter of fine judgement.

Finally, I have to apologise for any shortfall in my attempt to collate and simplify so many strands of a complex tale. I am not the first author on gout to have had this concern, and I defer to Dyce Duckworth (1840–1928) when writing his *Treatise on Gout*:

In the case of a malady like Gout, the task is, in my opinion, beyond the powers of any one Physician, if he seeks to write a complete work, and to bring to each part of it fresh contributions and new light. It would require no less than that he should be, at once, a good Anatomist, Physiologist, Pathologist, and Chemist, as well as a trained and accomplished clinical observer. One may well ask, therefore, who is sufficient for all this?[7]

That was written in 1889, and the task is even more difficult today. This is, therefore, the opportunity to highlight important limitations to the work.

I have omitted a vast amount of both scientific and medical detail for the sake of simplicity and clarity. This applies particularly to modern studies on the inflammation of gout and on the genetics. The book focuses on 'primary' gout and barely touches on more complex 'secondary' gout that can be a consequence of other problems such as kidney failure, psoriasis or cancer, or of taking certain drugs for other ailments. Furthermore, I have dealt only briefly on the large topic of uric acid as a direct agent of health and disease in the absence of gout. Much of this latter topic remains unresolved and the subject of ongoing research, and I do not think greater inclusion would add to the main narrative. Be that as it may, I do hope the reader finds enough to enjoy.

So, who is the readership intended to be anyway? The book makes no claim to any detailed dig into unmined historical archives, nor to any new scientific discovery. However, it contains many new connections providing context to the unfolding story, spiced by reports and advertisements from within contemporary public newspapers and magazines that give some idea of the importance that everyone attributed to gout and uric acid back in the day. Although written with lay readers in mind, I hope it will also be enjoyed by scientists and medics wishing to know more about the history and by historians wishing to know more about the science and medicine. Pitching the language and terminology for such a broad range has not been easy, and I am fully aware of the dangers of being 'all things to all people'. I have avoided technical terms as far as possible and mostly explained those that are there in footnotes and in a glossary at the end. Specialists will need to forgive this. Equally well, general readers will need to excuse the extensive referencing that is there for documentation. The book is intended to be read for pleasure and is not a textbook – if it reads like one or, worse still, a dry academic doorstop, it has failed.

I could not have completed this work without help, and I would like to give my heartfelt thanks to Mykola Baal, Jake Bransgrove, Aubrey Haskard, Luke Haskard, Skylar Haskard, Robert Jones, Cherry Lewis, Krystyna Marioudi, Henry Russell and Michael Wigan for invaluable critiques on various chapters. I particularly thank Brian Berenblut, who has been a constant source of feedback and support as the project has evolved. Lastly, it remains to thank my wife Kathleen for her enduring support, invaluable advice and extreme tolerance of my mental absence for the innumerable hours it has all taken.

Contents

Chapter 1

Introduction

The word 'gout' has its origin in the Latin *gutta*, meaning 'a drop' – and, yes, it shares its origin with the word for the channel that catches rain from the roof. The first to apply it to arthritis is said to be one Randolphus of Boking, a domestic chaplain to the Bishop of Chichester, in around 1200 AD, when describing the inflamed foot of a cathedral servant.[1] By all accounts, the sufferer was cured by being lent the bishop's boots but might just as well have been offered a handful of fried apple cores, as an acute attack of gouty arthritis, or 'a fit' as it was called, is self-limiting and usually resolves by itself over a week or two without any treatment at all.

Why apply a word meaning 'a drop' to an ailment? In the physiological system passed down from Hippocrates (see Preface), the Ancient Greek physician Galen of Pergamon (ca. 130–ca. 210) and others, health depended on a balance between four cardinal humours: blood, phlegm, black bile and yellow bile.[2] A surplus of humour was believed to drop by gravity down the leg and discharge as intense inflammation in the foot, like steam hissing from a pressure cooker. *Podagra*, which is the medical term still used, aptly captures the condition, originating from the Greek πόδοσ (*podos*, foot) and αγρα (*agra*, catch). Charles Scudamore (1779–1849), one of the first English physicians to quantify clinical observations, wrote in 1816 that 57 of the 71 first attacks that he had witnessed involved the ball of the big toe, a further eight were in other parts of the foot and just five elsewhere.[3] After the first attack, the illness can have a free-for-all around the joints, each affection decorated with equivalent names, such as *gonagra* for the knee and *chiagra* for the hand. The Greek-Latin mishmash of

1

old medical terminology served past physicians well in simultaneously boasting knowledge and hiding ignorance.

An acute attack of gout is said to be one of the worst pains one can experience. Illustrating this best is James Gillray's *The Gout* (1799), the most famous of gout images (see Figure 1.1(a)).[4] Gillray would have known about gout, as it is generally considered to have been common in his day, and the foot could well have been his own. His take on the problem is shown by his *Punch Cures the Gout, the Colic and the Tisick* (1799) (see Figure 1.1(b)), which offers up the gout-inducing but symptom-relieving punch as the treatment for a condition that doctors mostly believed to be untreatable.[5]

Gillray (1756–1815) (see Figure 1.2(a)) was a master entertainer and one of the most talented and productive satirical cartoonists of the Georgian era.[6] His legacy is a portfolio of sedition, poking fun at royalty,

(a)   (b)

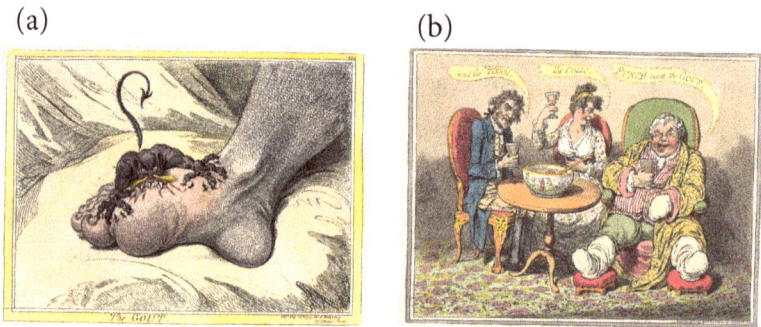

Figure 1.1.

(a) *The Gout* by James Gillray (1799). The gout demon sinks its teeth into a red and swollen forefoot, its waving tail held still for the artist. The ankle is extended on a cushion, as if the slightest movement would magnify the pain.

(b) Gillray's *Punch Cures the Gout, the Colic and the Tisick* (1799). 'Tisick' is an obsolete word for a cough but implies 'consumption', which would often have been due to tuberculosis. The words are from a popular tavern song, 'Landlord, fill a flowing bowl'. Note the swaddled feet resting on gout stools. The Georgian satirical cartoonists used the bandaged foot as a social pointer to much more than gout.

Source: (a) Courtesy of the Cleveland Museum of Art (bequest of Dr. Paul J Vignos, Jr. 2011.182), public domain; (b) courtesy of the Yale Center for British Art (Paul Mellon Collection), public domain.

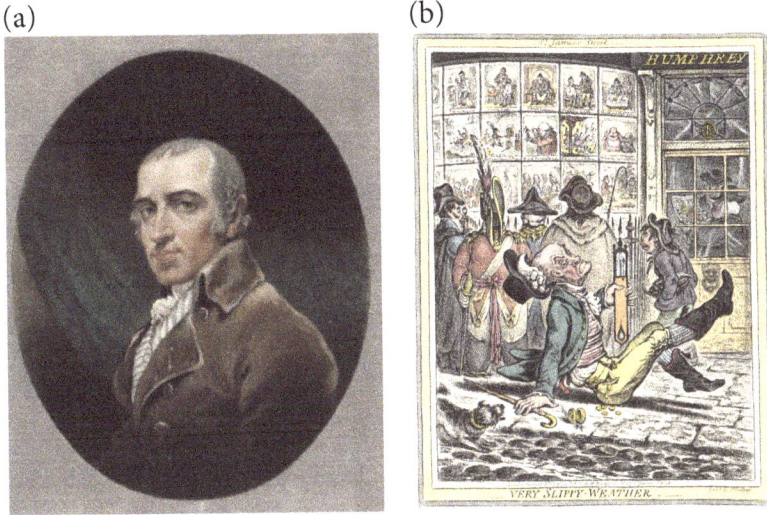

(a)

(b)

Figure 1.2.

(a) Hand-coloured mezzotint of Gillray's self-portrait, engraved by Charles Turner.

(b) Gillray's *Very Slippy Weather* (1808) (after John Sneyd), in which passersby are more interested in his work hanging in Hannah Humphrey's print shop window than in helping the old man who had fallen on the pavement. Such was the power of Gillray's cartoons.

Source: (a) Courtesy of the Yale Center for British Art (Paul Mellon Collection), public domain; (b) US National Gallery of Art (gift of the Arcana Foundation), public domain.

politicians, military men and other contemporary targets. *Very Slippy Weather* of 1808 (see Figure 1.2(b)) shows an old man upending onto the pavement outside the London printshop of Gillray's publisher and landlady Hannah Humphrey (ca. 1745–ca. 1818). Bystanders are too distracted by Gillray's prints in the window to notice or care about the fall.[7] Such was the draw of cartoons in a world in which most ordinary people seldom saw a painting; in which newspapers, magazines and billboards carried no photographs; and in which there was no cinema, television or even the internet. Humphrey's shop was in London at 27, St. James's street, well placed for gout-spotting, as this was, and still is, the land of smart private member's clubs, with Boodles (founded 1762) next door and White's (founded 1693) just beyond that. Humphrey's printshop was demolished long ago and has been replaced by a business plaza. Go there, and you will find bystanders on the pavement still avid for images and distracted instead by their smartphones.

Although acute attacks of gout resolve without treatment, the illness can progress to a chronic phase, in which hard chalky deposits form under the skin and eventually in and around internal organs (see Figure 1.3). These most typically occur around joints but can also form hard, telltale lumps on the rims of the ears or elsewhere. The concretions used to be called 'chalk stones', but are now referred to as 'tophi', or

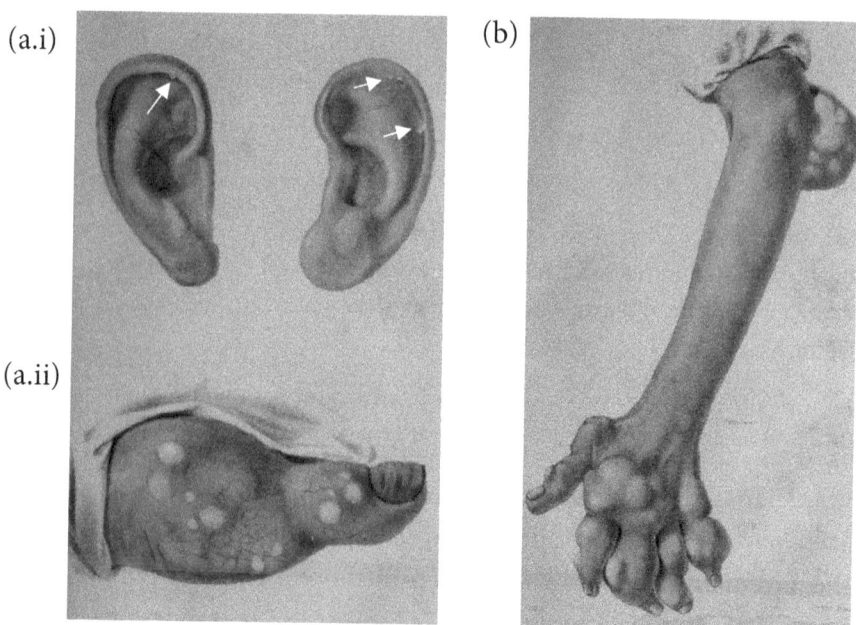

Figure 1.3.

Examples of gouty tophi taken from Alfred Baring Garrod's *The Nature and Treatment of Gout and Rheumatic Gout* (1859).

(a.i) Tophi on the helices of the outer ears (see arrows) and (a.ii) a complex tophus on the first interphalangeal joint (ball) of the big toe.

(b) White gouty tophi in the hand and around the elbow. With modern treatment, this shockingly extensive disease is fortunately vanishingly rare.

Source: Courtesy of the Wellcome Collection, public domain.

'tophus' if singular. They can be very extensive, destructive and disabling. In his *Modern Practice of Physic* (1821), Robert Thomas described their development as follows:

> The chalky liquid, when first secreted, gives to the finger, upon pressure with it, the feeling of fluctuation.... The consistency of the liquid becomes thicker and thicker, till at last nothing remains but a hard mass. The quantity at last accumulated becomes considerable, and seriously augments the sufferings of the patient; by its bulk, greatly distends the surrounding parts, and obstructs the motion of the tendons and joints.... The cutis, when distended to the utmost by frequent deposits of chalk, sometimes gives way, and an opening formed, through which a quantity of it is evacuated.[8]

They say nothing is useless, not even tophi. James Parkinson (1755–1824), famous for the disease that bears his name but also featured later in these pages as a perceptive author on gout and many other matters, wrote of a patient attending the Westminster Hospital in London who used the chalky lumps on his knuckles to write up the scores while playing cards.[9]

No one seriously doubts that gout was common in Stuart and Georgian times, but it is impossible to know just how common it really was. Although 'regular gout' has always been centred on the joints, the old 'gouty diathesis'[a] predisposed to much more than what we call gout today. Many a malady was put down to 'irregular gout', including whatever caused the demise of Lord Saltoun in September 1793:

> Yesterday morning died, of the gout in his stomach, at Baldwins, in Kent, the Right Hon. ALEXANDER LORD SALTOUN, in the 36th year of his age. His Lordship's indisposition lasted but a few days, which tenders the loss of so valuable a character the more severe and afflicting to his family and friends.[10]

---

[a] The word 'diathesis' is not used much now but means a tendency to suffer from a particular condition.

The seventeenth-century physician Thomas Sydenham (1624–1689), who features in the next chapter, would have considered this diagnosis entirely consistent with an insufficient discharge of gouty humour into the joints, perhaps caused by the thwarting of what he considered a salutary process through the administration of purgatives or bleeding:

> the sad catastrophe … the peccant matter lodges in the viscera, involves their structure, impairs the organs of secretion, leaves the blood stagnant, thick, and feculent, prevents the discharge of the gouty matter on the extremities, makes life worse than death, and finally brings death as a relief.[11]

Likewise, George Cheyne (ca. 1672–1743) wrote of 'an irregular gout, fix'd on these three great Instruments of human Life, the Head, the Stomach, and the Guts.'[12] Cheyne was an early advocate of psychological medicine and distinguished a 'nervous' or 'flying' gout, which he separated by means that are not entirely clear from the hypochondriacal symptom of 'windy gout'. Even William Cullen (1710–1790), a great disbeliever in the humours, taught the existence of 'atonic', 'retrocedent' and 'misplaced gout' affecting internal organs.[13] Other irregular gout categories, all loosely defined, were 'visceral', 'metastatic', 'anomalous' and 'repelled'.[14] French doctors talked of '*goutte larvée*' and '*goutte vague*'. All in all, it was like the 56 imaginary varieties boasted in 1896 by Henry J Heinz to market his pickle.[b]

Irregular gout did no harm to the lucrative medical practice of the preeminent Bath physician William Oliver (1695–1764), who taught that 'while this gouty matter is carried about in the body, mixt with the other fluids, it often occasions Head-achs, Vertigos, Sour belchings, Heart-Burns, Flatusses and wandering twitching pains in the limbs.'[15]

---

[b] The number '57' is thought to have been the combination of Heinz's own lucky number, '5', and his wife's, '7'. There was just the single variety at the start, and the others followed later, expanding to the 5,000 or so products sold by the Kraft Heinz Company today.

As gout mainly affects men, Oliver came up with a 'female gout', with manifestations such as hypochondriasis, failing appetite, imperfect digestion, prevailing flatus, wasting flesh and nervous atrophy.[16] All in all, 'irregular gout' served a general purpose by enabling more people to benefit from gout's social cachet and to have a calling card for a spell in Bath, a less fashionable spa in England, or even a visit to the Continent, both to relieve the aches and pains and to network socially. If they came to Bath, they could also partake of the original Bath Oliver biscuits, originally formulated by William Oliver for weight loss and improved well-being, strength and vigour. A silhouette of his head is still imprinted in the centre of each biscuit. He left the recipe to his coachman, a Mr. Atkins, along with £100 and 10 sacks of the best wheat flour. This was enough to set Atkins up with a shop in Green Street, Bath, and then to make a fortune.

As mentioned in the Preface, Hippocrates clearly recognised the maleness of gout, and indeed gout is the most common form of inflammatory arthritis in men. Thomas Sydenham added, 'Gout attacks women but rarely, and then chiefly the aged and the masculine. When you have symptoms of gout in slender females, they are really the symptoms of hysteria, or else of rheumatism imperfectly eliminated.'[17] Today, this sounds unsympathetic and even misogynistic; however, disease classification and diagnoses were not what they are today, and what Sydenham meant by 'rheumatism imperfectly eliminated' was most probably rheumatoid arthritis, which is three times more common in women. The protection of young women from gout was originally mostly put down to menstruation being a natural and healthy way of eliminating noxious material, although Cheyne had an alternative early eighteenth-century explanation: 'and this is one Reason, why Women are less subject to the Gout than Men; because of the known laxity of their Fibres.'[18] These theories, of course, reflect a complete ignorance of the scientific mechanisms of this and, indeed, any other illness. The central axis of this book is the slow journey of distilling modern gout out of the broad concept of 'the Gout' as a collection of supposedly integrated symptoms.

Gout is essentially caused by a buildup of uric acid, manifesting in the blood as monosodium urate (see Chapter 6). On the back of research into uric acid physiology came a better understanding of gender differences in susceptibility to gout, which we now know are largely caused by the contrasting effects of male and female sex hormones on the handling of urate in the kidney. Blood levels of male sex hormone levels rise in boys at puberty, and this coincides with a drop in urate excretion.[19] The same is seen when a woman self-administers testosterone or has ovaries removed, and a case has been described of gout following a female-to-male transition.[20] Conversely, administration of oestrogen, either to males reassigning in the other direction or as part of post-menopausal hormone replacement therapy, lowers urinary urate levels by increasing urinary urate.[21] Because of these hormonal effects, at a population level, males and females have equivalent blood urate readings up to the age of 10, after which levels are significantly higher in males for the next three decades. After menopause, urate levels climb in females towards those in same-age males and are accompanied by a similar predisposition to gout.

Where there is ill-health, there will always be someone willing to profit from it, and while the central story is about how science led to an understanding of gout, the first subtheme is how commercial treatment options changed as the concepts of disease developed. What comes out of this is the realisation that medicines have always been expensive, with prices driven up by market forces. We start in the seventeenth century with physicians offering purging, bleeding and other methods of physically evacuating toxic matter, backed up by unvalidated 'specific' herbal or metallic 'repercussives' and 'resolvers'. Developing health consciousness in the eighteenth century, matched by a widespread dislike and distrust of doctors, led to a boom in widely advertised proprietary self-help medicines, again usually containing herbal extracts and sometimes heavy metals, such as mercury or antimony (see Chapter 4). Initially, these medicines often just provided alcohol and opium, but eventually the trade delivered a nostrum from France that actually worked. Chapter 5 is devoted to the

French remedy, *L'Eau Médicinale d'Husson*, and then Chapter 10 covers the circuitous route that led to the purification of its active ingredient, colchicine, and understanding how it is effective.

The trade was not slow to pick up on uric acid once it was discovered and associated with gout, and it duly promoted it as a universal poison responsible for just about any malady. The second wave of proprietary medicines thus came in the nineteenth and early twentieth centuries, with pseudoscientific formulations of a more defined nature claiming to help uric acid elimination (see Chapter 7). Finally, there was the mid-twentieth-century era of rational drug discovery based on the emerging knowledge of how uric acid is formed and how it is eliminated. By that time, the pharmaceutical industry that had emerged had largely lost interest in gout and uric acid. The first means to reliably increase uric acid loss or reduce its generation thus came serendipitously from companies discovering drugs intended to fight infections and cancer (see Chapter 8).

The second subtheme deals with the nature *versus* nurture dimension of gout. This debate is as old as the hills and has always been confounded by social perceptions of gout as evidence of 'good breeding', on the one hand, and a life of misguided and ill-deserved luxury, on the other. Now that we understand so much more about genes and can rapidly sequence human genomes, we know that many small genetic differences exist that affect predisposition to gout, both by affecting uric acid levels and probably also by affecting inflammation (see Chapter 11). The simple take-home message is that experiencing attacks of gout usually requires both these and environmental or lifestyle triggering factors (see Chapter 12). The cause of one person's gout is never quite the same as another's, as we all differ in the precise mix of predisposing genes that we inherit, and of course, we all differ in the character and extent of our gout-provoking lifestyles. The same argument that applies to individuals applies to ethnic groups and under-scores the importance of moving away from a 'one-size-fits-all' approach towards more personalised medicine, not just for gout but for all diseases.

Leaving aside why one person rather than another gets gout, Chapter 13 addresses the humanness of gout. At the start of the book, living creatures were seen as discrete, perfect as God made them and driven by vital principles. This belief held up the biblical account of creation, which scholars had calculated to have occurred over six days (the seventh being for rest) and just five to six thousand years ago. There is a strong tradition of doctors being interested in geology. Several of the doctors who wrote on gout in the early years were fossil collectors and struggled with how the remains of marine creatures came to be petrified within hills and how different strata in a hillside came to preserve different examples of extinct species.[22] Doubts about biblical creation intensified with the new chemistry dismissing vital principles, as the organic compounds of living creatures turned out to obey the inorganic chemistry laws of matter. The biblical edifice finally tumbled, at least to the scientific mind, with the publication in 1859 of Charles Darwin's *On the Origin of Species by Means of Natural Selection, or the Preservation of Favoured Races in the Struggle for Life,* which set a new paradigm by which all life forms are connected by time but where species come and go according to their success in the environment.[23] This evolutionary framework helps us understand how uric acid's role in the elimination of surplus and potentially toxic nitrogen varies among animal species. Most mammals are protected from gout, as they biochemically degrade uric acid to soluble non-gouty urinary derivatives. Humans, however, along with chimpanzees, gorillas and orangutans, have lost the capacity during evolution to degrade uric acid, and this is the single most important cause of gout occurrence in humans, with individual genetic differences and lifestyles just topping up the uric acid level.

Coming on to the present time, the book ends with a look at gout in the modern world, with a focus on the strong link between gout and obesity. Chapter 14 takes an ecological look at uric acid and the international corporation-driven changes in farming practice and food distribution that have led to the global obesity epidemic, with all its adverse health consequences of not only gout but also related diabetes, high blood pressure and cardiovascular disease. Times and politics have changed since gout was exclusively a disease of the rich, and we currently need to explore the

Prevalent gout cases per 100,000 population

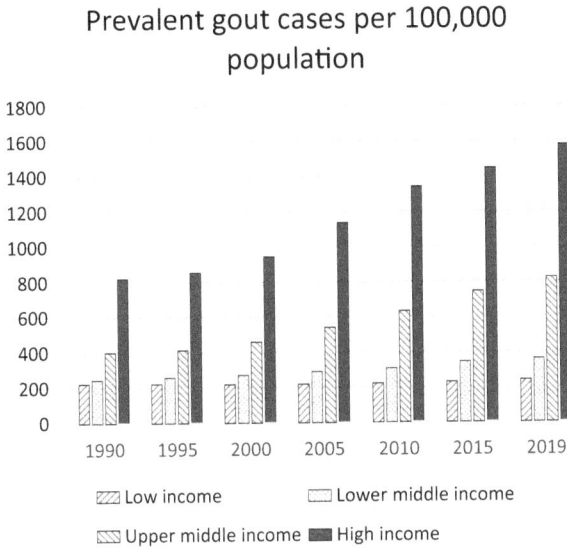

Figure 1.4.

Estimated increase in the prevalence of gout over 25 years, grouping countries according to World Bank income groups.

Source: Institute for Health Metrics and Evaluation. Used with permission. All rights reserved.

global economic and environmental reasons for the prevalence of gout increasing over the past 25 years (see Figure 1.4). It is estimated that in the order of 50 million people in the world today have gout, and this has risen dramatically since 1990 (see Figure 1.4).[24] While gout is still much more prevalent in high- and upper-middle-income countries, within those countries it is now as much linked to poverty as to wealth. Far from having vanished, gout and the associated diseases that together would have been contained within 'the Gout' remain with a vengeance.

Chapter 2

Thomas Sydenham and His Associates

Thomas Sydenham published his seminal *Treatise on Gout and Dropsy*[a] in 1683.[1] He was riddled with gout, and a secretary had to take dictation of what is now widely regarded as its definitive clinical description.[2] Sydenham thus provides a good basecamp for the long climb, taking 'the Gout' from a loosely defined concept to a scientifically delineated disease (called gout). He became revered as 'The English Hippocrates', largely on account of his rebelliously moving the focus of physicians from theory and speculation in the library to direct observation of patients (see Figures 2.1(a) and (b)). That said, Sydenham by no means shook off theory, and did little to discover underlying facts. Indeed, he established the enduring and misguided belief that attacks of gout are salutary and signify a healthy constitution.

Sydenham's Political Background

Before getting to Sydenham's writing on gout, I need to first explain the context in which he worked, both in terms of his own life story and the conventions that he found himself up against in contemporary medical practice. Sydenham came from landed-gentry stock that farmed at Wynford Eagle, a village in the pastoral county of Dorset in the south of England.[3] Schooled locally until 17, he travelled to Oxford in 1642 to

---

[a] Originally published in Latin as *Tractus de Podagra et Hydrope*. The obsolete term 'dropsy' referred to the accumulation of fluid, such as in the legs. This would often have been due to heart failure.

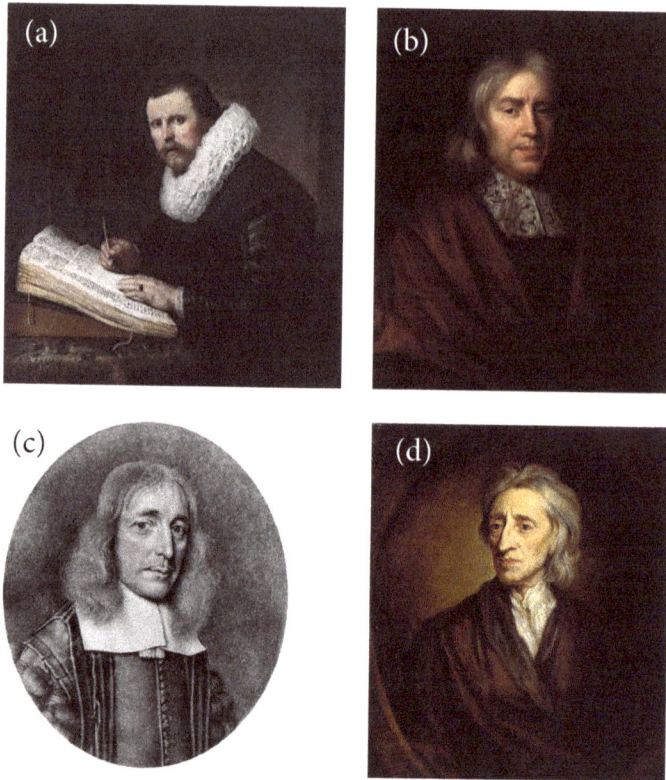

Figure 2.1.

Four types of seventeenth-century physicians:

(a) Academic medicine in the Middle Ages was a desiccated affair, bogged down in scholasticism and dependent on classical hand-me-down dogmas. The *Scholar at his Desk* by Rembrandt van Rijn (1631) may well have been a seventeenth-century physician, pouring over ancient texts and avoiding bedside learning.

(b) Thomas Sydenham, the 'English Hippocrates', marks the redirection of clinical medicine to the bedside. This portrait was painted in 1688 by his neighbour in Pall Mall, Mary Beale. Note the simple puritan attire rather than collegiate robes.

(c) Line engraving of Thomas Willis after David Loggan (1667). While Sydenham was a clinician with a scientific bent, Willis was a scientist in clinical practice.

(d) Sydenham's friend and intellectual collaborator John Locke. Although primarily known now as a moral philosopher, Locke trained as a physician with Sydenham. The portrait is by Godfrey Kneller (1697).

Source: (a)–(c) Wikimedia Commons; (d) courtesy of the Wellcome Collection, public domain.

study at Magdalen Hall.[b] He could not have achieved much by the time the Parliamentarians took up arms against the Royalists two months later. This led to him returning home to fight alongside his father and four brothers for the rebel cause. The background to the Civil War was complicated but included the dissatisfaction of provincial gentry with interference by the central bureaucracy of Charles I (1600–1649). Religion also came into it, as puritans like the Sydenhams resented the King as head of the Church of England. The war in Dorset was characterised by a series of local skirmishes rather than the pitched battles seen elsewhere; nevertheless, Sydenham lost three brothers fighting over the course of the war, and his mother Mary was murdered by Royalist dragoons outside the family home.[4]

The first phase of the Civil War ended in 1647, and Sydenham stopped off on the way back to Oxford to visit his elder brother William Sydenham (1615–1661) in an army hospital. There, he had one of those life-altering chance encounters.[5] The attending physician was Thomas Coxe (1615–1685), who was to become one of the original fellows of the Royal Society and president of the Royal College of Physicians. However, the latter was only for the year 1682, as he was quickly removed due to his anti-establishment politics and non-conformist religious views.[6] Coxe encouraged the young Sydenham to take up the 'Medical Art', a pursuit he seems not to have previously considered.[7]

Sydenham soon transferred to Wadham College, where the new master was the brother-in-law of the senior Parliamentarian Oliver Cromwell (1599–1659). The university was undergoing an administrative turnout, exchanging the Royalist old guard for the new political elite. The reconstituted faculty conferred degrees by 'creation' to allow preferred but underqualified candidates to be appointed rapidly to the vacated posts. Sydenham was thus favoured and, in 1648, became a bachelor of medicine after just one year of study – the usual requirement being six. He was soon made a fellow of the prestigious All Souls College and appointed the senior bursar – not bad progress for a 25-year-old bumped-up medical student.

---

[b] Magdalen Hall is now Hertford College.

It was at Oxford that Sydenham met Robert Boyle (1627–1691), the Anglo-Irish aristocrat and pioneer of Enlightenment science in Britain. It may have been through Boyle that Sydenham was introduced to the empirical philosophy of Francis Bacon (1561–1626).[c] A generation or two earlier, Bacon had proposed that no phenomenon was true unless it could be observed, documented and then reproduced. Sydenham would also have become aware at Oxford of the contemporary academic trendsetters and the disparate theoretical factions of medicine: the iatromechanical school of Santorio Santorio (1561–1636), Galileo Galilei (1564–1642), René Descartes (1596–1650) and Giovanni Borelli (1608–1679), which viewed the body as a machine; and the iatrochemistry school of Theophrastus von Hohenheim (Paracelsus) (1493–1541), Jan Baptist von Helmont (1580–1644), Johann Glauber (1604–1668) and Franciscus Sylvius (1614–1672), which considered physiology as a series of chemical reactions. Both approaches now seem as obvious and as complementary as bioengineering, biophysics and biochemistry are today, but at the time they were simply alternative forms of speculation. Despite the heady climate at Oxford, Sydenham does not appear to have involved himself in any laboratory research and may not even have realised its potential for medical progress.

The second phase of the Civil War broke out in 1651, when the Royalists invaded England from Scotland, having promised independence to the Scots. Sydenham returned to the army, this time fighting in the Scottish border regions and the English Midlands. He returned to Oxford after the invasion was repulsed, having been more than once wounded.

---

[c] The terms 'empirical' and 'empiric' are ambiguous. In its positive sense, 'empirical' means 'experimental', as in the philosophy of Francis Bacon. As we will see later, it was also used negatively to refer to an irregular, unlicensed medical practitioner who sold unconventional treatments. Physicians also tended to extend its use to licensed practitioners who had gone astray. Other words, even more negative, were quacksalver ('quack'), mountebank and charlatan, each implying secrecy and a lack of safety. The seventeenth-century empirics were a mixed group but survive in the popular mind as itinerant medicine men, selling from makeshift stalls with impressive theatrical sideshows in public places, as in *The Quack Doctor* by the Dutch artist Gerrit Dou in 1652, hanging in the Museum Boijmans Van Beuningen in Rotterdam. It is easy to imagine the impact of all this on naïve spectators at the time.

He remained there for a further three years until he married at the age of 31. As the monastic rules of the university did not allow him to remain a fellow, he now had to earn a living some other way. Life as a jobbing physician may not have been top of his mind, and he had anticipated a political career.[8] He thus moved to London, where he bought a house in Westminster, where the politicians lived. His brother William had been a senior Parliamentary army officer and had now risen to high office as Commissioner of the Treasury and a member of Cromwell's Council. It was through William that, in 1659, Thomas was made Comptroller of the Pipe in the Exchequer, a lucrative political appointment that was occupied many years later by the literary Horace Walpole (1717–1797). His job was to audit government income and expenditure, but it is hard to judge how much of Sydenham's time this required; it may have been something of a sinecure.[9] At that time, the Clerk of the Pipe, who was responsible for keeping the parliamentary accounts, was Henry Croke (1588–1660), one of incidental historical interest as the owner of Chequers, now the grace-and-favour country mansion of the UK Prime Minister.

Further evidence of Sydenham's political ambitions is his standing on two occasions for election as a member of parliament – both times in Weymouth and both times unsuccessfully. The first was in 1659, when the election had to be called off because Cromwell had just died. Sydenham's failure to be elected a year later must have been a setback, as this was home ground; however, the result was probably more due to the general weariness of puritan restrictions under Cromwell than anything personal. Soon afterwards, William lost his job owing to the restoration of the monarchy and the return of Charles II (1630–1685) from France. He became one of the 18 Cromwellian *persona non grata* denied a pardon by the *Indemnity and Oblivion Act* of 1660 and was thus banned from holding public office. The act officially forgave those who had committed crimes during the Civil War and subsequent interregnum but excluded those considered unsavoury,[d] as well as anyone who had contributed

---

[d] For example, having committed 'unlicensed murder, piracy, buggery, rape or witchcraft'.

directly to Charles I's execution. William was among the latter and died a broken man two years later, leaving Thomas isolated and politically tarred by his brother's brush.

Sydenham practised physic, as medicine was known, soon after he moved to London but only in a now-and-then manner. Without a political future, he had little choice but to become a full-time physician. Breaking into the competitive medical market was not easy. Seventeenth-century medical practice emphasised consulting with colleagues, and Royalist physicians, still full of post-Civil War rancour, preferred to mix with their own kind. Likewise, with the Royalist patients. Sydenham moved in 1664 to Pall Mall in St. James's, around the corner from where Hannah Humphrey later sold James Gillray's prints. It was a fashionable area full of aristocrats, but his past was not a good calling card for treating rich patients.

Sydenham and Fevers

This was an era in which fevers ruled the doctor's day, and it was with the fevers of the less well-off that Sydenham cut his teeth. The Great Plague of 1665 was the most recent of several similar epidemics. It has been estimated that in each of 1563, 1603, 1625 and 1665, 'plague' increased annual mortality by over fivefold, and each resulted in the deaths of around one in five of the population.[10] Although legend has it that rats and their fleas brought plague off ships from abroad, poor living standards, overcrowding, smoke pollution and malnutrition would certainly have contributed to its lethality. Daniel Defoe's *Diary of a Plague Year* (1722) is an imaginary reconstruction of what happened in 1665, but his account of the stampede to get out of town, which inadvertently spread disease to the countryside, is all too believable to those who witnessed events at the start of the COVID-19 pandemic in 2020.[11]

Sydenham left London himself to escape the plague and used the time to write his *Method of Curing Fevers*.[e] Encouraged by Boyle, Sydenham

---

[e] Originally published in Latin as *Methodus curandi febres*.

shifted the emphasis from individuals with supposedly unique fevers to epidemics, in which groups of patients had similar symptoms. He carefully recorded common manifestations and the natural courses of fevers and proposed a simple classification. There was smallpox, which was readily identified and in a category of its own. Then, there were continuous fevers and intermittent fevers. The latter, also known as 'agues', were probably mostly due to malaria, which was endemic in the southeast of England up until the beginning of the twentieth century.[12] Sydenham also recognised rheumatic fever, now known to be due to beta-haemolytic *Streptococcal* infection, and was the first to associate it with St. Vitus' dance, the involuntary movement of the face, hands and feet, which has since become known as Sydenham's chorea. His disciple, Richard Blackmore, had this to say about his contrary approaches to the treatment of fevers:

> Having taken a Resolution at his first entering upon the Practice of Physic, as himself assured me in conversation, to act contrary, in all Cases, to the common Method then in Fashion amongst the most eminent physicians (and he told me his reasons for it), in Conformity to the Design did in the Management of this Disease, as well as others, oppose the common Method of the Physicians of the Court and City.[13]

What Blackmore meant by 'the common Method' was the universal practice of treating illnesses by physically removing the hypothetical morbid humours. There were various means to achieve this, including purging with emetics or laxatives, heating the body to cause sweating, local suction (cupping), administering mercury to stimulate salivation or administering plant-based diuretics to stimulate the flow of urine.[14] Additionally, and more assertively, patients could be bled, either using leeches or through direct puncture of a vein. The physician would also have an apothecary make up his prescription of a 'specific' as a supplement. Although there were orthodoxies in the order of administering the various means of evacuation, the system basically stressed the uniqueness of a patient's illness and the need for a bespoke, personalised treatment regimen. Sydenham disapproved of purging, bleeding and the like, and he saw 'specifics' as particular to the common disease rather than the uniqueness of the patient. He observed that feverish patients who could not afford to see a physician or buy a prescription were not necessarily more likely to die; in fact, they often fared better. This led him to emphasise the body's intrinsic healing capacity and realise that doctors could make things worse. Accordingly, Sydenham's general approach to treatment was light touch and sometimes minimal intervention.

Unsurprisingly, many of his colleagues judged his omissions criminally reprehensible, and this particularly applied to his management of smallpox. This was a major killer before the introduction of immunisation, and those that survived it were often left with terrible scars. Standard methods were bleeding, purging and/or sweating (ideally with the patient wrapped in a scarlet cloth) to promote the release of the presumed toxic substance. Although not the first to try a cooling regimen instead, Sydenham takes the credit for popularising it.[15] Again, in Richard Blackmore's words:

> Dr. Sydenham, being … determined to oppose the whole Scheme of Practice, fell upon the cold Regimen, … and opened not only the Curtains around the Bed, but often the Windows likewise to let in fresh Air to the Room, and plied them constantly with diluting and attempering, or with acid and cooling Remedies.[16]

Sydenham and the College of Physicians

In 1663, Sydenham passed the examination at the Royal College of Physicians that licensed him to practice physic in London, but he was not eligible for fellowship status, which then required an Oxford or Cambridge doctorate. The *status quo* was rigidly hierarchical, and the social position, access to patients and fees of a physician depended on having a classical university education. This was lengthy and expensive, and it concentrated on library study rather than direct clinical experience. Sydenham's peers would have considered his meagre Oxford education as wholly inadequate a preparation for medical practice and demeaning of the profession, even though the brevity of his learning was in fact a blessing in leaving him unfettered by dogma. Peer disapproval of Sydenham's uneducated approach led to the College being lobbied by his colleagues to remove his licence. In this, Sydenham was not his own best friend, as he actively alienated those who did not share his puritanical values. In the preface to *Method of Curing Fevers*, he denounced his self-serving colleagues as follows:

> Whoever takes up medicine should seriously consider the following points: firstly, that he must one day render to the Supreme Judge an account of the lives of those sick men who have been intrusted to his care. Secondly, that such skill and science as, by the blessing of the Almighty God, he (the physician) has attained, are to be especially directed towards the honour of his Maker, and the welfare of his fellow-creatures; since it is a base thing for the great gifts of Heaven to become the servants of avarice or ambition…. Some are swollen up with pride, and puffed out with the vain conceit of their knowledge; so that these matters are small in their eyes. They can only come down to them negligently and contemptuously. They care nothing for the unfortunates committed to their charge. The Supreme Being they either disown or disregard. The others either gape or grow greedy for gain, or else are borne away by the hopes of some small celebrity; in either case looking to their purses or their fame.[17]

Munk's Roll, the Royal College's cumulative biography of fellows, is forgiving and maintains that the College held Sydenham in high esteem and that all he had needed to do to become a fellow after he obtained a Cambridge doctorate in 1676 was to apply.[18] Given as evidence is the College requesting permission to reprint Sydenham's *The Schedule of Symptoms of the Newly Arrived Fever*[f] and describing the work as 'most pleasing'. However, that was not published until 1686, by which time Sydenham had

---

[f] Originally published in Latin as *Schedula Monitoria de novae febris ingressu.*

just three years to live. If it took until then for the College to appreciate Sydenham, it was all too little, too late. Notwithstanding, it commissioned a posthumous bust of Sydenham for its premises in 1757.

Sydenham had hit a raw nerve at the College, as the educational system underpinned its place at the top of the medical trade. Apothecaries were there to make up and dispense prescriptions for physicians and were not entitled to consult with patients or initiate treatment for a fee. This subservience was based on their being trained by apprenticeship rather than tutored and degreed by a university. The College was legally tasked with examining apprentice apothecaries before they could be granted the freedom to work for physicians independently, as well as checking that the premises of apothecaries conformed to good practice. This was not going to last, and many apothecaries had their eyes on better things.[8]

Physicians and Apothecaries

One of the first apothecaries to stand out in revolt against the system was Nicholas Culpeper (1616–1654), who was the rebel to apothecaries that Sydenham was to physicians. After studying at Cambridge and then having undertaken seven years as an apprentice apothecary, he opened a shop in London's Spitalfields, from which he acted as an early general practitioner, dispensing free treatments to the poor. In 1652, he published his *English Physitian,* the first do-it-yourself medical manual written in English.[19] The author's name on the title page appeared as 'NICH. CULPERER, *Gent.* STUDENT in Physic and Astrology', which conveyed three things: first, that Culpeper was a Gentleman and therefore the social equal of physicians; second, that he considered himself to be a physician, if only a student; and third, his belief in links between medicine and astrology. Culpeper worked as a battlefield surgeon for the Parliamentarians in the

---

[8] In the British health system, apothecaries eventually became the general practitioners (GPs) of today, and GPs presently qualify by obtaining the same combined university degrees in medicine and surgery as hospital doctors.

Civil War and was seriously wounded by a musket ball in the chest, from which he died in 1654 at the age of only 38 – just before Sydenham came to London.

The *English Family Physitian* has survived as a best seller to the present day as *Culpeper's Complete Herbal*. It is an alphabetical compilation of indigenous medicinal plants, all itemised with their colloquial names[h] and was the product of an impressive knowledge of botany. Each plant mentioned comes with details on how to identify it, where to find it, the time of year it should be harvested, how to make an extract from it, what complaints it can help with and instructions on whether it should be swallowed or applied locally. Culpeper offered no explanation for gout (or indeed other conditions). Instead, there is a long list of herbals,[i] all recommended from experience or hearsay. By consulting with patients, Culpeper stretched his activities well beyond what was acceptable to the College of Physicians. Indeed, the College would have banned his book had it not been weakened into ineffectuality by the turmoil of the Civil War. But then, the Worshipful Society of Apothecaries did not care for Culpeper either, preferring to make up lucrative complex prescriptions to cheap everyday simples. The Society latched onto Culpeper's interests in astrology and accused him of witchcraft – he might not have fared well if he had not died of his war wound.

As far as the College of Physicians was concerned, the problem with apothecaries extended well beyond Culpeper. There was a flurry of pamphlets, with a Dr. Coxe, presumably Sydenham's mentor, publishing a catalogue of complaints, including apothecaries not understanding Latin, their knowing little about illness and their failing to make up prescriptions accurately.[20] Much in the same vein, the physician Jonathan

---

[h] This was before the Linnaean classification of plants.

[i] Including Hercules' All-heal, angelica, balm, barley betony, brank ursine, centaury, cuckow-point, dwarf elder, elm bark, endive, elecampane, fennel, flea-wort, flower-de-luce, stinking gladwin, goutwort, ground ivy, hemlock, hemp, henbane, hedge hyssop, black hellebore, houseleek, juniper, masterwort, mullein, mustard, nettle, pennyroyal, pepperwort, poplar tree, poppy, bastard rhubarb, English tobacco thyme and tumsole.

Goddard (ca. 1617–1675) published two essays encouraging physicians to make up prescriptions for themselves. [21] This Goddard certainly did, and he formulated the successful *Dr. Goddard's Drops*, recommended by Sydenham over other smelling salts for faints, apoplexy and lethargy.[j] They were so popular that King Charles II purchased the secret formula for the nation for an equivalent of about half a million pounds today, and that was despite Goddard having been Oliver Cromwell's doctor. When the King fell fatally ill (see the following), his doctors tried to revive him with the drops, but even these could not save him. [22] They turned out to be made up of a mixture of viper extract, human skull (the younger the better), ivory and the ammoniacal extract of hart's horn. [23]

Another physician joining the anti-apothecary campaign was Christopher Merrett (1614–1695). Merrett was entrusted with looking after the library that William Harvey (1578–1657) had left to the College of Physicians and was also one of the College Censors that Sydenham stood before to obtain his licence. [24] His pamphlet of 1670 is a window on poor seventeenth-century professional relations, complaining that the Society of Apothecaries was not regularly sending apprentices for examination to the College of Physicians and was snubbing the College's inspectors at Apothecaries' Hall dinners by not sitting them at the high table with the Master. [25] Merrett grumbled that apothecaries made money by extending the duration of treatment that physicians had prescribed, providing drugs for fabricated diseases and creating new illnesses and treatments. He concluded that they were trying to take over medicine and sided with Goddard that physicians should do their own dispensing. [26] However, Merrett was a bigger man than his sparring with apothecaries suggests. Like several other doctors that we will come across later, Merrett was fascinated by the history of the natural world. His *Pinax Rerum Naturalium Britannicarum, continens Vegetabilia, Animalia, et Fossilia*[k] was the most complete account to date of

---

[j] Apoplexy is an old term for stroke or cerebrovascular accident.

[k] Translates from Latin as *Register of British Natural Things Containing Vegetables, Animals and Fossils.*

plants and animals in Britain and was the first attempt to catalogue British insects.[27] It also has the first list of fossils found in Britain to date, bearing in mind that the word at that time was a catch-all for any stone or mineral found in the earth or in rocks. Merrett took a stab at explaining the enigma of how fossils, as we use the word today, came to be. Translated from Latin, this reads as follows:

> it is abundantly clear to me that many stones considered to be inorganic are fashioned out of animals or their parts through the action of some earthen fluid; that they had communicated their shape to the clay or soft earth and had then perished though their figure was preserved.

Merrett's *Pinax* is little more than an alphabetical index and precedes by many decades any thought of what fossils tell us about evolution.[28] The surviving version of the *Pinax* is actually a copy of the original, which was lost in the Great Fire of London in 1666. However, that was the least of Merrett's problems, as Harvey's library burned with it. Although the fire was considered by many to be an act of papist terrorism, Merrett was blamed for the loss of the books and duly lost his job as librarian.[29] He took the College to court, claiming that his appointment and the stipend that went with it were for life. After an extended legal wrangle, Merrett first lost the court case and then his College fellowship. He was an original fellow of the Royal Society, but having fallen on hard times, he failed to pay his dues and was expelled from there as well. It was rough justice.

Sydenham's Gout

Doctors have no professional protection from disease, and gout was Sydenham's serving from the common lot. He experienced his first attack while at Oxford, and by the age of 59 he was virtually housebound.[30] It was at this point that he wrote his classic, *Treatise on Gout and Dropsy*, which is additionally poignant in coming from his own suffering. He dedicated the work to Thomas Short (ca. 1630–1685), who was a successful London physician despite being a Roman Catholic. These were febrile times, and relations between Protestants and Roman Catholics were at a low ebb, fuelled in large part by Protestant fears of King Charles II promising to convert to Catholicism in return for subsidies from the King of France, the Catholic Louis XIV (1638–1715). Short was destined to die two years later, supposedly poisoned for spreading a tale that the King had been assassinated on account of his Catholic leanings.[31] A more likely explanation is that the King died because of his hands-on pursuit of chemistry in a laboratory that he had established in the basement of his living quarters at Whitehall. The King had a keen interest in the application of mercury for medicinal purposes but also held the alchemical dream of transmuting it into gold – which would have freed him from French handouts. That Charles II died from regularly exposing himself to mercury is supported by modern forensic analysis of a lock of hair said to be his.[32]

　　Sydenham apologised to Short in the dedication that his work might have been longer had not the very act of writing (or dictating) triggered a return of his gout. He then moved on, not for the first time, to his poor relationships with his colleagues:

> … if this dissertation escape blame both from you and those other few (but tried and honourable men) whom I call my friends, I shall care little for the others. They are hostile to me, because what *I* think of diseases and their cares differs from what *they* think. It could not be otherwise. It is my nature to think where others read; to ask less whether the world agrees with me than whether I agree with the truth; and to hold cheap the rumour and applause of the multitude.

Ben Welles' *Treatise on the Gout or Joint-Evil* (1669) had come out a few years before, and this provides a window on conventional thinking about gout and practice at the time.[33] Welles' work was almost entirely theoretical, with precious little evidence that he ever went near a patient. In contrast,

Sydenham reveals a wealth of clinical experience. Just as James Gillray gave us the best visual image of an acute gout attack a century later, Sydenham left us with what is widely regarded as the best written description:

> This pain is like that of a dislocation, and yet the parts feel as if cold-water were poured over them. Then follow chills and shivers, and a little fever. The pain, which is at first moderate becomes more intense. With its intensity the chills and shivers increase. After a time this comes to a height, accommodating itself in the bones and ligaments of the tarsus and metatarsus. Now it is a violent stretching and tearing of the ligaments – now it is a gnawing pain, and now a pressure and tightening. So exquisite and lively meanwhile is the feeling of the parts affected, that it cannot bear the weight of the bedclothes nor the jar of a person walking in the room. The night is passed in torture, sleeplessness, turning of the parts affected and perpetual change of posture; the tossing about of the body being incessant as the pain of the tortured joint, and being worse as the fit comes on. Hence the vain efforts, by change of posture, both in the body and the limbs affected, to obtain an abandonment of the pain.[34]

Sydenham not only precisely described the symptoms of an acute attack but also its timing, with the onset in the middle of the night and relief in the morning, only to recur the next night.[35] This rhythm of gouty inflammation has since been scientifically substantiated.[36] How this timing became a feature of gout has been a mystery until recent discoveries on the workings of the biological circadian clock. The basic principles were discovered in fruit flies, but the molecular mechanisms have remained preserved over evolutionary time and apply to humans. Not least is the important relationship between the circadian cycle and inflammation.[37]

Sydenham and Welles largely agreed on acute gout being a gravitational 'defluxion' of humours. Welles was distracted by which specific humour is involved and whether different humours could cause different forms of gout. Sydenham was not interested in that level of detail, sticking with the principle that gout was the same sort of internal detoxification process as he felt took place during fevers. He did not see the humours as abstract entities, as he referred to the offending material as 'morbific matter' or sometimes 'peccant matter'. Thus, in gout:

> ... we must remember, that it is the inviolable rule of Nature, interwoven with the essence of the present disease, to throw the peccant matter upon the joints. [38]

Treatments recommended by Welles were typical of the age, with the focus being on purging and bleeding. He particularly endorsed 'emptying of the antecedent matter' by 'opening a vein in a contrary part', by which he meant, for example, the right arm if gout was in the right foot.[39] In contrast, since an acute gout attack almost always resolves without treatment, Sydenham saw acute gout as performing a useful healing function by dispersing excess humour. Extrapolating from this, he regarded all the conventional methods for its removal with deep suspicion:

> ... all that can be done by purges or vomits, is to throw what Nature would eject through the extremities into the blood. Hence it happens that what was meant for the joints, takes hold of one of the viscera. Then the patients' life is in danger. This is often observed in those who, either to ward off a fit, or what is worse, to allay one, have used themselves to purgatives. Nature diverted from her own good and safe method of depositing the peccant matter in the joints, as soon as the humours are solicited towards the intestines, instead of acute pains with little danger, induces sickness, griping, fainting, and other irregular symptoms, which nearly destroy the patient.[40]

In other words, the body sacrifices the joints to spare the internal organs, and physical interference with this process could only make things more serious. The extension of this line of thought was that being able to mount an acute attack of gout was a sign of a sound, active constitution capable of correcting humoral derangements and preserving health generally. Conversely, an inability to mount an acute fit of gout risked developing chronic and more dangerous infirmities. Consequently, Sydenham's treatment was limited to the use of herbal medicines as 'digestives' and his own recipe for laudanum for pain relief.[1] This was a tincture of opium in alcohol that he probably resorted to a fair bit himself. Sydenham's view of herbal specifics was very similar to that of Nicholas Culpeper: the simpler, the better. Again, drawing from his experience with fevers, he favoured the use of 'Peruvian bark',[m] which he had helped introduce and which later turned out to contain quinine.[41] As for preventative treatment, Sydenham was very clear that this was all about lifestyle and particularly required a regimen of simple and judicious food and drink. Sydenham was a puritan, and regarding gout as a penance for indulgence probably coloured his views.

Sydenham brought to seventeenth-century medicine the much-needed moral mindset that doctors have an obligation to enhance the art of medicine:

> In all cases it behoves each and all of those physicians, who have the desire not only to *seem* but to *be* prudent and honest, to acknowledge and entreat the Divine Goodness, that from this they may look for wisdom and good fortune; and they ought not to be satisfied with simply giving health to the sick, but they should strive to add greater certainty to the art they administer; and they should so direct their experiments, that the science of medicine may grow

---

[1] The word 'laudanum' derives from the Latin *laudare*, meaning 'to praise'.

[m] This was the bark of *Cinchona* plants, which Sydenham referred to as 'cortex' or simply 'C'. It was first imported for medicinal use from Peru to Spain by Jesuits around 1632 and is believed to have first arrived in London in 1655.

day by day more clear and efficient. In this way the human race may reap the advantages thereof generally, and with safety, even after they themselves have been laid in their graves.[42]

However, this enthusiasm for experiments had boundaries, as Sydenham focused entirely on his patients and their lifestyles and had no interest in the laboratory. He compared himself to a plantsman who could easily harvest fruit without knowing much about the makeup of a tree. He especially disapproved of physicians studying anatomy or microscopy, dismissing these as only for surgeons.[43] That does not mean he rejected science and scientists, as he socialised in coffee houses with many of the brilliant natural philosophers who founded the Royal Society in 1660, including Robert Boyle, the physicist and microscopist Robert Hooke (1635–1703), and the architect Christopher Wren (1632–1723). Sydenham saw himself as primarily a physician rather than a natural philosopher and never became a fellow of the Royal Society. Nevertheless, *Method of Curing Fevers* was summarised in the first volume of the Royal Society's *Philosophical Transactions*, showing that Sydenham had the ear of the leading scientific circle if not of the College of Physicians.[44]

Even though he conducted no quantitative work himself and made no progress in understanding the mechanisms of diseases, Sydenham's insistence on the importance of direct clinical observation paved the way for clinical research to support what we now call evidence-based medicine. His disdain for the medical library was famously recounted by Richard Blackmore: 'when one Day I asked him to advise me what Books I should read to qualify me for Practice, he replied 'Don Quixote, it is a very good Book, I read it still''.[45]

Sydenham's response sounds flippant, but it has been pointed out that Miguel de Cervantes mentions over 100 medicinal plants in *Don Quixote*. Sydenham may therefore have genuinely thought he was offering good advice.[46]

Thomas Willis and Clopton Havers

If Ben Welles provides a clinical contrast to Sydenham, the anatomist and physician Thomas Willis (1621–1675) (see Figure 2.1(c)) provides a scientific one. Sydenham and Willis were at Oxford together; both moved to London to earn a living, and both came from country gentry families – but the similarity ends there. Willis was an orthodox Anglican and had fought in the Civil War for the University Royalist legion.[47] While Sydenham dismissed anatomy as irrelevant for medicine, Willis had a deep interest in anatomical detail and what it signified for physiology. Among his accomplishments was the discovery of the arterial arrangement that equitably distributes blood to the brain, which is now called the Circle of Willis. Two years after the publication of Sydenham's *Treatise on the Gout*, he published his *London Practice of Physick,* a broad-based textbook that illustrates well the entry of Enlightenment thinking into medicine. He modernised the humour responsible for gout as salt and converted supposed humoral diseases into disorders of the nervous system. A rather complicated arrangement, evocative of gender politics, incriminated the nerves in gouty arthritis:

> Therefore a saline or tartarous matter … is as it were the feminine Seed of this Disease; which nevertheless, tho heap'd together in a great plenty, is wholly unfruitful of it self, till the nervous Liquour growing turgid, sends acetous Recrements, falling from it, to the seat of the former, which, as the masculine Seed, presently renders the other prolifick: for, in as much as those two particles, which are of a different state and origine, meet, and mutually contest, they twitch the Fibres of the Membranes and Tendons, and so cause the Fit of the Gout.[48]

Willis' nervous theory of gout was challenged by the microscopist Clopton Havers (1657–1702).[49] This was the Havers of Haversian Canals, those tiny tubes in the outer cortex of bone that house blood vessels and nerves. Havers also described, for the first time, the microvillous synovial membrane, which forms the inner lining of joint capsules, and the synovial fluid released by its 'mucilaginous glands' into joint spaces. Havers pointed out politely that Willis' saline would excite the nerves directly without requiring an interaction with nervous liquor. He proposed instead that it was the mucilaginous glands that were irritated by viscous salt discharged from the blood into the joint. Nevertheless, versions of Willis' nervous theory lived on to be revived in the late 1700s by William Cullen (see Chapter 3) and then, in a sense, right up to the 1960s.

Whether the gout involved the nerves or the 'mucilaginous glands' was entirely academic for most practising doctors. Blackmore, fighting his own battles with medical imaginings 40 years later, reflected on the difference between Willis and Sydenham:

> Dr. Sydenham, who built all his Maxims and Rules of Practice upon repeated Observations of the Nature and Properties of Diseases, the Power of Remedies, has compiled so good a History of Distempers, and so prevalent a Method of Cure, by which he has improved and advanced the healing Art, much more than Dr. Willis, with all his curious Speculations and fanciful Hypotheses: For what can be expected but crude and unprofitable Conceptions, from Gentlemen, that imagine they have acquired great Attainments in the Art of Curing, and are accomplished Physicians, before they have had the Advantages of Experience and Observation?[50]

Sydenham was therefore, the prototype for the modern thoughtful clinician, and Willis the precursor of the academic clinician-scientist. Whereas Sydenham was outspoken on the uselessness of theory for medical practice, Willis was quite happy to speculate on disease mechanisms and mostly did so with some insight. Pointing to the tension between the clinician and the academic, the contemporary diarist John Ward recorded:

> Sydenham and some others in London say of Dr. Willis that hee is an ingenious man but not a good physitian, and that hee does not understand the way of practice.[51]

Versions of this are still repeated in modern times, with only the names changing. It behoves a clinical academic to be a good doctor.

Reflections on Sydenham's Legacy

Sydenham's conservative views on how to treat (or rather, how not to treat) gout had a huge influence on how patients and doctors alike saw the problem. His emphasis on acute gout as being salutary and protecting from ill health helps us understand *Dialogue with the Gout* by one of the founding fathers of the United States, Benjamin Franklin:

> Franklin: Ah! how tiresome you are!;
> Gout: Well, then, to my office; it should not be forgotten that I am your physician....
> Franklin: Ohhh! what a devil of a physician!
> Gout: How ungrateful you are to say so! Is it not I who, in the character of your physician, have saved you from the palsy, dropsy, and apoplexy? one or other of which would have done for you long ago, but for me.[52]

Such was the belief that gout is protective that, a century later, the physician William Heberden (1710–1801) wrote:

> people are neither ashamed, nor afraid of it; but are rather ambitious of supposing that every complaint arises from a Gouty cause, and support themselves with the hopes that they shall one day have the Gout, and use variety of means for this purpose, which happily for them are generally ineffectual.[53]

Likewise, in the words of the prominent London physician Charles Scudamore as late as 1825:

> I have known some gouty persons complaining of symptoms evidently threatening apoplexy, who have attempted a more than

usually stimulating plan of diet, with an increased quantity of wine, in the idea of forcing the gout; but the sensations in the head soon compelled them to desist from such improper proceeding. One gentleman actually suffered from apoplexy, in consequence of such hurtful excitement.[54]

Although the salutary nature of gout in protecting from other diseases has long since been consigned to history, Sydenham's emphasis on the body naturally healing itself was sound. After all, as I will discuss later, inflammation is fundamentally a corrective process as a response to injury or the threat of it. Sydenham anticipated the concept of internal physiological regulation, which was developed in the nineteenth century by the French physician Claude Bernard (1813–1878) and given the name 'homeostasis' in the twentieth century by the Harvard physiologist Walter Cannon (1871–1945).[55]

   Sydenham's treatise on gout was only a small part of his written output, but it is perhaps what he is best remembered for – at least by rheumatologists. He died in 1689, helped on his way by his own severe gout. His reputation for astute clinical observations and teachings is, to a large extent, posthumous, having been enhanced by those he trained. These included not only Richard Blackmore (as above) but also Hans Sloane (1660–1753), who became both president of the Royal Society and president of the Royal College of Physicians at the same time. Sydenham's legacy also owes much to his close friend and collaborator, the physician and moral philosopher John Locke (1632–1704) (see Figure 2.1(d)), who advertised his work more widely in Europe.[56] The great Herman Boerhaave (1668–1738), professor at the preeminent medical school of the times at Leiden in the Netherlands, supposedly raised his hat whenever he mentioned 'the shining light of England, that Apollo of the art'.[57] Boerhaave was, in turn, an inspiration for William Cullen and others who developed the Edinburgh Medical School, which was greatly influential in the eighteenth and nineteenth centuries. Lastly, Sydenham laid the foundation for the modern clinical art of medicine, which requires a detailed account from the patient of the history and nature of the symptoms as well as a meticulous physical examination. Only then should the appropriate laboratory tests and body imaging be requested, and only then can these be correctly interpreted.

Chapter 3

Some Gout Physicians of the Eighteenth Century

The eighteenth century has been referred to as the Gout's 'golden era', but that perhaps overlooks all the suffering. How much of 'the Gout' was what we now think of as true gout is debatable. In the long run up to scientific discovery, the century was rich in medical theories but short of new facts. Exercising his poetic nature, Richard Blackmore[a] lamented:

> The Colleges of Learning employed in enquiring into Nature, and searching after the Causes of Things, for many successive Ages, unhappily proceeded in such Ways and Methods, as rather obstructed than promoted the End they had in View: For they formed nothing but notional Speculation, falsly called Science, the trifling play of Fancy, and the idle Labour of the Closet. These curious Subtleties, for want of firm and solid Foundations to rest upon, hung in their brain, and floated in their Imaginations like fine wrought Cobwebs, or the loose Threads, that in the frosty Mornings are caught in Hedges, or hover in the Air; for this reason it is, that Natural Science has received so little Improvement and Augmentation since the Schools of Philosophers were first erected, even down to the last age.[1]

---

[a] Blackmore was primarily a physician. As an epic poet, he is sadly best remembered by the derision bestowed on him by contemporary wit poets, among whom he was not 'one of the gang'. He was particularly ridiculed by Alexander Pope in the *Dunciad* (1728), in which the poems Blackmore reads to a team of lawyers are so dull they fall asleep. Samuel Johnson is rather more forgiving about Blackmore in his *Lives of the Most Eminent English Poets* (1779–1781).

Although Blackmore wrote this in 1720, as far as gout is concerned, it is a reasonable summary up to the discovery of uric acid at the end of the century. This chapter looks at some of the eighteenth-century physicians who treated 'the Gout' and kept the bookstalls stocked with treatises, books, essays and pamphlets.

Archibald Pitcairne and Newtonian Medicine

'Sydenham versus the Establishment' moved to Scotland. The Edinburgh physicians had succeeded in obtaining a charter to establish their own Royal College in 1681, basing it on the London version and with a similar purpose of maintaining the medical hierarchy, policing conformity of practice and excluding apothecaries and other unlicensed practitioners. Andrew Brown (ca. 1640–ca. 1720) was not considered qualified for the fellowship but was given a license to practice physic, as he held an MD from King's College, Aberdeen. Having read Sydenham's work, Brown travelled to London to witness his practice firsthand. The visit convinced Brown of the success of Sydenham's methods for treating fevers, and he then applied these to his patients in Edinburgh. Just as Sydenham had experienced in London, this met robust local opposition, not helped by a prominent patient dying. Again, the issue was only partly medical. The Edinburgh physicians were mostly Catholics loyal to the deposed James VII of Scotland,[b] while Brown had backed the 'Glorious Revolution', which had brought in the English Dutch Protestant regimen under King William and Queen Mary. The issues with Brown were then sidelined as the Edinburgh College split into two internal factions related to medical theory of fevers, examination practice, political leaning, social status and religious belief, resulting in a riot in December 1695.[2]

The plethora of heated pamphlets leading up to the riot record different shades of orthodoxy within the Edinburgh College, with opinions being divided on why recognised treatment worked rather than whether it worked

---

[b] James VII of Scotland was James II of England.

at all or whether there was anything better to offer. A key participant was Archibald Pitcairne (1652–1713), who had recently returned from a year as professor in Leiden.[3] Pitcairne was on the losing side, and his fellowship was suspended until peace was resumed eight years later. Pitcairne' position derived from the then fashionable Cartesian[c] iatromechanical theory of physiology, which held the body to be a machine. The central driver of the fluidics of the system was the heart, and the central cause of disease was obstructions to fluid flow through blood vessels, a dogma adapted from ideas passed down from Galen.[4] Pitcairne was preoccupied with Isaac Newton, whose *Principia* had appeared in 1687. This led him to promote a stripped-down, modified Cartesian theory based on mathematics and the belief that the same laws that govern planetary movement apply to the movements of particles in the human body. Pitcairne provides a starting point for the mathematical approach to medicine, which, among other things, has ended up with computer-based modelling. His contribution to this story was to mentor and influence George Cheyne and Richard Mead (1673–1754), two quite different young physicians.

George Cheyne

George Cheyne was a larger-than-life character who started out fitting Pitcairne's Newtonian principles theoretically to diseases and ended up more interested in wellness and Christian mysticism (Figure 3.1). Along the way, he became a 'father of self-help' via a mass of popular publications for the public. At the age of around 14, Cheyne had entered Marischal College in Aberdeen[d] with a view to taking holy orders.[5] With his interest shifting to medicine, he moved his studies to Edinburgh, where he came under Pitcairne's wing, publishing his mathematical *A New Theory of Continual Fevers* in 1701.[6] This was dashed off at Pitcairne's request to help Pitcairne

---

[c] The word 'Cartesian' reflects the philosophy of René Descartes and indicates a rational mathematical approach to the body.

[d] Marischal College in Aberdeen merged in 1860 with King's College to form the present university.

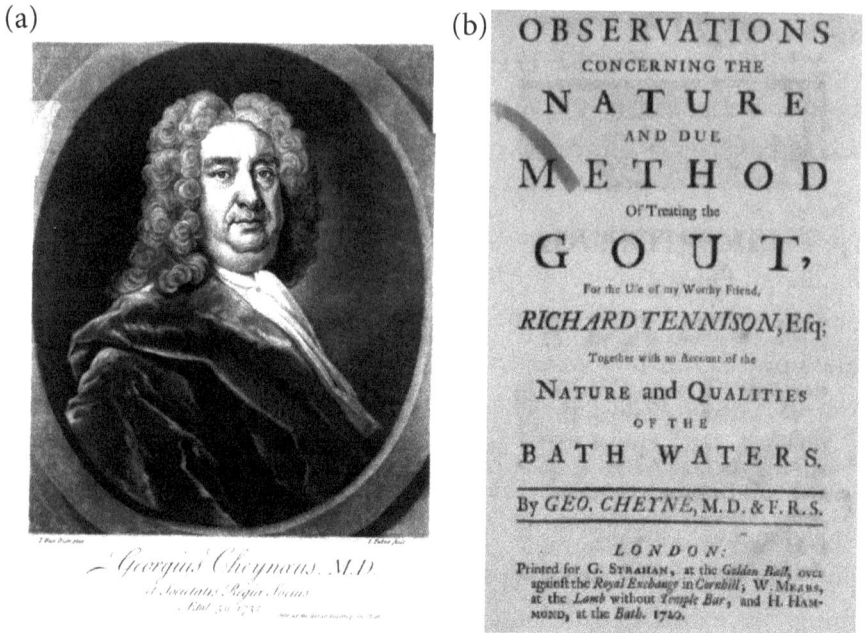

(a)

(b)

OBSERVATIONS
CONCERNING THE
NATURE
AND DUE
METHOD
Of Treating the
GOUT,
For the Use of my Worthy Friend,
RICHARD TENNISON, Efq;
Together with an Account of the
NATURE and QUALITIES
OF THE
BATH WATERS.
By *GEO. CHEYNE,* M.D. & F.R.S.

LONDON:
Printed for G. STRAHAN, at the *Golden Ball,* over
againft the *Royal Exchange* in *Cornhill;* W. MEARS,
at the *Lamb* without *Temple Bar,* and H. HAM-
MOND, at the *Bath.* 1720.

Figure 3.1.

(a) Mezzotint of the physician George Cheyne by John Faber Junior after Johan van Diest. Cheyne became one of the first authors of popular self-help medical books.

(b) Title page of the first edition of George Cheyne's *Observations Concerning the Nature and Due Method of Treating the Gout ....*

Source: Both courtesy of the Wellcome Collection: (a) CC BY 4.0; (b) public domain.

with his quarrel at the Edinburgh College.[7] To advance in life, Cheyne then obtained an MD from King's College, Aberdeen, and moved down to London. Highly recommended by Pitcairne, he was immediately elected a fellow of the Royal Society; however, his participation there was brief, as he soon fell out with the one man he needed to stay in with – Isaac Newton himself, the president of the Royal Society.

As for Sydenham 50 years earlier, the challenge of breaking into the highly competitive practice of physic in early eighteenth-century London must have been daunting. However, Cheyne was naturally affable and made a point of networking in taverns and coffee houses, where he built up a medical practice among the *bon vivant*. This was a common strategy; John Radcliffe (discussed in more detail later in this chapter) preferred the Bull's Head Tavern, then on the site where the London School of Economics stands today. Indeed, the practice persisted occasionally in London into the late 1970s, and I remember a general practitioner whose referrals to the Middlesex Hospital seemed to mostly come from a local public house. For Cheyne, this lifestyle was unsustainable as he became massively overweight, collapsed mentally and had to leave London.

Cheyne started practicing medicine in Bath around 1710, although we know that he initially split his time with London as, in 1714, he consulted there with the heavyweight metropolitan duo of Richard Mead and Hans Sloane.[8] He finally settled in Bath permanently in 1718.[9] It was from Bath that Cheyne published his *Observations Concerning the Nature and Due Method of Treating the Gout* in 1720 (see Figure 3.1(b)), branding it as an information pamphlet for his patron Richard Tennison.[10] This was the year the South Sea Bubble burst,[e] and many of his patients may have had good cause to feel unwell. Under Pitcairne's influence, Cheyne moved acute gout away from Sydenham's healthy discharge of humours to a local plumbing problem in which salts build up from high living. The salts 'by their plenty and nearness, uniting in great clusters, must necessarily form obstructions, and give pain, when, by the force of the circulation, they are thrust through narrower and stiffer small vessels (capillaries).'[11] Accordingly, gout attacks the joints mechanically because the 'quickness' of the circulation is diminished there and because small blood vessels are compressed by the protuberances of bones.[12] The fact that one person and not another suffers from gout could be explained by differences in the

---

[e] The South Sea Company was formed in 1711 to manage government debt. It obtained a monopoly to trade with South America and focused on the transport of slaves from Africa. The share price rocketed from around £100 to around £1,000 on the back of internal corruption and external hype. The bursting of the 'South Sea Bubble' in 1720 ruined thousands of investors, including the 'Quicksilver Doctor' Thomas Dover (Chapter 4), and it remains the prototype of all subsequent financial crashes.

narrowness and stiffness of these small blood vessels. These were still early days in the rise of Bath to eighteenth-century pre-eminence as Britain's foremost fashion and health spa. Thus, Cheyne's essay on gout doubled as an advertisement for visiting the city and implicitly as a call to consult Cheyne while there. The title had the suffix ... *together with an Account of the Nature and Quality of the Bath Waters*, and Cheyne explained that the sulphur and iron in the waters helped dissolve the gout salts by forming a kind of soap that cleared the obstructed blood vessels.

As he moved more and more towards a holistic approach, he increasingly saw gout as representative of the consequences of an ill-advised modern life, and by the fifth edition of his essay, he had added ... *and also of the Nature and Cure of Most Chronical Distempers, not publish'd before* to the end of the long title and explained in the updated preface, as follows: 'Physicians know how close a Connection, and near an Alliance Chronical Diseases have to one another.'[13] By 1724, Cheyne's transition from a Newtonian academic to a practicing clinician was complete, and he publicly said goodbye to his earlier mechanistic work, turning his approach from a Willis to a Sydenham (see Chapter 2). The preface to his *Essay of Health and Long Life* dismissed academia as little more than mental self-indulgence for those not needing a job.[14] Cheyne was the advance guard among popular health gurus, and his attempts to integrate the mind and the body and avoid gout through healthy living left a lasting legacy, even if ridiculed at the time:

DR. WINTER TO DR, CHEYNE, BATH
'Tell me from whom, fat headed Scot
Did thou thy system learn.
From Hippocrates thou hadst it not
Nor Celsus nor Pitcairn.

'Suppose we own that milk is good
And say the same of grass;
The one for babes is only good
The other for an ass.

'Doctor, a new prescription try –
A friend's advice forgive;
Eat grass – reduce your head- or die
Your patients then may live.'

DR. CHEYNE'S REPLY

'My system doctor, 's all my own,
No tutor I pretend,
My blunders hurt myself alone,
But yours – your dearest friend.

'Were you once more to straw confined,
How happy it might be -
Or would you, perhaps, regain your mind
Or from your *wit* get free

'I can't your new prescription try,
But easily forgive,
T'is nat 'tral you should bid me die,
That you yourself may live.' [15]

The poem refers to Cheyne's advocacy of a milky diet and vegetarianism, and he also espoused the temperate use of alcohol and frequent exercise. All good advice, but it did not help Cheyne, who, for whatever reason, continued to put on weight and at length achieved 32 stone,[f] with all the consequent physical restrictions.[16] Exemplifying Cheyne's holistic approach was the practical advice to have a hobby:

I would earnestly recommend to all those affected with nervous distempers, always to have some innocent entertaining amusement to employ themselves in, for the rest of the day, after they have employed a sufficient time upon exercise, towards the evening, to

---

[f] 448 pounds or 203 kilograms.

prepare them for their night's quiet rest. It seems to me absolutely impossible, without such a help, to keep the mind easy, and prevent it wearing out the body, as the sword does the scabbard; it is no matter what it is, provided it be but a hobby-horse, and an amusement, and stop the current of amusement and intense thinking, which persons of weak nerves are apt to run into.[17]

Richard Mead

Richard Mead (see Figures 3.2(a)–(c)) was brought up in the Netherlands, where his non-conformist father lived as a political refugee, and he was tutored by Pitcairne in Leiden. Having obtained a medical degree in

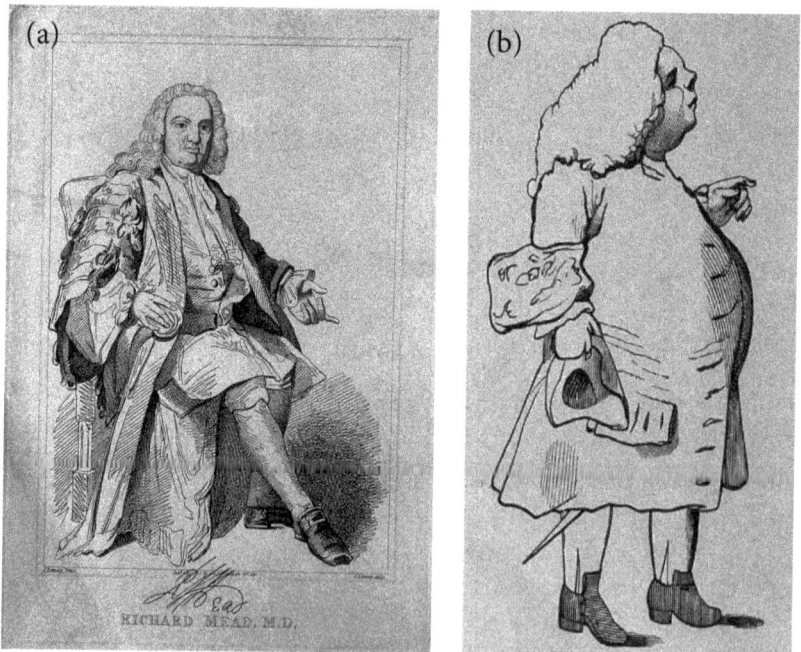

Figure 3.2.

(a) Richard Mead, an early proponent of a mathematical approach to medicine, etched by John Romney in 1817 after Allan Ramsay.

(b) A less official version of the portly Mead as a militia drill sergeant, reproduced in 1888 from a sketch by William Hogarth.

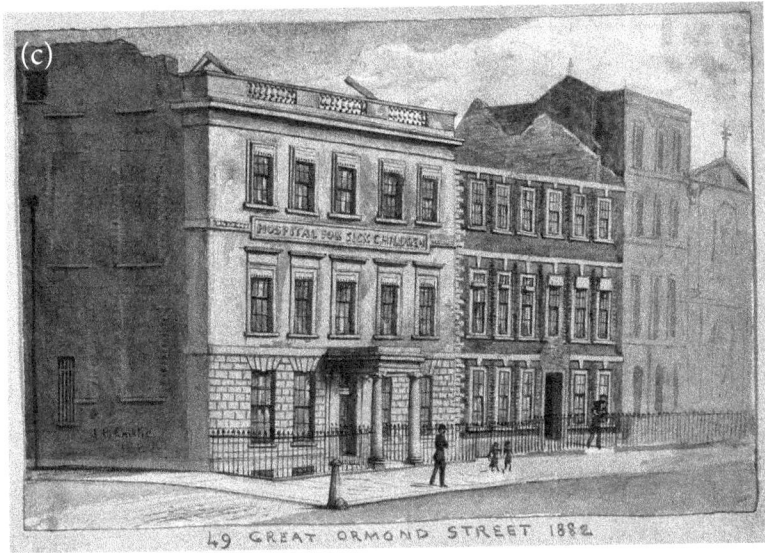

Figure 3.2. (*Continued*)

(c) Mead was highly successful as a physician and lived in style at 49 Great Ormond St., shown later in 1882 in watercolour by John Philipps Emslie, after the house had become the Great Ormond Street Hospital for Sick Children.

Source: All courtesy of the Wellcome Collection, public domain.

Padua, Mead moved to London, where he established his own medical practice. In 1702, he published his influential *Mechanical Account of Poisons in Several Essays*, in which he promoted a quantitative reductionist approach to medicine. Having mathematical learning would distinguish a physician from a quack and be as necessary as knowing Latin or Greek.[18] Physicians needed to:

> discover the footsteps of Mechanism in those surprizing phaenomena which are commonly ascribed to some Occult or Unknown Principle. But to unravel the Springs of the Several Motions upon which such appearances do depend, and trace up all the symptoms to their first causes, requires some Art as well as Labour; and that

both upon the account of the Exquisite Fineness, and marvellous Composition, of the Animal Machine in which they are transacted, and of the Minuteness of those Bodies which have the force to induce in it such Sudden and Violent alteration.[19]

Mead's essay on viper poisoning contains possibly the first written insight into the inflammatory potential of crystals. Upon examining venom under his microscope, he observed the formation of crystals capable of penetrating globules in the blood:

Upon the first Sight I could discover nothing but a Parcel of small salts nimbly floating in the Liquor, but in a very short time the Appearance was changed and these saline Particles were now shot out into *Crystals* of an incredible Tenuity and Sharpness, … and yet withal so rigid were these pellucid *Spicula*, or *Darts*, that they remained unaltered upon my Glass for several Months...[20]

In hindsight, the crystals Mead observed would have been an artefact of the venom drying on the microscope slide. Notwithstanding, Mead looked to see how they might affect the blood and observed:

that our Blood consisting chiefly of Two Parts, a simple Lympb, and an infinite Number of small Globular, containing a very sub-tle and elastic Fluid, these acute Salts, when mingled with it, do prick those Globules, or *Vesiculae*, and so let out their impris-oned active Substance, which expanding itself in every way, must necessarily be the Instrument of this speedy Alteration and Change.[21]

Bearing in mind that next to nothing was known at the time about the cellu-lar composition of blood or any other living tissues, Mead's deduction from seeing crystals penetrating 'blood globules' and causing them to discharge was an entirely novel way of thinking about the origins of inflammation.

In 1703, Mead was appointed to a staff physician post at St. Thomas' Hospital, then situated near London Bridge, close to where Guy's Hospital stands today. He prospered and became Royal Physician to Queen Anne (1665–1714), who has recently been featured cinematically with her gouty illness in *The Favourite*. Thomas Sydenham teaching the salutary nature of gout helps us understand a report in October 1712 from Windsor:

> Last Thursday Her Majesty remov'd to the Garden-House, on the South-Side of the Castle; the next Day She was seiz'd by a regular-form'd Fit of the Gout, which is looked upon as a Mark of great Vigour in Her Constitution; this Day the Fit is over, and her Majesty is very easy.[22]

The Queen is known to have been fond of her food and drink, to have taken little exercise and to have become seriously overweight. In 1712, she would have been 47 and presumably post-menopausal, and so her having had gout as a woman is certainly possible. However, there was more to Anne's medical portfolio than that. The physician John Radcliffe (1650–1714) (see Figure 3.3(a))[g] had been summoned to visit her some 17 years previously but had declined the invitation, spreading publicly his view that Anne's illness was 'nothing but the vapours'.[23] Nowadays, the 'vapours' summon up thoughts of psychosomatic ladies who lunch, but at the time, it referred to internal discharges assumed to emanate from a disorderly womb. This Anne clearly had, as her obstetric record was a disaster, with the majority of her 17 pregnancies ending in miscarriages, stillbirths or premature deliveries. Her failure to produce an heir left her succession in limbo and set the stage for the arrival of the House of Hanover and four successive King Georges. A limited post-mortem when Anne died found no evidence of gout.[24] Judging from her nickname 'Brandy-faced Nan' and what looks

---

[g] John Radcliffe was one of the most financially successful of the early eighteenth-century physicians. His will provided the legacy that enabled the building of the Radcliffe Infirmary, the Radcliffe Observatory and the Radcliffe Camera at the University of Oxford, as well as much else.

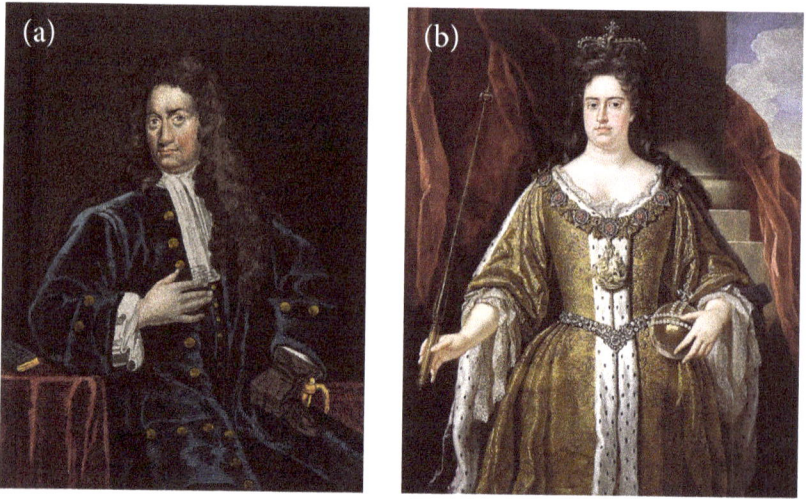

Figure 3.3.

(a) Coloured stipple engraving of John Radcliffe by M. Dahl after a 1710 portrait by Godfrey Kneller.

(b) Portrait of Queen Anne after John Closterman from around 1702. The subtle flush on the Queen's upper cheeks could well be the butterfly rash of systemic lupus erythematosus. Anne never forgave Radcliffe for suggesting that her illness was 'nothing but the Vapours'.

Source: (a) Courtesy of the Wellcome Collection, public domain; (b) Wikimedia Commons, public domain.

like a 'butterfly rash' on her upper cheeks in her portraits, such as the one by Godfrey Kneller (see Figure 3.3(b)), her primary illness may have been systemic lupus erythematosus (SLE).[25] This is an autoimmune condition first described much later in Vienna in 1872 by the Hungarian physician Moritz Kaposi (1837–1902).[h,26] If so, the Queen's miscarriages and stillbirths may well have been due to her having the associated anti-phospholipid autoantibodies.[27] Any gout that she may have had would also have been secondary to SLE.

---

[h] The same Kaposi that described Kaposi's Sarcoma.

As with Sydenham before him, Mead's major contribution was in the field of infectious diseases. When the plague broke out in Marseilles in 1720, Mead was asked to propose effective quarantine measures to prevent the spread of disease into and within Britain. He published these as *A Short Discourse Concerning Pestilential Contagion, and the Method to be Used to Prevent It*, providing the first public health report commissioned by the British government and written by a physician.[28] Mead was an early believer in contagion as a means for transmission of the plague at a time when this was still controversial, and the book could have been written today if one substitutes in bacteria or viruses for Mead's hypothetical contagious particles. Mead's arguments for and against quarantining and the focus on poverty, poor hygiene and overcrowding make it a salient read today.

Mead included his recommendations for gout among diseases of the liver in his *Pharmacopoeia Meadiana: Faithfully Gathered from Original Prescriptions, Containing the Most Elegant Methods of Cure in Diseases* of 1757. He held to Sydenham's views on the danger of treating acute gout and indeed took Sydenham's conservative approach even further by regarding even the pain as beneficial: 'It has been disputed among physicians, whether, or not, a vein may be opened, when the pain in the joint is extremely severe. Now, to settle this point, we ought never to forget, that this pain is highly necessary for tumefying the part and therefore ought to be borne with patience.'[29]

William Stukeley

The physician-antiquarian William Stukeley (1687–1765) (see Figure 3.4(a)) studied under Mead after completing undergraduate studies at Cambridge. He was an active fellow of the Royal Society and provides another example of the interest that doctors had in fossils. In 1717, he presented a large blue clay stone derived from cliffs around Fulbeck in Lincolnshire, containing what was previously considered to be an early human skeleton.[30] However, Stukeley concluded that it was the remains of an aquatic creature, either a crocodile or a porpoise. Not one to challenge Old Testament scholars, he

(a)

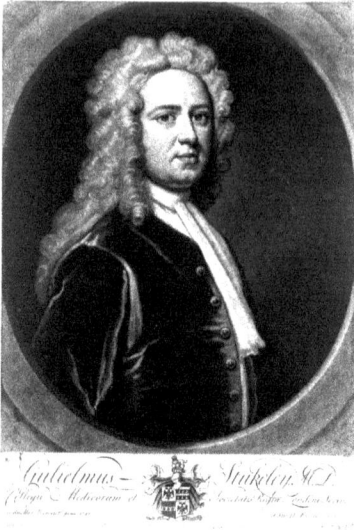

(c)

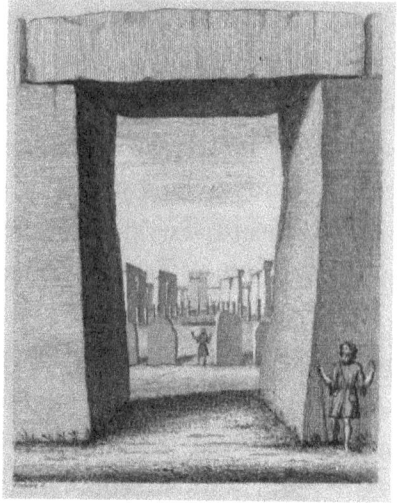

(b)

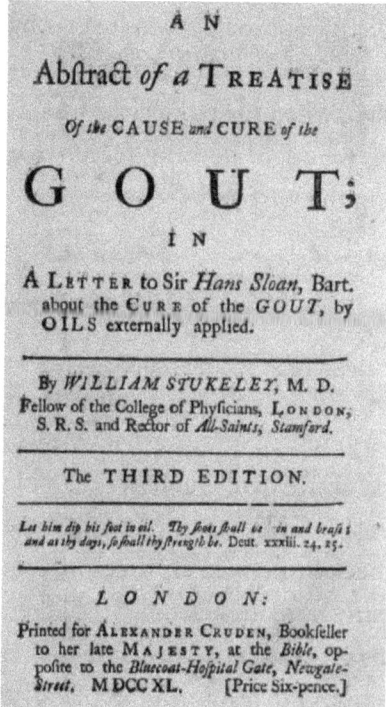

Figure 3.4.

(a) The physician and antiquarian William Stukeley, mezzotint by J. Smith in 1721 after G. Kneller in 1721.

(b) Title page of Stukeley's *Treatise on the Gout* (Third Edition, 1740), advertising *Oleum Arhriticum* and carrying the Biblical quotation '*Let him dip his foot in Oil. Thy shoes shall be iron and brass and as thy days, so shall thy strength be.*' Deuteronomy xxxiii. 24.25'.

(c) Drawing from Stukeley's *Stonehenge: A Temple Restored to the British Druids*. Stukeley systematically mapped the Stonehenge site and was instrumental in conserving the monument. He believed without much evidence that Stonehenge had been built by ancient druids, two of whom feature in the drawing and provide scale.

Source: (a) and (b) Courtesy of the Wellcome Collection, public domain; (c) public domain.

suggested that it was a relic of the Great Flood: 'upon retiring of the Waters of the Deluge from the Superficies of this Country into the Eastern Seas, these heavy Bodies met a full stop, and were intercepted by this Cliff, which retain'd such vast Quantities of them ever since.' Stukeley rationalised the predominance of fossilised aquatic animals in the hills and mountains by their being able to swim, whereas terrestrial animals just drowned and rotted away.

Suffering from gout himself, Stukeley tried and failed several times to finish a book on the subject. It was not until 1732, three years after becoming ordained and installed as vicar in Stamford, Lincolnshire, that he succeeded in doing so. If Cheyne's *Essay on the Gout* was, in large part, a plug for consulting him in Bath, Stukeley's aim was to advertise a proprietary blend of oils, *Oleum Arthriticum*, for rubbing on affected joints. The formulation had been devised by John Rogers, an apothecary in his parish.[31] Having tried the oil blend on himself, Stukeley decided it was a therapeutic breakthrough and encouraged Rogers to commercialise it. He announced the discovery in a public letter addressed to Hans Sloane and followed up the next year with his *Treatise of the Cause and Cure of The Gout* (1734) (see Figure 3.4(b)).[32] This slim and to-the-point volume was excused by Stukeley in the preface as not bothering the public with 'copious theories, long cases, and pompous nicetys upon a disease' if cure was now possible. This did not stop him from speculating on how *Oleum Arthriticum* achieved this, offering up a cocktail of reasoning based on Sydenham's elimination of morbific matter, Havers's mucilaginous glands, Pitcairn's microattractions and Mead's crystals.

Stukeley had a clear image in his mind of what the salts of morbific matter looked like. Evoking the Newtonian thinking passed down to him by Mead and indeed by Newton himself:

> from the smoothness of surface and solidity they strongly attract one another, and assemble too much together, from the sharpness and hardness of their points they lancinate; from their fiery malignancy they burn, and from nature's expelling them as much

as she can, out of the habit of the body, they cause what we call a fit of the gout.[33]

It is tempting to conclude from this that Stukeley was referring to the needle-shaped crystals the microscopist Anton van Leeuwenhoek (1632–1723) had earlier described under the microscope in a material from a gouty tophus (see Chapter 9). However, there is no evidence that Stukeley was aware of this discovery or, indeed, that he had actually seen any crystals for himself. He was probably merely extrapolating from Mead's work on snake venom:

> Would we then know the nature of the gout, we need only read Dr. Mead's book of poysons, and be fully appriz'd of the matter. I doubt not but the poysonous drop of the gout is similar to that of a venomous bite, as Dr. Mead observ'd it upon a microscope glass; a parcel of small salts nimbly floating in a liquor and striking out into crystals of incredible tenuity and sharpness, he calls them spicula and darts. Such likewise in the drop emitted by the sting of a bee, and in the common nettle.[34]

Stukeley proposed that Roger's *Oleum Arthriticum* worked by permeating the skin and then replacing a deficiency of natural oils normally released into the joints by Haver's glands. According to Stukeley, fiery salts and crystals in a joint would normally be enveloped and extinguished by the body's own oils; however, in gout, the glands become degenerate and cannot provide the oil for lubrication while walking or for preventing the morbific matter from causing a further attack.

Oleum Arthriticum made Rogers a decent sum and helped him purchase an Aberdeen doctorate and upgrade to physician.[35] On the other hand, Stukeley came in for severe criticism for promoting oils that would prevent the salutary disposal of humours, illustrating Sydenham's sustained influence. As usual, there was a political dimension, with a local Stamford physician, Thomas Wallis, writing to Sloane complaining that Stukeley had not divulged its composition and, just as bad, that the product was originally meant for horses. Wallis' attack was probably motivated partly by professional jealousy and partly by political rivalry – Wallis being a Tory and Stukeley a Whig. An unhappy Stukeley complained that:

> the use of these oyls has been generally decry'd at home, and it took its share even in party-contests. 'Tis not to be conceiv'd with what diligence and malice it was pursued here, as if the author of it had been a publick enemy to mankind when he recommended nothing but what he us'd first himself.[36]

Stukeley is much better known in other ways. While working with Mead, he became friends with Isaac Newton and ended up writing Newton's first biography, in which he related the story of Newton understanding gravity by watching a falling apple.[37] However, Stukeley is most of all remembered as the father of field archaeology. From his early 20s, he undertook equestrian expeditions into the countryside on the basis of the widely-held belief passed down from Sydenham that horse riding was a good gout preventative.[38] The main road taking the health-seekers from London to Bath passed by the ancient and ignored standing stones at Avebury. Stukeley became obsessed with Avebury and, in turn, with nearby Stonehenge and conducted the first detailed surveys of the two sites.[39] His interests strayed into their history and religious significance, and his *Stonehenge: A Temple Restored to the British Druids* (1740) and *Avebury: A Temple of the British Druids* (1743) contain not only maps of the stones and burial mounds but also wild conjectures on their symbolism (see Figure 3.4(c)).[40] He created the myth that Stonehenge was the work of druids who worshipped a pre-Christian version of the Holy Trinity. Although this led to his being viewed in scientific circles as a fanciful eccentric, his writings influenced romanticism. For example, Stukeley contributed inspiration for William Blake's poem of 1804[i] that was later set to music by Hubert Parry for

---

[i] *'And did those feet in ancient time'.*

Jerusalem. Most importantly, Stukeley helped save Avebury and Stonehenge from destruction by developers keen to break up the stones for use in their building projects.

John Hill

> For physic and farces
> His equal there scarce is
> His farces are physic
> His physic a farce is[41]

A new work on gout appeared in 1758, coming from the bestseller publisher Robert Baldwin. Entitled *The Management of the Gout, by a Physician from His Own Case. With the Virtues of an English Plant Bardana, not Regarded in the Present Practice; but safe and effectual in that Disease,* it was supposedly written by one George Crine.[42] This was presumably to protect sales, as, once the book had sold well, the sixth edition revealed the author to be John Hill (1716–1775) (see Figures 3.5(a) and (b)).[43] Hill was a prolific writer of weekly broadsheet political and social commentaries, pamphlets, books and plays, and was a mainstay of Grub Street.[j] He was famous for his self-promotion and antagonistic temperament, and he had so successfully alienated his peers that he failed to obtain even three signatures for election to the Royal Society.[44] By the 1750s, the Royal Society had somewhat run out of Enlightenment steam. They say revenge is a dish best served cold, and Hill served his up publicly by ridiculing the Society's activities in three satirical publications.[45] He mocked the preoccupation with curiosities and the focus on humdrum practical advice, as in papers such as 'A way to take off the fishy taste of wild fowl' and 'A Way to make Vines grow over the Roof of a House'. This was utterly self-defeating, as Hill secured for himself a lifelong ban from the Society's meeting rooms, then in Crane Court off Fleet Street.[46] Thenceforth, he depended on Stukeley, who

---

[j] Grub Street was home to tabloid-type journalists and low-end publishers and booksellers.

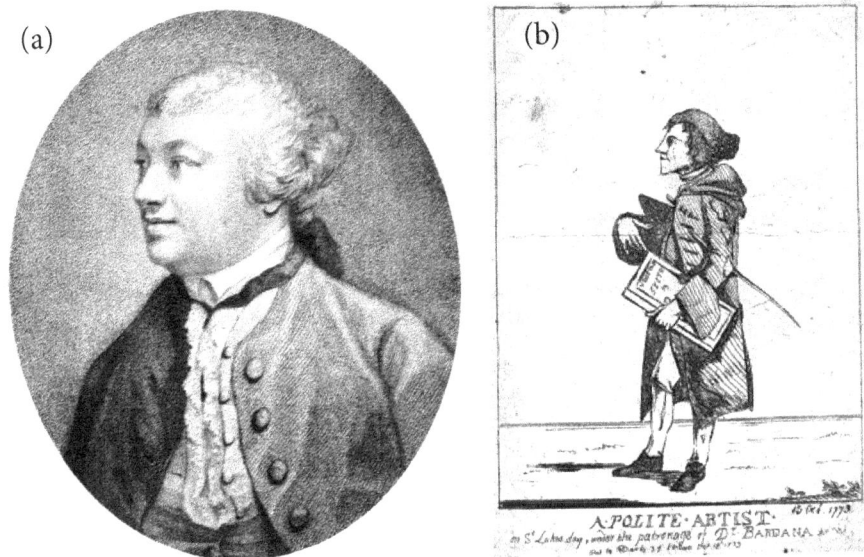

Figure 3.5.

The botanist physician Sir John Hill, an early tabloid-type journalist and author of theatrical farces.

(a) This engraving is by Giovanni Vendramini after a portrait by Frances Cotes. The caption (not shown) reads, 'Sir John Hill MD, Knight of the Polar Star, First Superintendent of the Royal Gardens at Kew'. The latter title may have been in anticipation, as, although Hill may have helped lay out the gardens, he was passed over for the position.

(b) Satirical print of John Hill published by Matthias and Mary Daly in 1773. Hill holds a volume of his twenty-six-volume *Vegetable System*. The title reads, 'A POLITE ARTIST on St. Luke's day, under the patronage of Dr. Bardana' and has four messages. First, Hill was not polite and was, in fact, renowned for being most impolite; second, describing him as an artist mocked him as a scientist; third, St. Luke's day celebrates the physician apostle and refers to Hill's pretensions as a healer; and fourth, Dr. Bardana is a reference to Hill's book on gout in which he recommended *Bardana* (i.e. common burdock) as treatment.

Source: (a) Courtesy of the Wellcome Collection, public domain (b) via Wikimedia Commons, public domain.

was a family friend, to keep him in touch. Hill would have been gratified years later by Isaac D'Israeli (1766–1848), father of the nineteenth-century British Prime Minister, attempting to repair his reputation in his *Calamities and Quarrels of Authors*:

> Sir John Hill, this despised man, after all the fertile absurdities of his literary life, performed more for the improvement of the *Philosophical Transactions,* and was the cause of diffusing a more general taste for the science of botany, than any other contemporary.[47]

D'Israeli was acknowledging Hill's genuine and knowledgeable activity as a naturalist, since he wrote several catalogues of plants, fossils and animals. Indeed, he has been referred to as the 'English Linnaeus'. His works included *Hortus Kewensis* (1768), the first catalogue of the 2,712 plant species that were already present in the nascent Kew Gardens.[48] Some of the new plants he described were added to a new edition of Culpeper's *English Family Physician,* published in 1792 after his death.[49] He did receive some recognition towards the end of his life, but not in London. King Gustavus III of Sweden made him a Knight of the Order of Vasa in recognition of his services to botany – and that is why D'Israeli referred to him as Sir John.[50]

Similar to the works on the Gout by Sydenham, Cheyne and Stukeley, Hill's gout book was centred on his own experience as a sufferer. His views on the causation of acute gout seem taken largely from Cheyne, with an emphasis on mechanical obstruction of small blood vessels. The *Bardana* in the title is common burdock (*Arctium*), and Hill's discovery was not that original, as Culpeper had recommended the juice of the leaves be mixed with honey to make a diuretic to help pass bladder stones and alleviate dropsy.[51] Although burdock root or its chemical derivatives have not been adopted by mainstream medicine, burdock root tincture remains on sale in the alternative medicine market. There is also ongoing research into the therapeutic potential of chemicals contained within burdock root for treating inflammation.

William Cadogan

The eighteenth-century elite keenly upheld as a birthright the hereditary origin of the Gout with all its supposed salutary benefits. Hill was not convinced. He had no lucrative medical practice to lose by refuting the creed and made the sensible point that children naturally live like their fathers.[52] The issue was taken up more assertively by William Cadogan (1711–1797) (see Figure 3.6(a)), who, in 1771, published his explosive *Dissertation on the Gout: and all chronic diseases, jointly considered, as proceeding from the same causes; what those causes are; and a rational and natural method of cure proposed. Addressed to all invalids* (see Figure 3.6(b)).[53] Hill thought Cadogan had stolen some of his ideas and contradicted others, so promptly rushed out a further edition of his own volume.[54]

Cadogan is best known for his pioneering work on the nursing and upbringing of infants.[55] He was probably born in Wales and studied in Oxford and Leiden. In 1746, he was appointed physician at the Bristol Infirmary. He then started working in an honorary capacity at the London Foundling Hospital (see Figure 3.6(c)), which had recently been established by the good graces of Richard Mead and others, near the present site of Great Ormond Street Hospital.[k] The *raison d'être* of the Foundling Hospital was to save abandoned babies left in the street by poor or unmarried mothers. Cadogan's experience there led to his publishing of *An Essay upon Nursing and the Management of Children from their Birth to Three Years of Age* (1748), one of the first medical texts on how to care for babies.[56] He expressed strong (and now modern) views on infant feeding, advocating breast feeding and challenging the prevailing wisdom that infants should be fed vigorously. He also encouraged light clothing of babies, contesting the rule that infants needed tight swaddling. On the strength of this work, he was appointed a governor at the Foundling Hospital in 1749 and to the staff as a physician in 1753.[57]

---

[k] Originally, the Hospital for Sick Children.

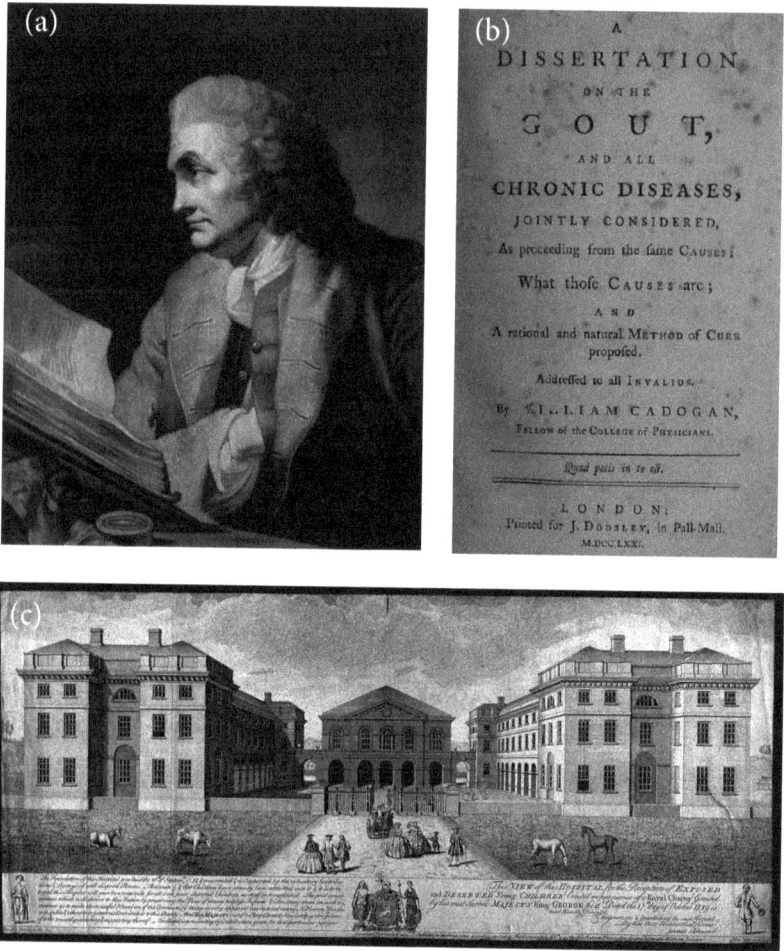

Figure 3.6

(a) Mezzotint of William Cadogan by William Dickinson after a portrait by Robert Edge Pine.

(b) Title page of Cadogan's contentious dissertation emphasising the Gout not being a proud family inheritance but due instead to 'Indolence, Intemperance and Vexation'.

(c) The Foundling Hospital in Guildford Street, London, where Cadogan came to work as a staff physician and developed the reputation of being the Father of Infant Care. Engraving by Henry Roberts after Jeremiah Robinson in 1749. Note the High Society men and women walking up the path.

Source: All courtesy of the Wellcome Collection, public domain.

The Foundling Hospital relied on charitable donations, and there was also an active fundraising campaign, which included exhibitions selling works by the top contemporary London artists, including William Hogarth, Joshua Reynolds and Thomas Gainsborough.[1] In addition, it staged benefit concerts, such as an annual performance of the *Messiah* by George Frederic Handel. Having moved to live in London in 1752, Cadogan may not have been able to keep his family in any style by solely treating unwanted babies, despite having a rich wife.[58] The social connections he would have obtained at these functions must have helped him build up a profitable medical practice, with all the gout that came with it. The house he built for his family in Fulham became the foundation for the present-day Hurlingham Club in West London. Despite his prosperity, a sense of exhaustion with professional pretensions seems to have overcome Cadogan, as manifested by his controversial dissertation. Rather like Sydenham, he started his *Dissertation on the Gout* with a long preface dismissing the ancient texts in the present age of natural philosophy and bemoaning the avarice and greed common among his colleagues. His main message was that not only gout but all chronic diseases are attributable to indulgence, specifically to what became his mantra of 'indolence, intemperance, and vexation'. Cadogan dismissed the notion that gout was hereditary, considering that to be a vanity and a psychological crutch.[59]

Cadogan's dissertation duly prompted a meteor shower of hostile pamphlets and poems, the precursors of the correspondence section of medical journals today and all in public.[60] At a purely medical level, the prominent Bath physician William Falconer (1744–1824) complemented Cadogan on its readability but baulked at the simplistic nature of the arguments.[61] However, there were further objections from elsewhere. First, Cadogan was a bastion of the College of Physicians, and his comments on

---

[1] The Foundling Hospital contained the first public art gallery in London, predating the Royal Academy (1768), the National Gallery (1824), the Tate Gallery (1897) and the Courtauld Institute Collection (1932).

expensive but useless doctors were considered hypocritical. This short poem links Cadogan's fondness for game shooting with the danger of physicians:

> Doctor, all game you either ought to shun,
> Or sport no longer with the unsteady gun,
> But like physicians of undoubted skill,
> Gladly attempt what never fails to kill,
> Not *lead's* uncertain dross, but *physic's* deadly pill.[62]

Second, his mantra was only new in wording and simply echoed earlier writers, such as Sydenham, Cheyne, Mead, Stukeley and indeed Hill. Samuel Johnson (1709–1784)[m] considered that Cadogan's essay was 'only Dr. Cheyne's book told in a new way'.[63] Third, some practicing doctors with patients to keep saw writing a book for the public with a focus on bad living while denying the inheritance of gout as seriously breaking ranks by stating the unstable. All in all, Cadogan was judged to have shown a distinct lack of discretion and constraint. Nevertheless, the book appealed to the public and did have some impact by persuading the gouty to change their ways.[64] However, the view that gout was inherited was unshakeable, with the physician William Grant lecturing five years later that 'The gout is hereditary … a contrary opinion has done a great deal of mischief'.[65] Forty years on and after the dust had settled, the surgeon John Ring (1752–1821) wrote, 'Cadogan, who is fond of being singular, denies that the gout is a hereditary disease: as well he might deny that the crown of England is hereditary; because there are occasional exceptions to the general rule.'[66]

Although Cadogan was wrong about heredity (see Chapter 11), his views on gout as a representative chronic disease caused by lifestyle were prophetic of our current age (see Chapter 14). At the age of 60, he was in the latter stages of his career, and perhaps he was bored with the demands made by patients lacking the insight or motivation to improve their own health. Maybe he just felt that he was old enough not to care what people

---

[m] Dr. Samuel Johnson, the eighteenth-century literary celebrity.

thought, and many senior doctors may feel the same today. Possibly, Cadogan was simply overstating the lack of a hereditary basis of gout for effect, and what he really meant was not so much that gout is not inheritable but that it is not inevitable.

William Heberden

William Heberden (Figure 3.7(a)) was one of the outstanding English physicians of the mid-late eighteenth century. He was educated at St. John's College, Cambridge, and lectured there on *Materia Medica*[n] for 10 years before establishing a successful medical practice in London. He was a respected classical scholar as well as a physician who still wrote in Latin. Samuel Johnson considered him 'the last of our learned physicians'. *Commentaries on the Course and Treatment of Diseases*[o] is a compilation of Heberden's most influential medical writings and was published shortly after his death by his son William Heberden the Younger in 1802.[67] Apart from his views on gout and arthritis, Heberden's medical accomplishments included being the first to distinguish chickenpox from smallpox and being the first to describe in detail the night blindness that would most likely have been due to Vitamin A deficiency. He was also the first to describe in Western literature *angina pectoris*, the central chest pain that comes on with exercise or stress. We know now that this is attributable to insufficient blood supply to the heart, but nothing was known then about coronary artery diseases, and Heberden regarded it as an ominous form of asthma.

Heberden joined Cadogan in casting doubt on gout being salutary and agreed about its association with other chronic diseases. Referring generally to gouty afflictions, he wrote:

> I find by the notes which I have taken, that the patients in whom they have supervened other distempers without relieving them, or where they have been thought to bring on new disorders, are at

---

[n] *Materia medica* is the old Latin collective term for therapeutic substances.

[o] Originally published in Latin as *Commentarii de morborum historia et curatione*.

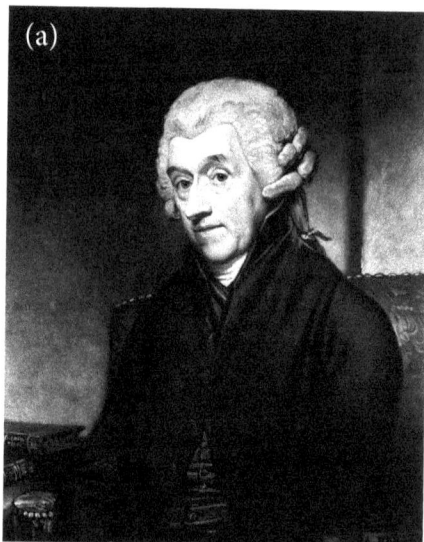

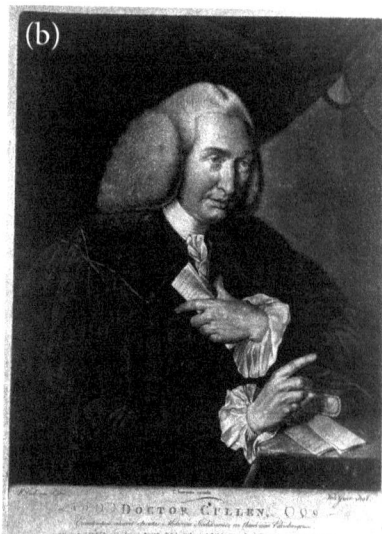

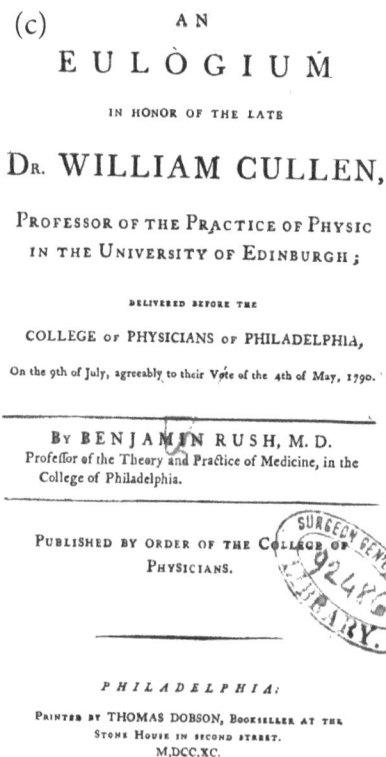

Figure 3.7.

(a) William Heberden by James Ward after William Beechey.

(b) The great Edinburgh medical teacher William Cullen, mezzotint by V. Green in 1772 after W. Cochran.

(c) Title page of Benjamin Rush's eulogy to Cullen, commissioned by the American College of Physicians. Cullen was adamant that the orthodox humoral theory of gout was incorrect, although his contention that gout is a primarily a nervous disorder was also wide of the mark.

Source: (a) and (b) Courtesy of the Wellcome Collection, with (a) public domain and (b) CC BY 4.0; (c) courtesy of the US National Library of Medicine, public domain.

least double in number to those in whom they have been judged to befriend the constitution; and it has appeared to me, that the mischief which has been laid to their charge, was much more certainly owing to them, than the good which they had the credit of doing.[68]

Heberden was also not a believer in gout as a catch-all explanation for ill health, writing that it was common but not as common as imagined.[69] We can see in his writing a genuine attempt to separate out cases of arthritis that did not show the classic features of gout in the joints. For instance, he described 'Heberden's nodes', which are the bony outgrowths on the terminal joints of the fingers in osteoarthritis.

William Cullen

Meanwhile, in Scotland, the Medical School at Edinburgh was flourishing, 75 years after Pitcairne. The professor of medicine there, William Cullen, had become an educational centre of gravity (Figure 3.7(b)).[70] He developed a large consulting practice, much of which was through 'prescription by post', enabling him to treat patients far afield from Scotland.[71] The Royal College of Physicians of Edinburgh houses the invaluable archive of these distant consultations. Cullen had an international influence as a teacher, particularly in the new United States of America. Benjamin Rush (1745–1813), a founding father of the United States and professor of the theory and practice of medicine at the College of Philadelphia, had studied under Cullen in Edinburgh for two years from 1766 to 1768. When Cullen died, Rush delivered a eulogy to the American College of Physicians[p] (see Figure 3.7(c)):

His learning was of a peculiar and useful kind – he appeared to have overstepped the flow and tedious forms of the schools, and,

---

[p] The old College of Philadelphia is now incorporated into the University of Philadelphia.

by the force of his understanding, to have seized upon the great ends of learning, without the assistance of those means which were contrived for the use of less active minds.[72]

Cullen's teaching sits at the origins of American medicine that becomes so prominent as our story progresses.

Early on in his career, Cullen taught chemistry in Glasgow, and one of his students was Joseph Black, the discoverer of carbon dioxide and, in turn, a mentor to several others mentioned as we proceed. Cullen moved to Edinburgh as a professor of chemistry and medicine in 1755. By the 1770s, he was bucking the system by lecturing emphatically against the humours and in favour of gout and other illnesses being due to disturbances of the nervous system.[73] He held that:

> The supposition of a morbific matter being the cause of the gout, has been hitherto useless, as it has not suggested any successful method of cure. Particular suppositions have often corrupted the practice, and have frequently led from those views which might be useful, and from practice which experience had approved.[74]

The chapter therefore closes with two authorities, William Heberden in England and William Cullen in Scotland, heralding a move away from Sydenham's century-long domination of the contemporary understanding of gout. On the one hand, Heberden had serious doubts about the salutary effects of the condition and the umbrella nature of 'the Gout' as the cause of arthritis, while, on the other hand, Cullen was teaching at one of the forefront medical schools that the entrenched humours were not worth the theory. The deaths in 1790 of Cullen and in 1801 of Heberden coincided with the arrival into medicine of the new chemistry that would transform our understanding and treatment of gout, albeit ever so slowly. Whether Cullen was right or wrong on the humours having nothing to do with gout is the subject of subsequent chapters.

Chapter 4

Pills, Powders and Other Potions

Physicians held the power in medicine during the eighteenth century, with apothecaries and surgeons playing second fiddle. However, their scarcity in the countryside, not to mention their expense and sometimes tarnished reputations, meant that self-help and traditional home remedies sufficed for the majority. Salisbury Cade was a St. Bartholomew's Hospital physician and censor at the Royal College of Physicians. A notice in the *Stamford Mercury* on 5 January 1721 announcing his death from 'gout in the stomach'[a] illustrates a common view of doctors:

> We are credibly inform'd, that Dr. Cade, the eminent Physician, who dy'd last Week at his House in the Old Bailey, dying of the Gout in his Stomach, was really found to expire for Want of a Doctor: So well has that happy Thought of a late merry Poet been made good.[1]

The sad sentiment that Dr. Cade's life could have been saved if a colleague had been nearby turns on its head once one realises that the 'merry Poet' was none other than Ned Ward (1667–1731), who had

---

[a] No one dies of 'Gout in the Stomach' these days: this was a case of 'the Gout' not being gout.

recently lampooned doctors and their offerings in his *The Delights of the Bottle; or the Compleat Vintner: A Merry Poem* (see Figure 4.1)[2]:

Thither[b] Physicians fly, to save
Themselves from the devouring Grave;
And, to preserve themselves, imbibe
Much safer Draughts than they prescribe.
What Doctors or Dispensors care
To take the Physick they prepare?
Or, when themselves are out of Order,
Will run the Hazard of Self-Murder?
But are, it seems, too wise to Sport
With Nature, by the Rules of Art;
They've no recourse to damn'd Emeticks, Cathaerticks,
Opiates, Diarroheticks,
They'll turn not up their Bums to Clysters,[c]
Nor flea their Backs with Spanish Blisters,
or will themselves depend on this Course, or that Catholicon:
But their declining Health repair,
With cordial Wines and wholesome Air.
So cunning Guides that lead their Hearers,
for Int'rest, into dang'rous Errors,
Renounce the Cheat, in their decay,
and seek the Lord a safer way....

Ward was the one-man *Private Eye*[d] of the age, regularly publishing satirical articles and poems on topical issues. Highly conservative, he was publicly humiliated in pillory for attacking Queen Anne's failure to support the Tories. Over the years, he ran various taverns in which doctors

---

[b] To the tavern.

[c] 'Clyster' is an old term for an enema.

[d] *Private Eye* needs little introduction to the British. It is a popular weekly satirical magazine that has run since 1961.

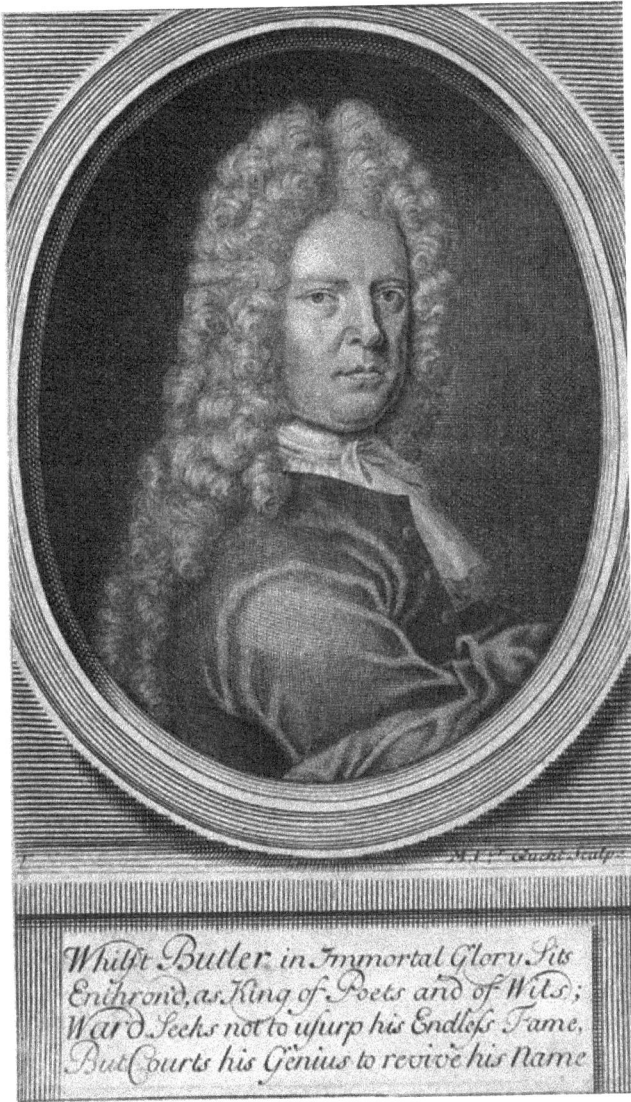

Figure 4.1.

Engraving of Ned Ward by Michael Vandergucht.

Source: Via Wikimedia Commons, public domain.

worked the rooms. His best-known piece, *The London Spy*, was published in 18 monthly parts from 1698 and showed how low he held the Royal College of Physicians, which he renamed the 'Anti-mortal Society', with 'the privilege of making by-laws, of interest to themselves, and injury to the public'.[3] As Ward put to verse what many people felt, it is fair to say that the huge expansion of health and sickness consciousness during the 1700s cannot be attributed to a perception that regular doctors had become more effective.

The Royal College of Physicians in London was supposed to regulate the quality of physicians locally, but it had little to no control over the provinces, where permission to practice medicine more often needed to come from the local bishop. Provincial physicians were a mixed bag, some educated at Oxford or Cambridge while others had studied, however briefly, at one of the Scottish medical schools or on the Continent. Apothecaries, such as John Rogers (see Chapter 3), could upgrade to physicians quite easily if they could afford to purchase a doctorate from Aberdeen or St. Andrews, and this fuelled the antipathy to Scottish graduates harboured by English physicians. Richard Blackmore took a dim view of the motley crew treating illnesses that they so poorly understood with methods they understood even less:

> When I reflect on the great Number of these unfortunate Men, that enter upon a difficult Profession, in which for want of Sagacity, and good Sense required on Nature's part, they are unable to succeed, and are likely to be more detrimental than beneficial to their Patients, of whom they serve best, whom they least visit; ... I am doubtful whether the whole Faculty might not be spared without any Damage to Mankind in general.[4]

The Proprietary Medicine Trade

Widespread doubts about the safety of physicians' treatments, not to mention their expense, fostered a climate of self-help as the emerging 'middling sort'ᵉ was increasingly willing and able to pay for whoever or whatever else promised well-being and longevity. Trade was happy to step in, and innumerable unregulated formulations sprung up, which were pitched at avoiding or treating the Gout and much else. Although often referred to as 'quack medicines', the manufacturers mostly operated from physical premises and were quite distinct from travelling empirics selling concoctions on the village green. Some of the manufacturers took out a patent, with one of the first being granted to the apothecary Richard Stoughton (1665–1716) in 1712 for his *Restorative Cordial and Medicine*, or, as more grandly marketed, *Elixir Magnum Stomachicu*.[5] However, reading Stoughton's patent today makes one none the wiser about what it was for, other than as a general pick-me-up. Actually, most of the many products on sale were not patented and were instead commercially protected by secrecy, similar to how the composition of *Coca-Cola* was held under lock and key.[6] In fact, a patent was often the last thing needed, as it would have revealed the disparity between the exorbitant price of the medicine and the cheap, mundane ingredients. 'Proprietary Medicine' is therefore a more fitting general term.

The purveyors of these self-help medicines made full use of the developing maritime trade, which exchanged manufactured goods for exotic plants and spices, such as cochineal, sarsaparilla, cinnamon, cardamom, rhubarb root and, of course, opium, for inclusion in cordials, elixirs, powders and tinctures.[7] Aided by improvements in printing and travel, the proliferation of regional newspapers carried countless advertisements for medicines on their front pages – the papers were the internet of the age. Today, these advertisements, with their claims of infallible effectiveness, often against just about everything, make one laugh. Many newspapers relied on advertising revenue. Alternatively, some manufacturers partnered with publishers, and the advertisements came free. One such publisher was John Newbery (1713–1767), who created the literary market for children's

---

ᵉ The middle class.

books but became wealthy from being the sole agent for *Dr. James' Fever Powder* (discussed later in the chapter). His bestselling *History of Little Goody Two-shoes* (1765), attributed to the novelist Oliver Goldsmith, opens with a subliminal advertisement: 'CARE and discontent shortened the days of Little Margery's father – He was forced from his family and seized with a violent fever in a place where Dr. James' powder was not to be had, and where he died miserably.'[8]

The boundaries between the proprietary medicine trade and ortho-dox medicine were blurred.[9] Physicians were not expected to disclose the composition of their prescriptions, nor their conflicts of interest; we have seen earlier how Jonathan Goddard sold the secret recipe for his drops to King Charles II for a fortune and Thomas Sydenham did not reveal the precise ingredients of his laudanum.[10] It was not until the early 1700s that the dictate mandating the contents of a physician's prescription be entirely open appears to have entered professional medical ethics. In 1725, the Newtonian physician John Friend (1675–1728), a close colleague of Richard Mead, wrote his *History of Physick* while incarcerated in the Tower of London as a political prisoner.[11] His theme that physicians were often no better than quacks for protecting their nostrums was not universally welcome. In return, a College of Physicians fellow, Clifton Wintringham (1710–1794), wrote a public pamphlet espousing the right of a physician to keep prescriptions secret and to profit from them.[12] However, by the 1730s, the tide was turning, and William Stukeley was heavily criticised for promoting John Roger's secret *Oleum Arthriticum* (see Chapter 3).

Thomas Daffy's elixir

Proprietary medicines would not have survived long if no one bought them, and no one would have bought them twice if they did not think they worked. Besides the obvious placebo effects, many provided a good purge. One of the first and best known is Reverend Thomas Daffy's *Elixir Salutis*, the Elixir of Health.[13] Daffy put together the mixture around 1650, claiming it was 'found out by the providence of the Almighty' and marketed it on a small scale. After he died, his nephew, Anthony, stepped up the distribution of the *Elixir* at home and abroad as a panacea.[14] The sales pamphlet especially commended it for the Gout:

> For this my *Drink* stifles the *Gout* in its *birth*, and kills it in its strength; extracting out of all parts of the *Patient's Body* these crude and viscous *humours*, which are the *Spawn* and nourishing source of this *grievous Disease*, and frees the joints of all other Diseases and Pains to *Admiration*.

The elixir was originally based on brandy and contained senna, as found in laxative products today. The additional ingredients varied over time and included caraway, cardamom, coriander, guaiacum, raisins and rhubarb. These may have supplemented the laxative effects but probably served mainly to add extra taste and protect the cocktail from unwelcome imitation.[15] After Anthony Duffy died, different pirated versions of the Elixir sold well into the twentieth century.

Advertisements for *Daffy's Elixir* recommended it as 'a noble Cordial after hard Drinking',[16] but this must sometimes have merely appeased the alcoholic with another drink. Elixirs, cordials, tinctures and the like were, of course, mostly alcohol based. Ideally, this was brandy from France, but often London gin or proof spirit was used due to the recurrently poor relations with neighbours across the Channel.[17] The alcohol served two purposes: chemical and psychological; on the one hand, it extracted the medicinal compounds out of whatever plant matter was added, and on the other hand, it warmed the mind.[18] Daffy's came to be mixed with gin for all ages, most famously in fiction by Mrs. Mann, the poorhouse superintendent in Charles Dickens' *Oliver Twist*:

> 'Why, it's what I'm obliged to keep a little of in the house, to put into the blessed infants' Daffy, when they ain't well, Mr. Bumble.'

replied Mrs. Mann as she opened a corner cupboard, and took down a bottle and glass.

'It's gin. I'll not deceive you, Mr. B. It's gin.'

'Do you give the children Daffy, Mrs. Mann?' inquired Bumble, following with his eyes the interesting process of mixing.

'Ah bless 'em, that I do, dear as it is,' replied the nurse, 'I couldn't see them suffer before my very eyes, you know, sir.'[19]

In time, 'Daffy's' became a euphemism for gin itself.

Thomas Dover's safe opium powder

Alcohol was not the only feel-good factor in proprietary medications, as many also contained opium. People viewed opium in a very different way in the seventeenth and eighteenth centuries than they do today. It was legal, and addiction was not considered a disease. Opium was a mainstay for physicians treating patients in pain – indeed, it was the routine resort for acute gout. A doctor was not required to obtain it, and druggists and grocery store owners legally sold their own preparations or even raw opium.[20] Large numbers in every social class used opium, and like gin, it was routinely given to infants. Proprietary syrups containing opium that were pitched at mothers with fractious babies included *Godfrey's Cordial, Dalby's Calminative, Atkinson's Infants' Preservative, Mrs. Winslow's Soothing Syrup* and *Street's Infant Quietness*.[21] Unfortunately, infants not infrequently became quiet forever.

Sudden deaths due to opium were considered a greater problem than the social issues of using opium as a 'stimulant' and of opium dependency.[22] Thomas Dover came up with a special formulation to make opium safer, devising this originally for acute gout attacks, which he certainly knew about having been a house-pupil of Sydenham's. Sydenham had used his cooling regimen on Dover when he was stricken with smallpox. Formulating *Dover's Powder* containing opium was in no sense morally reprehensible, as judged by the standards of the time. Some of the rest of Dover's life certainly was, although again, many, if not most, of his contemporaries would have defended him. Coming originally from Warwickshire, he had set up practice as a physician in Bristol.[23] He found time to make several voyages to the Caribbean and fell in with some of the local shipping magnates in Bristol. They were 'privateers' – essentially state-sanctioned pirates encouraged by the government to sail their well-armed vessels across the seas to capture foreign shipping. Privateering had become attractive as the 1708 Prize Act allowed ship owners to keep all the proceeds from their adventures. It was a convenient, low-cost way for the government to denervate Spain and Portugal, whose ships were considered fair game as the treasures they carried home from South America were looted anyway. Dover invested substantially in two frigates, the *Duke* (320 tons, 30 cannons and 117 men) and the *Duchess* (260 tons, 26 cannons and 108 men), which together set sail on 2 August 1708, with Dover serving as third in command and styling himself 'Captain Dover'. The adventures of the *Duke* and the *Duchess* were recorded by the Captain, Woodes Rogers.[24] The most memorable event occurred in February 1709, when they rescued a castaway from the Juan Fernandez Islands some 400 miles off the coast of Chile (see Figure 4.2(a)). This was a Scottish sailor named Alexander Selkirk, who 'was clothed in goat skins and look'd wilder than the first owners of them'.[25] He had been marooned for four years, living off fish and wild goats. Selkirk was taken onboard and used to advantage by being given command of a captured Spanish vessel being used as the hospital ship. The island Selkirk was found on is now called Robinson Crusoe Island, as Selkirk's adventure formed the basis for Daniel Defoe's bestselling tale, written in 1719, three years before his *Journal of the Plague Year* (see Chapter 2).[26]

The *Duke* and *Duchess* returned to England in 1711 with £170,000 worth of booty.[f] This was the most successful of all the eighteenth-century British privateering ventures and was used as evidence the following year to support investment in the South Sea Company (see Chapter 3), into which Dover put most of his profits.[27] He was subsequently employed by

---

[f] Worth £50 million or more today.

(a)

(b)

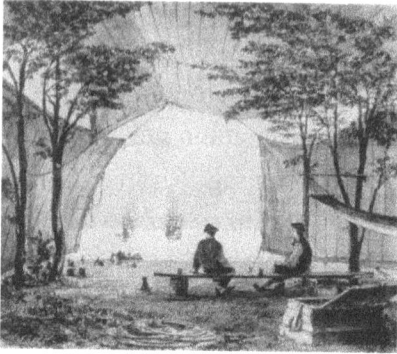

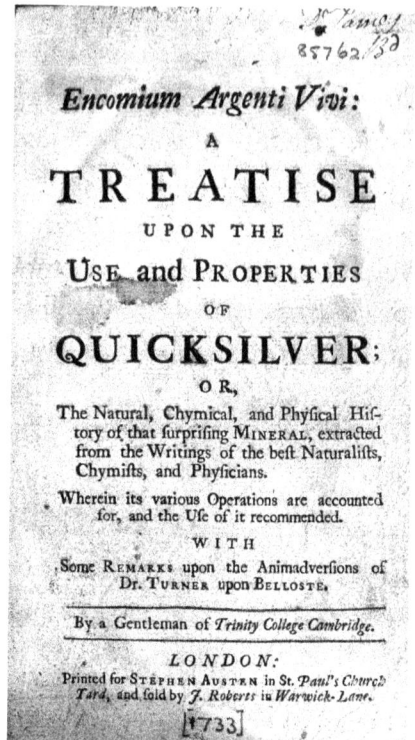

Figure 4.2.

(a) 'Captains Rogers and Dover under the Piemento Trees' in the Juan Fernandez Islands, where they rescued Alexander Selkirk, the original Robinson Crusoe. The *Duke* and the *Duchess* are afloat in the background. This is as close an image as we have of Thomas Dover, who one assumes is on the right.

(b) Title page of Dover's book on mercury. His prescribing crude mercury in substantial quantities for gout and other various ailments earned him the title 'Doctor Quicksilver'.

Source: (a) From Captain Woodes Rogers's *Life Aboard a British Privateer in the Time of Queen Anne,* first published in 1712, public domain; (b) courtesy of the Wellcome Collection, public domain.

the company as its president in Buenos Aires, but was then sacked because of his short temper and private trading. His losses were heavy when the 'South Sea Bubble' burst in 1720, and he was forced back into practicing medicine. He passed the licentiate examination of the College of Physicians in London and set himself up in practice in London. His use of Sydenham's cooling regimen led to the survival of a patient deemed unsavable by Richard Mead, which marked the beginning of a flourishing practice.[28] His relations with the College of Physicians were even more strained than those of Sydenham.

With old age looming, in 1732, Dover published the bestselling *The Ancient Physician's Legacy to His Country* for general readership.[29] Within the chapter on the Gout, he disclosed his recipe for his opium powder, which was then prescribed by doctors and made by apothecaries as *Pulvus Ipecacuanha Compositus*:

> Take Opium one ounce, Salt-Petre and Tartar vitriolated each four ounces, Ipecacuana one ounce, Liquorish one ounce. Put the Salt Petre and Tartar into a red hot mortar, stirring them with a spoon until they have done flaming. Then powder them very fine; after that slice your opium, grind them into powder, and then mix the other powders with these. Dose from forty to sixty or seventy grains in a glass of white wine Posset going to bed, covering up warm and drinking a quart or three pints of the Posset–Drink while sweating.[30]

Dover did not explicitly give the reason for having ipecacuanha in the formulation, but it is such a powerful emetic that vomiting was no doubt how his patients survived the opium. The opium dose was so high that apothecaries would advise patients to settle their affairs when dispensing the prescription. *Dover's Powder* was still being recommended for the treatment of acute gout at the start of the twentieth century.[31] It survived occasional deaths by overdosing and control by the Dangerous Drugs Act of 1920, which tightened the regulations of opiates available in Britain without prescription.[32] It was still being recommended in British regional newspapers in the 1950s for treating the common cold.[33]

Dover was an enthusiast for mercury, with his publication on the subject (see Figure 4.2(b)) gaining him the nickname 'Dr. Quicksilver'. He recommended it for prevention in the intervals between acute gout attacks, seeing it as providing physical protection against abrasive gout-causing acids:

> The Gout in its infancy, the Rheumatism, the siatica, all Diseases of the Same Nature, though differently named the different Parts of the Body Affected, are all to be cured by swallowing mercury, as frequent Experience has Assured this Author on many occasions; and the mechanical Solution of its operations very obvious; to wit, by its Percussion, Friction, shaking, dislodging, and taking off the points of acids.[34]

Joanna Stephens' cure for urinary stones

Selling a secret remedy recipe to the nation, as Jonathan Goddard had done to Charles II (see Chapter 2), was always a hope. Urinary stones are somewhat peripheral to gout now, as only some are chemically connected to it. However, this was before anything was known about their chemical composition, and stones were considered a central part of the 'Gouty Diathesis'. Attempts to dissolve them date back to ancient times, but in the eighteenth century, the standard treatment was painful and dangerous surgery. Mrs. Joanna Stephens' *Nephritick Medicines* for dissolving stones without surgery were believed to be worth a try and became so popular that she offered to make the ingredients public in return for a compensation of £5,000.[g] Initially, this was to be raised by subscription, but the large sum could not be achieved, and so her supporters lobbied Parliament with boxes of stones voided by her satisfied customers. A bill was then voted through Parliament (Yeas: 91, Nos: 60) to the effect that Mrs. Stephens would receive her fee once the formulation had been put to the test by a committee of physicians and surgeons.[35] In March 1740, a majority of the evaluation committee wrote to Parliament that it was satisfied, and Mrs. Stephens was duly paid off.[36] The cost was high,

---

[g] Nearly £600,000 today.

but, bear in mind, the government had no National Health Service to support.

When Mrs. Stephens revealed her recipes and how they should be used, it turned out that, first, there was a powder made from baked and finely ground egg and snail shells, and to this, she added some burnt and finely rubbed swine-cress 'only with a view to disguise it'.[37] The powder was to be taken three times a day, mixed with white wine, cider or punch. Then, there was a decoction that was needed to wash down the powder. This was prepared by boiling a ball of Alicante soap with parsley, camomile, burdock, fennel or other herbs, along with some honey added as a sweetener. Stephens accepted that drinking the decoction was not enjoyable and offered the option of taking her pills instead; these were made by mixing the ingredients of the powder with the decoction.

There were objections. One correspondent to the *Stamford Mercury* found that the treatment did the opposite of what was needed and cemented excretable gravel into impassable stones. The correspondent could not 'help thinking that the same Effects would follow upon taking of the like Quantity of common Lime, viz. a great Thirst, a Costiveness, an Ice-like Scum upon the Urine, with a turbid Sediment, which upon Evaporation, produces an impalpable Powder in Colour and Taste like Lime'.[38]

We do not know much more about Mrs. Stephens other than that she died 34 years later, in 1774, ostensibly of fright, having been burgled and relieved of £5. Her supposed assailants, Henry and James McAllesterm, were acquitted at their trial at the Old Bailey.[39] Mrs. Stephens is mostly remembered as a clever quack who made a fortune, but it has been pointed out that she merits rather more positive posthumous recognition for stimulating early biochemical research into urinary stones and how to avoid surgery.[40] Needless to say, 'me-too' formulations soon appeared on the market after Mrs. Stephens' disclosure, such as one made at a cut price by Archibald Eagle, merchant and seedman to the Honourable Society for Improving Agriculture in Edinburgh.[41] Another was 'Baron' William Schwanberg's *Liquid-Shell*, which was advertised in regional newspapers from 1746 for 50 years.[42]

Robert James' analeptic pills

Schwanberg claimed to have been the real inventor of *Dr. James' Powder and Pill*, which I touched on earlier. Robert James (1703–1776) was a leading mid-eighteenth-century physician and author of successful medical texts, including *A Dissertation on The Gout and Rheumatism* of 1745.[43] The main pitch of this tedious work was recommending treatments with antimony and mercury, setting the stage for his commercial venture. James patented 'A Powder and Pill, which in a few Hours, and with very few Doses, most effectively cure Acute Fevers of all Kinds.[44] He then took out a further patent for his 'Analeptic Pills', which were a modification for those with 'Gouty Habits' or for any of many other complaints.[45] James died in 1776, but the Analeptic Pills were marketed posthumously as:

> … contrived to prevent the bad effects of free living, and to pro-mote longevity; of which their celebrated inventor is a memorable instance; for he is well known to have preserved his life many years by the use of them, and he died at the age of 75 – they are equally efficacious in rheumatic and gouty cases; and likewise in those disorders which arise from a sedentary life.[46]

The upright physician Nicholas Robinson lamented about Robert James and his ilk:

> 'tis no Crime, now to Quack It for Advantage, and turn Empiric for Profit, we have so many brave Men, and some, those of Char-acter and Note too, to bear us out in this Practice, those that may be asham'd to impose their specific Arcana's upon a credulous World, and vend them after such a Quacking Manner, for such extravagant Prices. This covetous Temper, in Physicians, is not only a downright Affront to the Profession, but a lessening of their Dignity, and deserves the Censure of that noble College, these unworthy Gentlemen have the honour to be Members of. In vain do they stigmatize Quacks and Empiricks with opprobrious

Names, whilst themselves, by their Actions, are guilty of the same Facts they condemn in others.[47]

Seven years after James took out his first patent in 1747, he received an affidavit from the executor of the deceased William Schwanberg.[48] This maintained that James had befriended Schwanberg, purchased a third share in the profits from his Fever Powder and his *Aurum Horizontale* pill for curing Gout and other diseases and then claimed the 'Powder and Pill' as his own inventions. It might well have been true; however, the petition to have the patent reversed was not successful, and both the powder and the pills lived on commercially. The powder had a setback when it was believed to have killed Oliver Goldsmith but still enjoyed sufficient reputation to be given to King George III to help with his madness.[49] An analysis of *Dr. James' Powder* by George Pearson was presented to the Royal Society in 1791 (see Chapter 6).[50] Both powder and pill were still being advertised in the 1850s by the Newbery Publishing House, as above.

Portland powder

Another proprietary medicine for gout was so much appreciated by William Bentinck, Second Duke of Portland, that he purchased the secret for £2,000[h] and generously bequeathed it to the public, naming it 'Portland Powder'. Actually, his Grace might have saved himself the expense, as the formulation, being a mixture of birthwort, gentian, germander, ground-pine and lesser centaury, had been recommended by Galen.[51] Davey and Law's *Lady's Assistant: Family Physician* of 1755 had nothing but good to say about its sustained use for preventing the Gout:

> This disease is well known, and needs no description. The best cure for it is the Duke of Portland's powder, which is now sold in most apothecaries shops in London.... The patient must not be discouraged if he perceives no great amendment at first. It works

---

[h] Approximately £380,000 today.

slow, but sure, and it may be sometimes two years before he receives any benefit.[52]

It is certainly possible that the cocktail of plant materials in Portland Powder had beneficial effects. However, the craze fell out of favour, as crazes do. William Heberden suggested that the product's decline in popularity was actually due to the maintained belief of gout being salutary rather than the powder not working:

> Nor indeed was its disgrace owing to its doing too little, but to its doing too much. The dread of being cured of the Gout was, and is still, much greater than the dread of having it; and the world seems agreed patiently to submit to this tyrant, lest a worse should come in its room.[53]

William Cullen was more circumspect:

> In every instance which I have known of its exhibition for the length of time prescribed, the persons who had taken it were, indeed, afterwards free from any inflammatory affection of the joints; but they were afterwards affected with many symptoms of the atonic Gout, and all, soon after finishing their course of the medicine, have been attacked with apoplexy, asthma, or dropsy, which proved fatal.[54]

Similarly, the Bath physician William Falconer considered that it:

> certainly prevented the return of the paroxysms, but never failed, at the same time, of putting an end, in a few years, to the life of all those who made a trial of it.[55]

Looking back and knowing now how gout is associated with other serious chronic diseases rather than protecting against them (see Chapter 14), the sober Thomas Beddoes, who we will meet again in Chapter 6, was probably correct in his view that 'Gouty people die exactly in the same manner, whether they take Portland powder or not'.[56]

Abraham Buzalgo's physical regimen

Not all unlicensed gout practitioners sold medicines. Abraham Buzaglo was considered a quack in his day; however, if we look at him through a modern lens, we see an early physiotherapist. He was the son of a rabbi in Essaouira, a pleasant seaside town on the Atlantic coast of Morocco known to tourists nowadays for its traditional medina, a long sandy beach and a reputation as a 1960s hippie hangout frequented by Jimmy Hendrix. Having trained in iron-foundry work and with an entrepreneurial bent, Buzaglo moved to London in about 1762. He developed a series of flamboyantly elaborate cast iron 'warming machines' for heating large buildings and patented a stove that warmed the feet of passengers in horse-drawn carriages.[57] Long suffering from gout, he understandably saw the illness as a thermal problem, in which, as we will see in Chapter 9, there may be some truth. According to Buzaglo, poor circulation of the blood led to cooling, the deposition of sediment around the joints and the formation of chalkstones. Now doing well in business, he developed a system aimed at reducing this sedimentation through profuse sweating and vigorous exercise (see Figure 4.3(a)).[58] During 1770–1771, he advertised his 'warranted Proposol For the CURE of the Gout and Rheumatism' widely across the country in the regional newspapers. The *Northampton Mercury* published an editorial, probably written by Buzaglo himself:

> The very extraordinary Efficacy of Mr. Buzaglo's Practice in the GOUT and RHEUMATISM, being much the Subject public Conversation, and the concurrent Testimony Numbers, who have been almost miraculously cured by him, furnishing a strong Probability his having discover'd an absolute specific for the total Eradication of these dreadful Disorders, we have here procured an authentic Copy of his warranted Propo'als for the more ample information

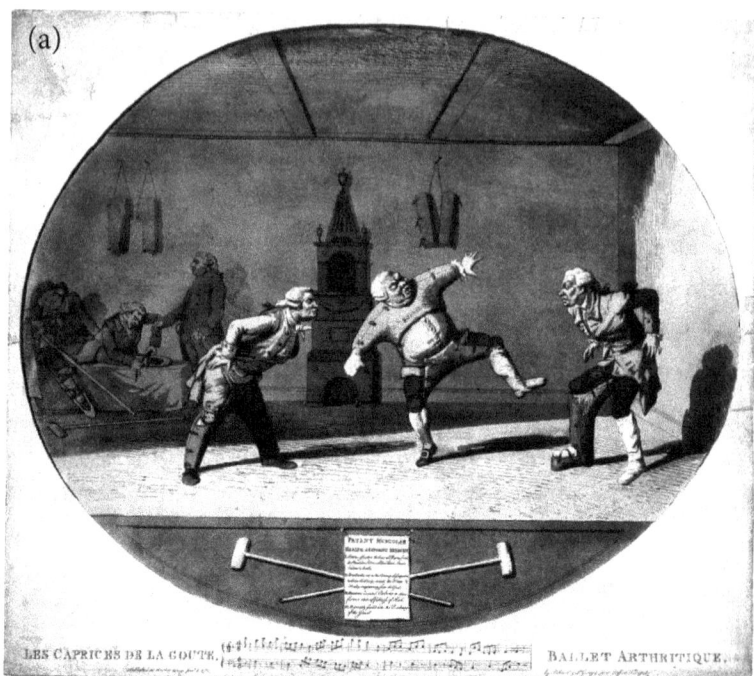

Figure 4.3.

(a) *Patent Exercise, or Les caprices de la goutte, ballet arthritique.* Three men are exercising whilst another is being strapped into leg braces The central figure's shirt has the word 'BUZAGLO'. It is not clear whether this is Abrham Buzaglo himself or a client. The notice over the crossed crutches reads 'Patent muscular Health-Restoring exercise' and explains the many benefits. A short music score is within the title at the bottom. Note also the Buzaglo multi-tiered stove against the far wall. The aquatint is attributed to Paul Sandby, a founder member of the Royal Academy, 1783.

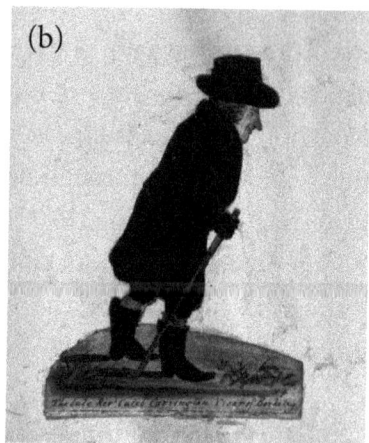

(b) The Reverend Caleb Carrington, vicar of Berkeley in Gloucestershire and originator of Reverend Carrington's *Life Pills*. Watercolour and ink painting of 1864 by Stephen Jenner, great-nephew of Edward Jenner of vaccination fame.

Source: Both images courtesy of the Wellcome Collection: (a) CC BY 4.0, (b) public domain.

of our Readers, especially as we are assured that his Method has not failed in a single instance, and that none his Patients have had the slightest return of their Complaint.[59]

Buzaglo's head became swollen. Dismissive of doctors, he published his own *Treatise on The Gout* in 1778. Anyone wishing to know more about the condition would have found the book disappointing. It started with an apology for the author being an immigrant and falling short in his English, and then proceeded to deride the shortcomings of doctors and standard treatments:

> The Prescriptions of the Faculty, consist generally of *Flannels*, *Patience* and *Sleeping Draughts*: the first to keep the patient warm, the second to make him bear his torments without Complaint, and the third to deaden his Feelings from Time to Time.... After Years of Study; after all the Assistance drawn from the Universities; after numberless pretended Discoveries, *Flannel*, *Patience* and *Opiates*, constitute the only relief that the Ingenuity of the Faculty has been able to produce. Pity so much Time and Study should have been bestowed to so little purpose![60]

There followed an extremely brief outline of his thermal sedimentation theory, a long list of semi-anonymised well-known figures whom he alleged to have cured and then a claim that if his cure was made public, it would banish the Gout from the world. He hoped for a grant from Parliament to allow this to happen; however, unlike Mrs. Stevens, he was not so rewarded, and his secret, whatever it was, has been lost.

James Mounsey and the introduction of rhubarb

Rhubarb has been used in traditional medicines since the Ancient Greeks and was imported into Britain during the eighteenth century for its purgative properties. It was the root that was prized – eating the cooked stalks only began in the nineteenth century. George Cheyne considered that rhubarb prevented the absorption of gouty salts and recommended it for the intervals between acute attacks.[61] There were several proprietary panaceas that included rhubarb in their ingredients, the best remembered being *Dr. Gregory's Stomachic Powder*. The original source was the Shaanxi province of China, where it grows high up on Mount Taibai.[62] From the time of Marco Polo, rhubarb roots passed along the Silk Trading Routes to the Turkish port of Scanderoon, from where they were distributed.[63] The trade was then monopolised in the mid-eighteenth century by the Russians, and St. Petersburg became the sole distribution hub. It was very expensive in Britain; by 1775, it was selling for 1 guinea a pound.[i] Supply was managed in London by the Russian Ambassador, the poet Prince Anteoch Cantemir, and it was Cantemir who was responsible for recruiting the physician James Mounsey (1710–1773) in 1736 to work at the St. Petersburg Naval Hospital. Mounsey did well and climbed the ranks to become First Physician to the Empress Elizabeth. After the Empress died in 1762, Mounsey became personal physician to her nephew and successor, Peter III; however, the appointment was a poisoned chalice, as Peter was soon imprisoned following a palace coup. Fearful of a lethal cleansing of the old guard, Mounsey fled back to Scotland, illegally taking *Rhubarb palmatum* seeds along with him. He gave these to the professor of botany in Edinburgh, John Hope (1725–1786), who succeeded in germinating them and eventually introducing the plant throughout Britain. Mousey then spent the rest of his life watching his back. Having built a retirement house near Dumfries that supposedly had a secret underground escape corridor, he slept with a loaded gun at his bedside.[64] Dating back well before the pickaxing of Leon Trotsky and the radiation poisoning of Alexander Litvinenko, the threat of assassination by Russian agents abroad is not that new.

Reverend Carrington's Life Pills

The proprietary medicine manufacturers did not tend to position their wares as alternatives. On the contrary, they often went to great lengths

---

[i] Approximately £370/kg today.

to convey respectability, and it was common for advertisements to feign links to the aristocracy, often conveniently foreign and unavailable. An association with Holy Orders could also be helpful. Advertisements warned those foolish enough not to take *Reverend Caleb Carrington's Life Pills* of a self-inflicted grim future:

> FOR COLDS, Rheumatism, Gout, & c. – LIFE PILLS, entirely vegetable, discovered by the Rev. C. CARRINGTON, Vicar of Berkeley, one of his Majesty's Lieutenants, & c. for the county of Glocester: to alleviate the tortures of spasm, gout, rheumatism, cholic, and nervous afflictions, with superb success, by giving fresh life and energy to the efforts of nature, is not the only merit of CARRINGTON'S LIFE PILLS: on the same principle they are adapted to female complaints, rouse the dormant constitution, and with gentle exercise in the open air, soon spread the bloom of health on the palest cheek; they strength the digestive organs, and expel wind; they cherish and prolong life in those debilitated by years or pleasure: they restore the powers of imprudent youth; and they prevent the attack of many fatal acute diseases, if resorted to on the first sensation of chill, pain or morbid lassitude; on which account no person should ever be without them: a large portion of the human race is hurried to an untimely grave by inflammations, consumptions & c. the effect of neglected colds; but a recent cold is certainly cured by these pills, invigorating the torpid arteries of the skin, and thereby restoring the perspiration, that whoever throws away his life by omitting them, dies little better than a suicide. Sold in boxes at 1s 11/2 and 4s 6d each, by Barry and Son, Bristol, without whose name on the stamp, they cannot be genuine.[65]

Reverend Carrington was the vicar of St. Mary's Church in the Parish of Berkeley, Gloucestershire, from 1799 to 1837 (see Figure 4.3(b)) and had had a chequered career, leaving him in need of funds. We do not know exactly what was in his *Life Pills* other than chili pepper, which gave a welcome sensation of an instant effect. In an answer to a complaint condemning Rev. Carrington as a quack more concerned with personal gain than the spiritual welfare of his parish, the Bishop of Gloucester replied that the advertisements were 'grossly unbecoming the clerical character' but not punishable in the ecclesiastical court.[66] If Carrington took his own pills, they could not have harmed him, as he lived to the age of 80. They were less helpful for his pocket, as it seems that he was swindled by Mr. Barry, the distributer, and he died in the Gloucester Debtors' Gaol.

Stamp Duty

The stamp referred to in the advertisement for *Rev. Carrington's Life Pills* signified the payment of the stamp duty on proprietary medicines that had originally been introduced in 1783. By the time of its revision in 1812, there were 550 specific proprietary medicines so listed.[67] This might be considered similar in intention to the high taxation that King James I wisely imposed on tobacco in 1604 on the basis of his regarding it as unhealthy[68] – but that was not the case. The country was broke, and the new tax was introduced not so much to protect the public from dangerous medicines as to pay the debts incurred from the financially disastrous American War of Independence. The tax was then maintained to pay for the ongoing wars with France.[69] It was only the unlicensed vendors who were being taxed, as the sometimes equally questionable prescriptions of physicians were judged to be respectable and made exempt. Nevertheless, as far as the proprietary medicine manufacturers were concerned, the tax was money well spent, as the Crown stamp on the bottle implied official approval. This unintended consequence did not go unnoticed, and in 1830, a strongly worded petition was presented to the House of Commons in Parliament ending as follows:

> Was there ever a more monstrous absurdity exhibited in the most barbarous country and the most uncivilized age, than that empirics and imposters of the most detestable description should be legally

and authoritatively enabled to rob mankind of their health, their property, and their lives, and to announce that they practice their impostures under the sanction of a government Stamp Duty, and vend their nostrums as prepared and sanctioned by His Majesty's august authority, and that all this mischief should be allowed to be inflicted on society merely for the sake of the paltry and disgraceful revenue, arising from the pest, to the Exchequer?[70]

The stamp duty on proprietary medicines survived well into the twentieth century and is now replaced, of course, by the generic value-added tax.

Adulteration of Opium and Other Products

It was generally accepted that medicines of all sorts were widely adulterated. This was initially flagged by the chemist Fredrick Accum (1769–1838) in the 1790s and then highlighted in a report in 1838 by the toxicologist Robert Christison (1797–1882) for the Royal College of Physicians of Edinburgh.[71] The matter, together with the quality of food and drink, came to a head with *The Lancet*'s Analytical and Sanitary Commission of the early 1850s.[72] This was initially a collaboration between the surgeon and founding editor of *The Lancet*, Thomas Wakeley (1795–1862), and the physician Arthur Hill Hassall (1817–1894) (see Figure 4.4(a)). While Hassall was responsible for purchasing and then analysing everyday items around London, Wakeley was responsible for the cost and significant legal liability of publishing the names of the unhappy vendors whose items were adversely publicised.[73] Hassall had taught himself microscopy as a student and had already published several illustrated works on its use for studying marine invertebrates, pollen and freshwater algae.[74] He had also recently published the first textbook on the histology of the human body, containing the original description of 'Hassall's corpuscles' in the thymus.[75] This was before the days of precise analytical chemistry, and Hassall brought his skills with the microscope to bear as a powerful tool for visualising adulteration. He employed an artist, a Mr. Miller, to provide incriminating images for public view. Although he

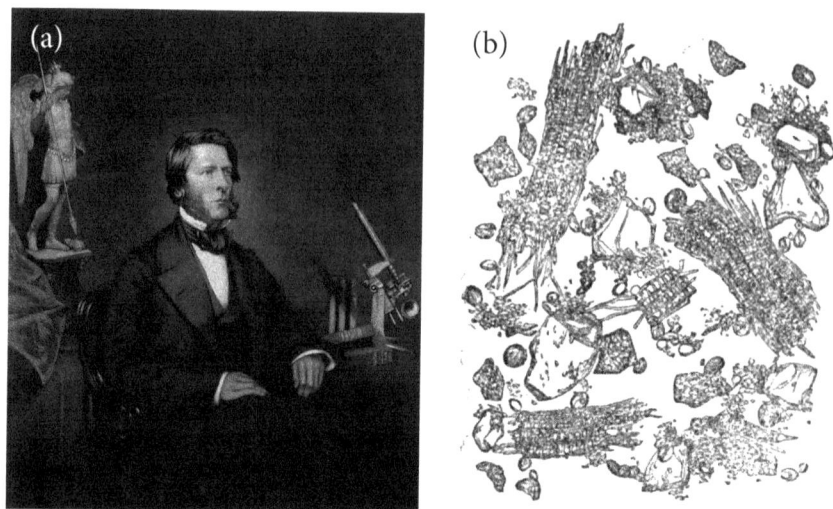

Figure 4.4.

(a) Arthur Hassall, whose analyses led to government legislation to prevent the sale of adulterated food, drink and drugs. Mezzotint by S. Marks after John Mayall. To Hassal's left is a microscope, which was his principal means for detecting contamination, and behind him on his right is the statuette presented to him at a celebratory dinner in May 1856. It depicts the discovery of adulterators' falsehoods and frauds by a touch of the spear of science. The statuette alludes to John Milton's *Paradise Lost*.

(b) Drawing of an opium sample from Egypt analysed by Hassall, containing powdered gum, wood fibre and wheat flour.

Source: (a) Courtesy of the Wellcome Collection, public domain; (b) used with permission of Elsevier Science & Technology Journals, from *The Lancet*, The Analytical Sanitary Commission, 63 (1509) 11 February 1854. p. 168.

performed some of the accessory chemical analyses himself, many were conducted in collaboration with the chemist Henry Letheby (1816–1876) of the London (now Royal London) Hospital. Hassall received most of the public approbation once the results of the venture appeared in *The Lancet*, leading to an unseemly public squabble with Wakeley and Letheby.[76]

As mentioned, opium was the mainstay for pain relief from gout and was ubiquitous in proprietary medicines. *The Lancet*'s commission found opium to be extensively adulterated by suppliers, and Wakeley allocated 17 journal pages for the matter, spread over five weeks.[77] Contaminants included variable amounts of poppy capsule, wheat flour, rye flour, miscellaneous woody fibre, sand, sugar and gum, giving rise to very uncertain potency (see Figure 4.4(b)). Preparations of laudanum were found to vary dramatically in opium content, and this was attributed additionally to the different techniques that pharmacists used for preparing the tincture, despite directions specified in the *London Pharmacopoeia*.[78] Considering that the commission was dealing with drugs sold by pharmacies and incorporated in the prescriptions of physicians, proprietary formulations could only have been worse.

The Lancet was instrumental in sparking the public outrage that resulted in the passing of the UK Adulteration of Food and Drink Act of 1860, which made it illegal to knowingly sell adulterated products. While this initially focused on food products, it was amended in 1872 to include drugs and was a precursor to subsequent drug regulations.[79] Selling opium openly became illegal in Britain with the passing of the 1868 Pharmacy Act, but this excluded proprietary medicines.[80] The decline in opium in these was largely at the instigation of the manufacturers, who recognised a rising tide of opium phobia, some including its absence in their advertisements as a distinct benefit. By 1909, no proprietary medicines advertised for gout were found to contain opium when systematically analysed by a British Medical Association survey, although opium and morphine were still being used in cough medicines.[81]

Reflections on the Safety of Proprietary Products Today

It has been estimated from the records of stamp duty revenue that around 2.2 million bottles and boxes of proprietary medicines were sold in Britain in 1810.[82] The trade was still in full swing, with advertisements unchanged in nature, when investigated in the early twentieth century by the British Medical Association.[83] Indeed, revenues rose 25%, from £266,403 in 1899 to £334,141 in 1908 (approximately £44 million and £55 million equivalent in 2023). In the latter year, 42 million proprietary medicine articles were sold, totalling around £2.4 million (approximately £369 million today). The same British Medical Association survey analysed 24 proprietary remedies marketed for Gout and Goutiness (although usually not only), which variously contained *Colchicum* corm, salicylate, lithium and piperazine, as well as various herbs and spices (see Chapters 5 and 7). All were being sold at exorbitant markups on the cost of the ingredients. It was not until the Medicines Act 1968 that the contents of proprietary medicines and what could be sold over the counter fully came under state control in the UK. Vestiges of the trade live on with cough syrups and so on, which in some countries are still seriously contaminated and unsafe.[84]

The old proprietary medicine trade preyed on a client base which was attracted to the mystery of secrecy and the possibility of discoveries from the great unknown, say from the exotic Himalayan mountains or from the heart of Africa. Nowadays, 'alternative' remedies and supplements appeal to a public equally suspicious of doctors, whereas the romance of distant parts has faded with globalisation, and the appeal is now often more of pseudo-science. Moreover, the menu has vastly expanded since moving from the newspapers to the internet, where there are even more options. The dietary supplement trade of vitamins, proteins, minerals and other choices has been estimated to have yearly sales globally of US$94 billion in 2023 and is estimated to expand to around US$200 billion over the next 10 years.[85] Some are innocuous, while others, such as body-building anabolic steroids, are potentially very dangerous. In the United States, over 57.6% of adults over 20 years of age were reported to have taken at least one health supplement over the previous 30 days, with 13.8% having taken four or more.[86] Although many supplements help avoid genuine nutritional deficiencies, many can make you ill enough to result in hospitalisation.[87] The old issues of unregulated supply chain provenance, questionable quality and a lack of side-effect monitoring remain.[88]

It is worth pointing out that attempts to regulate the over-the-counter proprietary medicine trade have not simply been a matter of controlling the safety of medicines, as the developing pharmacy and medical professions have had powerful vested interests.[89] Added to that were the commercial ambitions of the emerging pharmaceutical companies. With respect to opium and its modern synthetic derivatives, despite good intentions, the problems have not gone away by requiring a doctor's prescription to treat pain, be it physical or mental. First, the current international 'opioid crisis' depends as much on the pharmaceutical industry and doctors for its existence as it does on illegal drug dealers[90]; second, prescribed medicines currently account for around 18% of the coroner's Prevention of Future Death reports in the UK, and of these, around one in five are due to opioids[91]; and third, and most importantly, current legislation is ineffective in stopping people taking drugs and instead has the unintended consequence of fuelling both petty and organised crime. Not surprisingly, variable quality due to dilution and deliberate or unintentional contamination remain common and serious in the illicit drug trade.[92] In the UK, deaths due to drug misuse are on the rise, accounting for 84.4 deaths per million population in 2022 according to Government statistics, with roughly fifty percent due to opiates.[93]

It is not all bad news for proprietary medicines, as in the following chapter, we come on to one that transformed the treatment of gout – indeed, it established, for the first time, that gout could be treated at all. Then, in Chapter 12, I briefly touch on dietary supplements for gout in the modern age.

Chapter 5

The French Remedy

The untreatable *Opprobrium Medicorum* – the Disgrace of Physicians – was how the physician Nicholas Robinson viewed gout in 1755. Robinson reflected on how the circulation of the blood was so obvious that it should have been apparent long before William Harvey published it in 1628, and he predicted that a treatment for gout would likewise one day stare everyone in the face:

> And who knows but that a specific Remedy, as effectual in the Cure of the Gout, as the Peruvian Bark is in intermittent Fevers, may lie as obvious and visible in the Surface of Nature, as the Circulation did before its Discovery, and only want some superior Genius to rise up in the present Age to make the invaluable Secret known, for the Benefit of those, that suffer under the Tyranny of the Gout.[1]

There was indeed a breakthrough, but not in Robinson's lifetime. To the great embarrassment of the Faculty, the 'invaluable Secret' was just that, as it came from the despised proprietary medicine trade.

L'Eau Médicinale d'Husson

Lieutenant Nicholas Husson had retired from the army of Louis XVI – the same Louis who ended up under the guillotine. Sometime in the early 1780s, he was living on a pension and presumably feeling the pinch, so he launched his *L'Eau Médicinale d'Husson*,[a] together with a testimonial-packed pamphlet (see Figure 5.1(a)). He marketed his product for just about anything wrong, including mad dogs and illnesses of cattle.[2] Having presumably purchased it as a laxative or an emetic, many found that it had a singularly useful effect in settling their acute gout attacks. Despite its ensuing popularity, or perhaps because of it, French physicians considered the product a poison. They had more political clout than their British counterparts and secured a police ban; however, this was reversed after only five days due to a public outcry.[3] Some French physicians adopted it, despite its unknown composition. Dr. Dejean, the regius professor of medicine in Caen, wrote:

> In spite of prejudices, the gratitude due to M. Husson increases daily. Above all, patients afflicted with gout look upon this precious remedy as a present sent by Divine Providence, to relieve them from the severities of their sufferings. I have not met with one who has not experienced the happiest effects from it.[4]

England and France were off and on at war, and it was 20 years before *L'Eau Médicinale* made its way across the Channel, for which we have the Scottish aristocrat John 'Fish' Craufurd (ca. 1742–1814),[b] Laird of Auchinames in North Ayrshire, to thank.[5] Choosing not to live in Scotland, Craufurd joined London's metropolitan elite and had himself elected a member of parliament representing Old Sarum near Salisbury. This was an old Iron Age hill fort, and the few in the constituency allowed to vote consisted of less than 10 vicars and landowners who apparently held elections in a cornfield. It was dissolved with the 1832 Reform Act, along with many other 'rotten boroughs'.[6] Craufurd was somewhat beyond being a career backbencher and probably more of a party whip. His oratory in the House of Commons consisted of just three speeches over 22 years.

---

[a] 'Husson's Medicine Water'.
[b] Craufurd has also sometimes been spelt Crawfurd or Crawford.

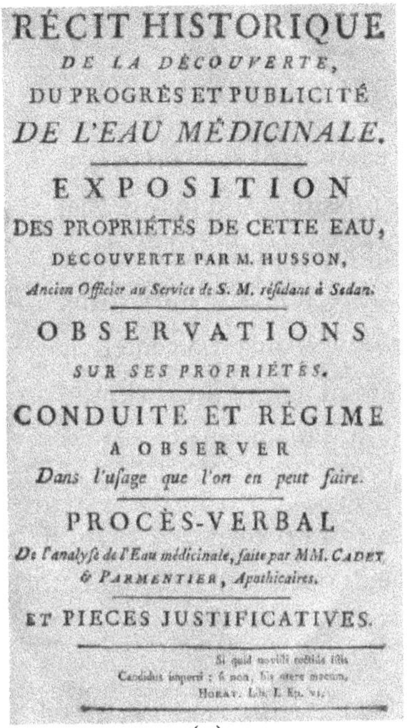

RÉCIT HISTORIQUE

DE LA DÉCOUVERTE,

DU PROGRÈS ET PUBLICITÉ

DE L'EAU MÉDICINALE.

EXPOSITION

DES PROPRIÉTÉS DE CETTE EAU,

DÉCOUVERTE PAR M. HUSSON,

Ancien Officier au Service de S. M. résidant à Sedan.

OBSERVATIONS

SUR SES PROPRIÉTÉS.

CONDUITE ET RÉGIME

A OBSERVER

Dans l'usage que l'on en peut faire.

PROCÈS-VERBAL

De l'analyse de l'Eau médicinale, faite par MM. CADET & PARMENTIER, Apothicaires.

ET PIECES JUSTIFICATIVES.

Si quid novisti rectius istis,
Candidus imperti : si non, his utere mecum.
HORAT. Lib. I. Ep. vi.

(a)

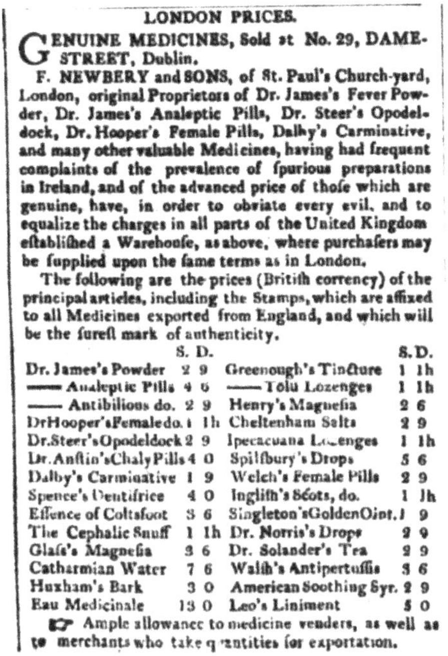

LONDON PRICES.

GENUINE MEDICINES, Sold at No. 29, DAME-STREET, Dublin.

F. NEWBERY and SONS, of St. Paul's Church-yard, London, original Proprietors of Dr. James's Fever Powder, Dr. James's Analeptic Pills, Dr. Steer's Opodeldock, Dr. Hooper's Female Pills, Dalby's Carminative, and many other valuable Medicines, having had frequent complaints of the prevalence of spurious preparations in Ireland, and of the advanced price of those which are genuine, have, in order to obviate every evil, and to equalize the charges in all parts of the United Kingdom established a Warehouse, as above, where purchasers may be supplied upon the same terms as in London.

The following are the prices (British currency) of the principal articles, including the Stamps, which are affixed to all Medicines exported from England, and which will be the surest mark of authenticity.

	S. D.		S. D.
Dr. James's Powder	2 9	Greenough's Tincture	1 1h
—— Analeptic Pills	4 6	—— Tolu Lozenges	1 1h
—— Antibilious do.	2 9	Henry's Magnesia	2 6
DrHooper'sFemaledo.	1 1h	Cheltenham Salts	2 9
Dr.Steer'sOpodeldock	2 9	Ipecacuana Lozenges	1 1h
Dr.Anstie'sChalyPills	4 0	Spilsbury's Drops	5 6
Dalby's Carminative	1 9	Welch's Female Pills	2 9
Spence's Dentifrice	4 0	Inglish's Scots, do.	1 1h
Essence of Coltsfoot	3 6	Singleton'sGoldenOint.	1 9
The Cephalic Snuff	1 1h	Dr. Norris's Drops	2 9
Glass's Magnesia	3 6	Dr. Solander's Tea	2 9
Catharmian Water	7 6	Walsh's Antipertussis	3 6
Huxham's Bark	3 0	American Soothing Syr.	2 9
Eau Medicinale	13 0	Leo's Liniment	5 0

☞ Ample allowance to medicine venders, as well as to merchants who take quantities for exportation.

(b)

Figure 5.1.

(a) Title page of Nicholas Husson's promotional booklet on his *L'Eau Médicinale* (1783).

(b) By November 1810, *L'Eau Médicinale* was being widely distributed. This price list was printed for the Irish market and intended to show equitable pricing throughout the United Kingdom (as it was). At 13 shillings a bottle, *L'Eau Médicinale* was easily the most expensive proprietary medicine being distributed by Francis Newbery, son of the publisher John Newbery, who had originally teamed up with Dr. Robert James to market *Dr. James' Powder*. Note the relatively low cost of *Dr. James' Analeptic Pills* (four shillings and sixpence) also marketed for Gout. From Sander's News Letter 28 November 1810.

Source: (a) Courtesy of the Wellcome Collection, public domain; (b) kindly provided by The British Library Board. All Rights Reserved. With thanks to the British Newspaper Archive (www.britishnewspaperarchive.co.uk).

His insight into his performance in his final speech is food for thought for dull speakers:

> It was a prepared speech, ill-timed, ill-received, ill-delivered, languid, plaintive, and everything as bad as possible. Add to this, that it was very long, because being prepared and pompously begun, I did not know how the devil to get out of it.... The only thing I said which was sensible or to the purpose, was misrepresented by Burke.... Certainly it was not the intention of nature that I should be a public speaker and I shall never attempt it anymore.[7]

The description of Craufurd's gout by his physician, Edwin Godden Jones (d.1842), is a reminder of just how bad gout could become before treatment was possible:

> ... as he advanced in age the paroxysms increased in severity and duration; the joints were injured and gradually disorganized; and chalk stones, as they are called, were everywhere formed about them. He at length entirely lost the use of his feet, and his hands, fingers, and elbows, were also considerably crippled. The paroxysms continually thickened till at last he was hardly ever tolerably free from them....[8]

Not surprisingly, therefore, having gout was something of a parallel career for Craufurd. He was a close friend of the great letter writer Horace Walpole, who recorded his taste for unlicensed practitioners:

> Poor Mr. Crawfurd is laid up with the Gout, but will not be so long, for in spite of my wisdom he has sent for a fashionable empiric, who has clapped a plaster to his foot and removed the pain in one night.... I shall not have recourse to the quack, though he should not kill Crawfurd.[9]

Two weeks later, things did not look so good:

> I left poor Mr. Crawfurd flayed alive, that is, his foot – I never saw
> so horrid a sight. The quack brought off the whole coat of his foot at
> once, and it looks like a leg anatomized and thrown on a dunghill;
> yet the man made him walk a mile on it the day before I set out.[10]

Craufurd was also one of the prominent people Abraham Buzaglo
claimed in his book to have cured (see Chapter 4), despite his managing
very little of the harsh physical regimen: 'J—n C—d, Esq. just recovered
from a Fit of the Gout; exercised *three Days* only, and though his Exercise was next to Nothing, yet the third Day he walked from Somerset
House to New Grafton Street, with Pleasure.'[11]

In 1802, Craufurd had retired from politics and was overwintering
in Montpellier, taking advantage of the brief suspension of hostilities with
France allowed by the Treaty of Amiens. A local physician, Dr. Chretien,
told him about *L'Eau Médicinale* but hesitated to recommend it on account
of Craufurd's frailty. Nevertheless, Craufurd was introduced to a stout but
fit-looking 90-year-old who had walked two miles to visit, having been
gout-free for years on a daily dose of the remedy.[12] He declined to try it at the
time as he felt better in the Montpelier air, but three years later, he received
a letter in London from Chretien further praising the medicine. His gout
attacks had resumed, and he managed to obtain four dozen bottles from
Paris, which must have taken some doing, as the French coast was lined
by Napoleon's soldiers waiting to invade – a threat only disbanded later
that year by Admiral Nelson's ships destroying the French fleet off Trafalgar.
A further three years passed by before another severe attack of arthritis in
both hands led Craufurd to put the medicine to the test in the summer of
1808. He found the results miraculous and generously shared his remaining
bottles with his appreciative London friends.

Craufurd had taken Edwin Godden Jones with him to Montpellier
as his physician and subsequently retained him. Unfettered by modern

patient confidentiality, Jones publicised Craufurd's improvement in a pamphlet containing the names of other public figures of 'considerable rank and consequence' who had also benefited: 'It seems now to be ascertained, almost beyond a doubt, that this medicine has the power of relieving a disease, which has hitherto held all medicines at defiance.'[13]

Trade frenzy

The genie was out of the bottle, and tradesmen rushed to obtain the new treatment. There was a touch of *déjà vu* in the price, as 30 years previously, a Frenchman, suitably named Doctor Le Fevre, had charged each patient a hundred pounds to receive his proprietary cure.[14] He had returned to France after just one season with around £5,000[c] – and it seems with just one fatality. Compared to Le Fevre's attentions, *L'Eau Medicinale* was good value but still dear; indeed, Newbery and Son's November 1810 London price list (see Figure 5.1(b)) shows that it cost over double that of *Dr. James' Analeptic Pills* (see Chapter 4), which also would have lasted longer.[15] Depending on the supplier, a bottle of *L'Eau Medicinale* cost between 10 and 22 shillings,[d] and the instructions were to take half the contents at once for an acute attack and then the other half 4–6 hours later. The accompanying pamphlet on its virtues cost two shillings and sixpence.

The *Bristol Mirror* announced in March 1811 that fresh stocks had arrived in town, so demand must have exceeded supply, rather like weight reducing drugs today.[16] Considering the profit margin, it was good public relations for one purveyor, a Monsieur Delcroix, to advertise that he was.

> happy to leave it in his power to afford relief gratis to the Poor afflicted by the Gout, if they will apply at his house, 56, Poland Street under the recommendation of any Gentleman of the Faculty, or any other person of known respectability, on Mondays and Fridays, between the hours of twelve and two.[17]

---

[c] Translates to around a million pounds today.
[d] 10–20 shillings translate to approximately £40–85 today.

The advertisement made no mention of poor patients having to pay to consult a 'Gentleman of the Faculty', so the number qualifying for free treatment was perhaps manageable. In any case, the poor rarely suffered from gout.

Many other advertisements for *L'Eau Médicinale* appeared in British newspapers between 1810 and 1812, and it is now hard to judge which were for the genuine article. The suppliers mostly had French names, made strident claims to authenticity and issued stern warnings on the consequences of buying counterfeit brands. A Monsieur Befort had set up a supply shop at 18, St. James', near where Thomas Sydenham had lived and across the road from Hannah Humphrey's printshop. He went to substantial trouble and expense to state his superior claim, as well as threatening legal action against his competitors.[18] Versions of Befort's advertisement came out in different towns on dates spread out over 14 months, and each may have been to see off a local trade challenge:

IMPORTANT ADVICE to all those persons who are subject to the Gout, on the most effectual means of distinguishing the GENUINE EAU MEDICINALE DE HUSSON from spurious compositions – The Commissioners of the Stamp Office, convinced by the official acts produced by Mr. B. BEFORT, that he is solely appointed by Mr. F. Chardron to have and hold in London the only depot for the sale of the EAU MEDICINALE DE HUSSON, and on account of the attestation of some of the most eminent physicians of the well known efficacy of that extraordinary Medicine, have granted the particular favour of having a plate engraved purposely for the Stamp, with his name and the direction of the Depot. Mr. B. Befort, in order to fulfil the object he had in view, to put the public on its guard against all spurious compositions, has thought it expedient, for the safety of the community as well as his own, to give a particular form to the bottles of Medicine now vending at the Depot. – In order to prevent the fermenting medicine from uncorking in summer, the cork is tied by a bit of thread, and covered with bladder-skin. Secure as they will then be, Mr. B Befort will no more, on any pretext whatever, take back any of the medicine, once out of the Depot. The neck of the bottle is enveloped in brown paper, so as to render it of the same size as the body of it; over the whole there is a wrapper of white paper pasted, on which are printed the following words – 'The Genuine Eau Medicinale De Husson.' – The stamp is black, on it is the inscription 'B. Befort, 18, St. James' street.' – its crown covers the cork, and its extremities meet at the bottom of the bottle and are concealed by a red seal, on which are the following words – 'Only Depot, 18, St. James' street. B. Befort.' – By all these minute, though necessary and expensive precautions, Mr. B. Befort is in hopes of having quieted the fears of those persons who abstained from taking Eau Medicinale De Husson, and preferred suffering from the excruciating pains of the gout to the certain risk of endangering their health as well as their life, by making use of those spurious compositions, which have for the last six months infected most parts of the United Kingdom.[19]

Danger featured prominently in advertisements for *L'Eau Medicinale*, but upon closer inspection, the danger was less that of the product to the purchaser than that to the vendor of the purchaser obtaining the medicine from another supplier. 'GOUT – A CAUTION' appeared in the *Morning Post* on 2 November 1810 with a stern warning from one of Befort's rivals:

M. DESGENETTE, finding that imitations of the true EAU MEDICINALE are sold under pretended authorities in London, begs … the public to understand that it was not the *Eau Medicinale*, sold under the sanction of his name, that the late Mr. Hughes, of Covent Garden Theatre took.[20]

All that is left to help us know what had happened to the unfortunate Mr. Hughes is a masterpiece of understatement in the *Morning Chronicle*:

'The late Mr. Hughes. Treasurer of Covent Garden theatre, has long been a victim of the Gout. He took the celebrated French medicine, and it did not agree with him'.[21]

Initial reactions

A tongue-in-cheek safer but more painful alternative to *L'Eau Medicinale* was announced by *The Examiner* on 5 May 1811:

> *Eau Medicinale* – this most powerful enchanter, which compels the complaint to move off, sometimes with and sometimes without the complainant, has it seems met with a rival, equally powerful, though of a very different nature. Nothing indeed can be more opposite. The *Eau Medicinale* acts inwardly; being poured down the throat, it sweeps away the disorder in its irresistible course; while the new discovery is an external application, beginning its work in the opposite quarter, yet acting, according to report, with equal celerity and certainty. Conforming to this mode, you have only to procure a slip of wood, of about two feet in length, and flattened on one side. With this instrument the patient is to receive two or three smart strokes on the soles of the feet, and the disease is immediately put to flight. Though this matchless remedy has been boasted of as a 'New Discovery', yet … this identical cure has long been known in the East.[22]

Reception of *L'Eau Medicinale* by the Faculty was predictably cool, as its members were not inclined to endorse a proprietary medicine of unknown composition, particularly one coming from France. The surgeon and classical scholar John Ring rushed out his *Observations on The Eau Medicinale* the following year, noting that 'At present the *Eau Medicinale* swallows up all other remedies for the Gout, as the rod of Aaron swallowed up the rods of the magicians'. Ring was appalled by Jones' pamphlet, which he considered 'an unmerited reflection on other medicines, and a slander on the healing art'.[23]

Unsurprisingly, the spa resorts had mixed feelings about the prospect of curing a mainstay of their income. The *Cheltenham Chronicle* published a poetic address on 1 November 1810 to England's John Bull:

L'EAU MEDICINALE.

TO JOHN BULL

Oh John thou are surely the greatest if Ninnies!
Why still send to Frenchmen such heaps of thy Guineas?
Do prythee thy senses recall!
Know'st thou not, honest John, that all curable ills,
Are quickly dispell'd by fam'd *Cheltenham's* bright rills?
Come then John and try,
And thou'it not deny,
That here's the EAU MEDICINALE!

E.J.

The writer, E. J., is thought to be the inventor of vaccination, Edward Jenner (1715–1798), who lived nearby.[24]

False starts at cracking the secret

What was in *Eau Médicinale* was, of course, closely guarded. If the active ingredient(s) could be identified, then the members of the Faculty could be spared the indignity of recommending a secret nostrum, and the public might be offered the treatment at a lesser cost. The contents had been tested in 1782 by the Parisian pharmacists Antoine-Alexis Cadet de Vaux (1743–1828) and Antoine-Augustin Parmentier (1737–1813), the latter being better known for elevating potatoes from food fit only for pigs into the French national cuisine. They concluded that *L'Eau Médicinale* did not contain minerals or metals and that it was composed of wine infused with some unknown vegetable matter.[25] There were many rumours as to what this was, and one mocking report, published in the *Medical and Physical Journal* of November 1810, came from 'The Great, Great, Great Grandson of JOSHUA SYLVESTER'[e].[26] This determined *L'Eau Médicinale* to be an infusion of tobacco in sweet wine, bittered by columbo root. A boy and a girl were chosen for not having previously tasted wine and asked to compare the new concoction with the original. They agreed that the two looked, tasted and smelt the same, and the importance of the outcome was covered in newspapers across the country.[27] It seems absurd now, but appearance, taste and smell were still the gold standard of pharmacological methodology.

A plausible composition was suggested by James Moore, an army surgeon in the King's Lifeguards who had recently been appointed direc-tor of Edward Jenner's National Vaccine Establishment. Moore proposed that *L'Eau Médicinale* was a tincture of white hellebore (*Veratrum album*) in white wine, with opium added for pain relief. He hit upon *Veratrum album*, as it had been widely prescribed by the classical physicians for gout as well as for mania and depression.[28] Its use in those days seems to have been something of a last resort due to its powerful cathartic properties, although it was revived in seventeenth-century France for administration to horses.[29] Satisfied that his tincture passed the look, taste and smell test, Moore tried it on some patients and published in two open letters to Edwin Godden Jones his conclusion that he had prepared a *L'Eau Médicinale* equivalent.[30] The news was of international importance, with the first ever issue of what is now one of today's top medical journals, *The New England Journal of Medicine*, praising Moore's work for ingenuity and accuracy and rating it peculiarly worthy of commendation.[31] A clinical scientist today would dine out forever on such high-level praise.

---

[e] Joshua Sylvester was a minor late-sixteenth-century poet.

John Want and His *Colchicum* Tincture

Despite the early optimism that a cheap 'generic' was now available, druggists priced their versions of Moore's formulation just as highly.[32] Anyway, it did not succeed in the market, as most people found that it was certainly a strong laxative but not nearly as helpful for gout as the French original.[33] The London surgeon John Want[f] decided instead to make a tincture from the roots of the lavender-pink autumn crocus *Colchicum autumnale* (henceforth *C. autumnale*), and once again, this looked, tasted and smelt about right. When tried on 40 patients, it gave results of 'the most satisfactory nature, the paroxysms being always removed, and, in several instances, no return of disease having taken place after an interval of several months'.[34] Want's discovery was reported unattributed in the *Medical and Physical Journal*, and the same piece was then republished in the lay press under Want's name, 'less to recommend the medicine than to point out to those who have experienced its beneficial effects – a cheap and easy way of preparing it'.[35]

At this point, the old evacuation controversy resurfaced. Want was aggressively challenged by the Greenwich physician Thomas Sutton (1767–1835), a committed purger. The previous year, Sutton had published his *Tracts on Delirium Tremens, on Peritonitis, and on Some other Internal Inflammatory Affections, and on the Gout*, in which he introduced the term 'delirium tremens',[g] the severe withdrawal symptoms of alcoholics.[36] Sutton's view was simple: 'However unpleasant it may be for the profession to confess obligations to a secret medicine, it cannot be denied, that the most ample experience of purgatives has been derived from this source'. As far as Sutton was concerned, any purgative would do the trick, and whatever Want had discovered was of no particular interest or importance.[37] The two then embarked on a good old-fashioned Georgian public quarrel. Want retaliated that, in Sutton's writing:

---

[f] Want was active in the early 1800s but birth and death dates are unknown.
[g] The 'DTs'.

the sentiment is so diffused that it is difficult to fix upon a sentence sufficiently decisive to afford matter fit for quotation.… The assertion that all purgatives will cure gout, is so obviously unsupported by common experience, that our readers will scarcely require its refutation. It only requires for me to show that the curative powers of *Colchicum autumnale* are quite unconnected with its purgative operation.[38]

To press home the point, Want subsequently published descriptions of two patients whose acute gout had improved after taking his tincture before any bowel disturbance.[39] He concluded that 'the colchicum, although it has generally a purgative and often an emetic property, appears to have some specific operation in the treatment of gout, which it remains for future experiments to develop'.

Sutton then sent in a second, longer paper to the journal reiterating his position, but Want had already somewhat clinched the controversy.[40] Nevertheless, the last laugh was perhaps on Want, as Sutton then rolled in a grenade by publishing an anonymous letter he had received casting doubt on Want's claim to the discovery in the first place:

Sir, On perusing Mr. Want's answer to your remarks upon the preparation of a medicine which he conceives to be the true eau medicinale, he says, he is perfectly convinced, from the united testimony of several distinguished literary characters, that the two compositions are identically the same. Mr. Want needed not their testimony, if he had acknowledged the having obtained a specimen of the plant from which the French remedy was prepared … it having been given him by the housekeeper of the preparer or vendor of that medicine, during his attendance upon her. This, I think, is conclusive, as to the identity of the two remedies.[41]

The editor, who may have been Want himself, responded that a refutation would appear in the next number of the journal, but this seems not to have appeared.[42] Supporting Sutton's version of events is a later account from a pharmacist, a Mr. Bushell, who had been apprenticed in London in 1816.[43] He described how a Mr. Grimley, one of the herbalists in Covent Garden, had told him that, years ago, Mr. Want had asked him for help in identifying a plant root which he said he had obtained from his wife's maid. Want told Grimley that the maid lodged in a house in which 'a little Frenchman' lived behind a locked door at the top, where he prepared a secret remedy for gout. Grimley duly informed Want that the bulb was *Colchicum* and that he had only one recent customer for it: a Frenchman, who purchased hundred-weight quantities and refused to tell him what they were for.

Enlisting Joseph Banks

Remember that this all happened at a time when medical belief usually depended on eminent opinion rather than experimental evidence. One of the distinguished persons that Want enlisted in support was Joseph Banks (1743–1820) (see Figure 5.2(a)), whose opinion and physique could each hardly have been heavier. Banks was in his 36th year as president of the Royal Society and duly played his part in having *Colchicum* taken up by orthodox medical practice.

Banks had decided to become a botanist while still in school. The large fortune he came into at a young age enabled him, as an Oxford undergraduate, to hire a lecturer from Cambridge to augment what he considered inadequate teaching on plants. After Oxford, Banks accompanied James Cook (1728–1779)[h] on his first voyage to the South Pacific, paying his own expenses and those of his eight-man team. This consisted of Daniel Solander (1733–1782), the Swedish protégé of the botanical taxonomist Carl Linnaeus, three illustrators and four servants. The expedition left England in 1768, explored New Zealand and the Australian Great Barrier Reef and returned in 1771. The only survivors in Banks' group were Solander and Banks himself. Once back in London, Banks rather stole

---

[h] The author's great (×6) uncle!

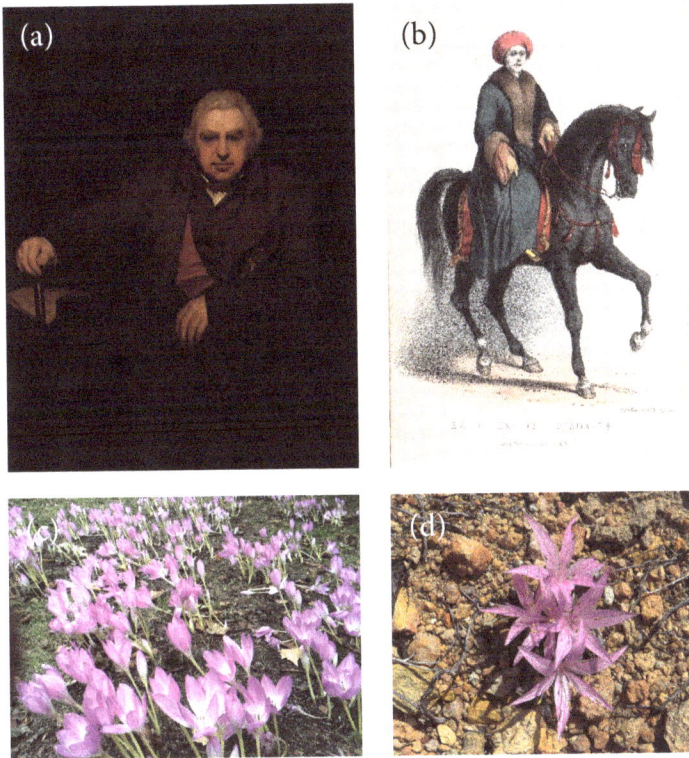

Figure 5.2.

(a) Joseph Banks, painted by Thomas Phillips in 1810, the year *L'Eau Médicinale* 'hit town'.

(b) Banks wrote to his cousin, Lady Hester Stanhope, at Mount Lebanon, asking her to send him *Hermodactyl*. The image of her riding in men's clothing is from *Memoirs of the Lady Hester Stanhope* by her doctor and travelling companion, Charles Meryon.

(c) A patch of *Colchicum autumnale* caught flowering by the author in Saint James's Park, London, in September 2019.

(d) While it is highly likely that the Hermodactyl of the Greek and Byzantine physicians was a *Colchicum* species, the preferred habitat of *Colchicum autumnale* is damp meadows, which is not a good fit for the Middle-Eastern climate. *Colchicum variagatus* with pink-purple chequered petals is a more likely candidate for being one of the old medicinal hermodactyls.

Source: (a) Image licensed from the National Portrait Gallery, London; (b) Wellcome Collection, public domain Mark; (d) courtesy of Ed Allen, via Wikimedia Commons, CC0 1.0 Universal Public Domain Dedication.

the show from Cook, who did not mix in the same high social circles. Cook had been promoted from a humble ship's master to lieutenant to give him the necessary authority to lead the expedition, and he was only made captain after the voyage. Banks never went back to the Pacific but supervised the large-scale importation of plants from there and elsewhere for the developing botanical collection at Kew and to test their ability to grow in the British Isles.

Medical politics were not new to Banks, as, in 1794, he had been lobbied unsuccessfully to financially support Thomas Beddoes' Medical Pneumatic Institution (see Chapter 6). More recently, he had helped Edward Harrison (1766–1838), an Edinburgh graduate and his physician in his home county of Lincolnshire.[44] Concerned about the safety of local doctors and their medicines, Harrison had conducted a survey of the county in 1802, which had revealed that there were nine 'empirical pretenders' for each member of the 'regular faculty'. Banks took up Harrison's cause and invited him to London, offering up his house at Soho Square for further discussions. These went nowhere, as the Royal College of Physicians had its own plans and was not inclined to give over to an outsider – and certainly not to a provincial doctor who had graduated in Scotland. Harrison was treated roughly, with a memorable slight being the president of the College offering him help with his Latin.[45] However, he did well afterwards, going on to become a pioneer in treating spinal deformities and founding the first infirmary in London for that purpose[i].[46]

We know that Banks suffered his first attack of gout at the age of 45, as he received a letter from George III: 'The King is sorry to find that Sir Joseph is still confined; and though it is the common mode to congratulate persons on the first fit of the Gout, he cannot join in so cruel an etiquette.'[47] The usual congratulations, of course, reflected Sydenham's view that acute attacks of gout were a sign of a robust constitution and promised good health (see Chapter 2). As it happened, Banks was a good example of this not being the case, as his health steadily deteriorated and he was confined

---

[i] In Stanhope Street.

to a wheelchair for his last 15 years. Earl Spencer[j] visited him on 17 February 1810 and found him in a terrible state.[48] Straight afterwards, he sent him a bottle of *L'Eau Médicinale* along with a lengthy encouraging letter on the medicine, writing of gout as 'the inveterate enemy to half aristocratic mankind' and ending, 'God Bless you d[r] Sr Jos. & prosper the bottle'.[49] Banks may have been a little sheepish as president of the Royal Society, taking *L'Eau Médicinale* behind the back of his surgeon and friend Everard Home (1756–1832) but not withstanding that he was impressed, and he started using the remedy on a regular basis. An article in the *Edinburgh Medical and Surgical Journal* reported that:

> noblemen and philosophers concurred in sounding its praises, if not dancing hornpipes, in testimony of the agility and flexibility of toe with which it has endowed them; and the President of the Royal Society, Sir Joseph Banks, who experienced the most extraordinary deliverance from his arch enemy, is said to have made it almost his pocket companion.[50]

In an undated letter, most probably written in the summer of 1814, Banks somewhat pompously informed Home that he wished to test Want's tincture of *Colchicum,* in part for the good of the public:

> I have a great desire to try the Vinum Colchici. I have little, if any, doubt of its efficacy; &, in case of it not doing for me what Housson has never failed to do, I can, hours after taking it, have recourse to Housson as usual.
>
> I consider a trial of the Vinum Colchici as a duty due from me to the Public: if I am cured by it & think it proper to change Housson for it in future, the credit for the medicine will be established, and no doctor afterwards object to prescribe it on pretence of not knowing the ingredients of which it consists.

---

[j] Ancestor of Lady Diana Spencer, Princess of Wales.

I am well aware that you have never recommended this trial to me, but I cannot suppose that you hold any disinclination to my trying this experiment which is wholly & entirely of my own suggestion and originated in a wish of doing good.

If you think, as I do, that the experiment may produce an important result, do me the favor to procure for me some Vinum Colchici of which I mean to take as dose 130 drops.[51]

Banks became satisfied that *L'Eau Medicinale* was based on *Colchicum*. In August 1814, regional newspapers carried the following story:

MR. WANT is authorised by Sir JOSEPH BANKS and Major REN-NELL,[k] to publish their decided conviction that his medicine ... and the *Eau Medicinale* are the same, as far as they have been enabled to judge from the appearance, taste, and smell. Several gentlemen conversant with the latter, who have seen Mr. Want's at Sir Joseph's house, are of the same opinion.[52]

All the same, Banks hedged his bets and, in October, wrote to Charles Blagdon, his ambassador in Paris, asking him to send him two dozen bottles of *L'Eau Médicinale* and local information on how it worked.[53]

Are Colchicum and Hermodactyl the same?

John Want thought *C. autumnale* could be the same as *Hermodactyl*, so named from the fingers of the protecting Greek God, Hermes. This had been used for gout by Byzantine physicians, such as Alexander of Thralles (c. 525–c. 605 AD) and Demetrius Pepagomenos (thirteenth century), and was also used in Britain up to the Middle Ages.[54] *C. autumnale* is, in fact, listed under *Hermatoactyl* in Sydenham's *Materia Medica* but followed by a query, so he must have been unsure whether or not they were identical.[55] Anyway, Sydenham does not seem to have written about the use of either

---

[k] James Rennell, the pioneer geographer and oceanographer. See also Chapter 9.

plant for gout, probably because of his distrust of laxatives. Forwarding to December 1814, the botanist James Dickson[l] sent Banks bulbs of the 'true' *Hermodactyl* to compare with *C. autumnale*, writing that he considered them the same plant.[56] His cover note came from Covent Garden, suggesting he purchased them in the market there. We do not know whether they were imported from abroad or what they would have been used for. Banks remained unconvinced that *C. autumnale* was the same as *Hermodactyl* used by the Byzantines and took steps to acquire plants from the Middle East by writing to his cousin Hester Stanhope (1776–1839) in Lebanon (see Figure 5.2(b)).

Stanhope led a life worth remembering. She had kept house for her bachelor uncle, the gouty Prime Minister William Pitt (1759–1806). When Pitt died in 1806, the government honoured him by granting Stanhope a handsome annual pension of £1,200.[m] She had hoped to marry the surgeon James Moore's brother, Major-General John Moore, a friend of her own brother Charles, but both were killed in 1809 at the Battle of Corunna during the Peninsular War. At the age of 33, she had a slim prospect of marriage, so she set out by boat to tour the Mediterranean. A woman travelling in this way was unheard of in Constantinople,[n] where she disguised herself in male clothing. She subsequently moved on to Egypt and then the Near East, eventually settling in what is now Lebanon. Her adventures were faithfully recorded by her physician and travelling-companion Charles Meryon (1781–1877).[57] Stanhope organised the first modern stratified archaeological dig in Palestine. Having come across a mediaeval manuscript locating the site of buried Crusader treasure in Ashkelon, she obtained permission from the Ottoman authorities to explore the site and bring the treasure back to the Sultan. Her excavation demonstrated the changing ownership of Palestine, passing through the floors of a mosque and then an underlying church before coming to a Roman temple. If there

---

[l] This was the Dickson that the *Dicksoniaceae* family of tree ferns is named after.

[m] About £90,000 a year today.

[n] Now, Istanbul.

ever had been treasure, it was gone. All that was left was some columns and pavements and a colossal headless statute, which she destroyed to avoid being accused of relic collecting.[58]

Stanhope wrote back from Lebanon to Banks in June 1815, saying that she had made enquiries and 'I must wait until I can get some of the plant from Mesopotaemia,° where, I am told, it is to be found in large quantities, & used internally for pains in the joints & for humours'.[59] Then, in September, she wrote that she was sending Banks some roots and added that the local doctors knew nothing of the meaning of the gout as it 'is certainly nearly unknown'.[60] We do not have a record of Banks receiving the dispatch, and it is possible that it did not survive the long sea voyage. Nevertheless, on 13 March 2016, the *Hereford Journal* informed its readers:

> *Eau Medicinale* – Amongst numerous instances which might have be advanced of the neglect and oblivion, and of the future revival, of useful medicines, one of the most striking in the history of physic, is that of the Remedy for the Gout, which, within these few years, has acquired considerable celebrity; and through it has been found not to answer its original character, yet it still regarded as a remedy of very singular and decided power. Demetrius Papigomenos, a medical Byzantine writer of the 13th Century, in a work professedly on the gout (*de podogra*) ascribes to the *Hermodactyl* the same virtues as belong to the secret medicine vended under the name of *Eau Medicinale de Husson*. It is sufficiently ascertained that it is to this plant that the medicine in question owes its virtue. The public is indebted to Sir Joseph Banks for a knowledge of these particulars.[61]

Colchicum autumnale, the only *Colchicum* species native to the British Isles, prefers damp and partly shady pastures. The plant is erect and bulbar, with lanceolate leaves that rise around 25 cm high from the base

---

° A region in modern Iraq.

(see Figure 5.2(c)). The botanical genus *Colchicum* takes its name from the fertile ancient kingdom of Colchis, on the eastern side of the Black Sea – now part of Georgia. This was where the Argonauts travelled to in Greek mythology in search of the Golden Fleece. There are now known to be around 160 *Colchicum* species, and which exact *Colchicum* species was the *Hermodactyl* of the ancients remains unclear. In 1856, Jules-Émile Planchon, a student at the L'École de Pharmacie in Paris, defended his doctoral thesis entitled *Des Hermodactes au point de vue botanique et pharmaceutique*, with the conclusion that *C. variegatum* (see Figure 5.2(d)) is the best fit.[62] That said, there may have been more than one *Hermodactyl*, as modern analysis suggests that all *Colchicum* species contain colchicine, the critical chemical ingredient which we will encounter in Chapter 10.

Great effort was put into determining the relative merits for treating gout of the *Colchicum* corms *versus* the seeds, as well as at what time of year these should be harvested and how they should be dried. Corms were strongest if selected in late July or August, just before their vigour was sapped by flowering.[63] It is worth mentioning that although *C. autumnale* is colloquially called the Autumn Crocus, it is much larger and genetically distinct from the common Spring Crocus (*Crocus vernus*). Another colloquial name is 'Naked Lady', as it flowers in the autumn after the leaves have died away; yet another is 'Meadow Saffron', reflecting its superficial similarity to the Saffron Crocus (*Crocus sativus*).

Entering Orthodoxy

C. autumnale does not feature as a treatment for gout in the 1792 edition of Culpeper's *English Family Physician*, nor in William Heberden's *Commentaries on the History and Cure of Diseases* of 1806, testifying to its not being in general use at either end of the medical market in Britain when *L'Eau Médicinale* first appeared.[64] The pioneer pharmacologist Baron Anton von Störck (1731–1803) had described its use in Austria, but that was as a diuretic for dropsy.[65] We also know that extracts were probably being used in France in the late 1700s, as Benjamin Franklin took corms

back to the United States from Paris following his stint there as ambassador. Most likely, at that time, it was seen as a useful laxative rather than as
a 'specific' for gout.

That *L'Eau Médicinale* was based on *Colchicum* has not since been
seriously questioned, but it would be good to settle the matter with modern
chemical analyses if a bottle could be found. By March 1815, *Colchicum*
tincture was in regular use at St. George's Hospital, as shown by Banks
writing to Edward Smith,[p] saying it was 'found to be a more efficacious
medicine with inflammatory rheumatism than any in the Pharmacopoeia'.[66]

Banks' doctor, Everard Home, shortly to become first president of the
Royal College of Surgeons, then published his own *Colchicum* formulation,
voicing his views that low doses of *Colchicum* extracts did indeed provide
successful treatment of gout without upsetting the bowels. He wrote that he
was 'desirous of putting an end to the quackery respecting that medicine,
and to restore it to the place it held in the pharmacopoeia in the time of
the Greek Physicians'.[67] It took longer for some others to be convinced.
The society physician Charles Scudamore was generally dismissive of both
L'Eau Médicinale and *Colchicum* in his *Treatise on the Nature and Cure of
Gout* of 1816; however, he then converted and, nine years later, published
the *Observations on the use of the Colchicum autumnale in the treatment
of Gout*, writing:

> I am convinced that the colchicum autumnale, administered in
> its mildest form, and in conjunction with other medications, is a
> valuable auxiliary in relieving the symptoms of gout. Ample expe-
> rience enables me to assert, that, if properly used, it is innocent in
> its immediate effects, and does not in the smallest degree injure
> the constitution.[68]

---

[p] James Edward Smith (1759–1828), founder of the Linnean Society of London. In the
same letter, Banks wrote a postscript, 'Shocking work in France', referring to news
that Napoleon Bonaparte had escaped from exile in Elba and was rallying the army
that would result in the Battle of Waterloo.

On 22 August 1819, *The Scots Magazine* announced that *C. autumnale* had come into flower. This was meant literally, but it could just as well have been metaphorical, as *Colchicum* had entered everyday language. The fourteenth of October 1823 was the presumably gouty Sir Thomas Mostyn's bumper day at the Hollywell Hunt races, as his chestnut colt *Colchicum* won the Chieftain Stakes (50 sovereigns entry, with 6 runners) and the Taffy Stakes (25 sovereigns entry, with 3 runners). This was big money, as the prize pot for the two races was the equivalent of approximately £45,000 today.[69]

Safety Concerns

L'Eau Médicinale soon vanished, superseded by cheaper commercial and home-made *Colchicum* tinctures. That was all for the good, but John Want was worried about their unregulated use:

> I cannot too often caution the public against the use of this insidious and potent drug; and feel the more regret, as I was the first to make known its powers in the removal of the paroxysm of gout: though the readers of the *Monthly Magazine* must ever bear in mind, that I have stated, in the most distinct terms, that it was a medicine not to be trusted in the hands of the public. The tinctures sold by Wilson, Reynolds and Hyden, are prepared according to my pre-scription for making the French Medicine, and possess the power of relieving the pain of gout, but, sooner or later, bring innumerable evils to the credulous patient.[70]

He was right to worry, as *C. autumnale* was known to be poisonous: farmers might find their horses or cattle dead on a patch of the plants in a damp field, and country walkers occasionally died from mistaking it for wild garlic. Very much as Want predicted, the public got wind of the dangers and panicked. The *Wilson's Tincture* that he mentioned came from Charles Wilson, a provincial surgeon working in the small Suffolk town of Yoxford.

Seeing how the wind was blowing, Wilson changed tack by asserting his tincture was *Colchicum* – free anyway (Figure 5.3 (a)). Banks suspected that this was a lie, as it was 'most unlikely two drugs should produce effects so exactly similar'.[71] Not bargained for by Wilson was William Williams, a physician at the nearby Ipswich Public Dispensary. Williams was an ex-army surgeon and had distinguished himself in the war with France by inventing the 'Williams Field Tourniquet', a simple and efficient device that the army adopted for reducing bleeding from sword, bayonet and gunshot wounds.[72] He took great exception to Wilson's activities (Figure 5.3(b)):

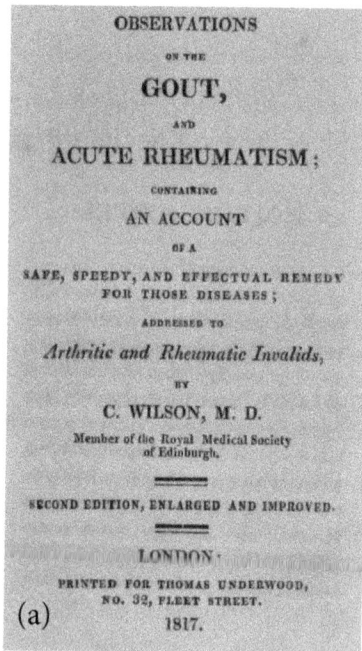

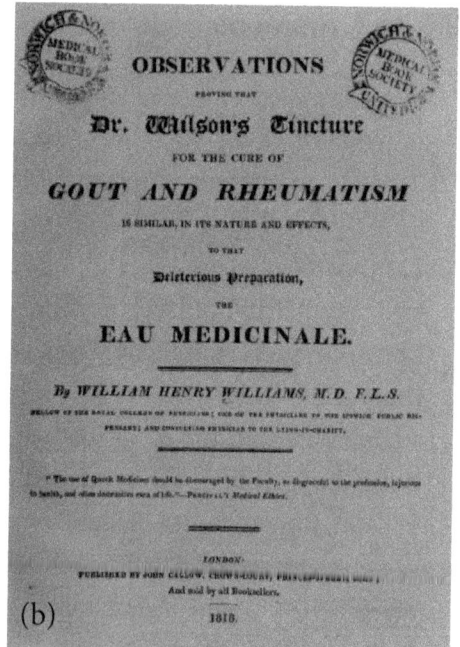

Figure 5.3.

(a) Title page of the 1817 edition of Charles Wilson's book, promoting his tincture and claiming it was altogether distinct from *L'Eau Mèdicinale* and *Colchicum autumnale* preparations.

(b) Title page of William Henry Williams book 'outing' Wilson for his tincture being based on *Colchicum* after all.

Source: Both courtesy of the Wellcome Collection, public domain.

At what time did Dr. Wilson announce to the public the discovery of his Tincture? At the very period when, by a general conviction of the pernicious effects of Eau Medicinale, its sale, *by that name,* became comparatively nothing. Immediately Dr. Wilson had recourse to the ingenious strategem of discarding the Medicinal Water, and strenuously recommending a Tincture, which is a similar preparation, and, *bona fide*, the Eau Medicinale.[73]

Williams discovered that Wilson had secretly been obtaining deliveries of locally grown *C. autumnale* and worked out that the case reports described in an 1813 publication by Wilson espousing *L'Eau Medicinale* were clearly the same as his previous reports illustrating the results of his own tincture.[74] The squabble that ensued involved several to-and-fro public newspaper letters and eventually exhausted at least one of the readers:

A PILL FOR A POETASTER

Whate'er the comparative merits may be,

of WILLIAMS and WILSON, we all must agree,

That thy Muse, while she means to be witty,

Inflicts on thy readers a penance, that few

Will ever forget, should they chance to go through

Thy delectably dolorous ditty.

I ne'er had *the gout ;* and I never yet took

WILSON's *Tincture,* or look'd into WILLIAM's *Book;*

So I cannot decide which the worse is; -

But I think I would rather *of Gout* have a fit,

WILSON's *quackery* gulph down, *read *all* WILLLIAMs,

has writ; -

Than yawn o'er thy asinine verses!

DEMOCRITUS

*This is not said in disparagement of the Doctor's publications, which, I have understood, are very interesting to professional readers; but, for my own part, I would almost as soon take physic, as read about it.[75]

Nevertheless, Wilson weathered the storm. He was asked to divulge the formula by the physician Henry Halford (1766–1844) to enable him to prescribe it to his patient, the Prince Regent (see Chapter 14), but declined and then unsuccessfully tried to negotiate a parliamentary reward in return for the disclosure.[76] It seems that the Regent ended up buying it for himself anyway, telling his physicians, 'Gentlemen, I have taken your measures long enough to please you' and making it his 'never ending resource, when attacked by the Gout'.[77]

Wilson was not alone in camouflaging *Colchicum*. Some 20 years later, Bartholomew De Sanctis, a licentiate of the College of Physicians, decided to commercialise his *Rheumatic and Gout Pills*. He advertised their particular advantage thus: 'Suffice it to say, that these pills do not contain Colchicum or any other deleterious drug, they are perfectly innocent, and may be administered to the most delicate individuals'.[78] De Sanctis' pills were still on sale well into the twentieth century. The American Medical Association had them analysed in 1919 as part of its efforts to suppress quackery and established the main ingredient to be powdered *Colchicum* seed.[79]

Old-fashioned empirics also peddled *Colchicum*. In 1855, the *Staffordshire Advertiser* reported the deaths of two countrymen who died from medicine provided by an elderly itinerant salesman. The medicine responsible was judged to be from 'meadow saffron' and the salesman, a Mr. Morris, was sent by the coroner to the assizes on a charge of manslaughter.[80] The jury found him guilty of being grossly ignorant of the medicine he was administering:

The learned judge, after observing on the important nature of the prosecution, and that the age of the prisoner, and the disgrace, which would be itself a punishment, prevented him passing a more severe sentence, ordered the prisoner to be kept in the House of Correction for six weeks. If a few of these quacking gentry be treated to a week or a fortnight's diet on their own filthy concoctions, the result might be helpful to society at large. Scarce an assize takes place without the trial of some ignorant fool, who takes upon himself the doctoring of his fellow creatures, without the slightest knowledge of medicine or the human frame.[81]

The safety issue was not restricted to misleading advertisements and travelling salesmen. Many people bought *Colchicum*-based tinctures prepared by local druggists or simply made them up at home by soaking *Colchicum* corms or seeds in brandy or port. Fatalities due to overdosing, poor labelling or misidentification were common. For example, in 1826, the *Bury and Norwich Post* reported a 'melancholy accident',[q] as follows:

> COLCHICUM, OR MEADOW SAFFRON – A melancholy accident has occurred in Birmingham, in consequence of a female taking a quantity of the tincture of the seeds of colchicum, under the following circumstances: Mrs. Larkin, of the Garrison Lane, having requested her son to give her a small quantity of spirits, he directed her to a number of bottles, and she took one containing the tincture, from which she drank half a wine glass, thinking it was brandy, the seeds having being steeped in brandy, and kept as a cure for gout and rheumatism. The mistake was laughed at, as it was not supposed any serious consequences would result, but in about four or five hours afterwards she was seized with violent evacuations, which continued till Monday last, when she expired .... The use of this dangerous drug is stated to be very common, but it is perhaps not generally known to be so strong a poison; the public are therefore cautioned against ignorantly administering what requires the greatest care even in the hands of the Faculty.[82]

Lastly, there was murder. The nurse Catherine Wilson appeared in the Old Bailey dock in 1862, charged with trying to poison her patient with a

---

[q] 'Melancholy accident' was a much-used journalistic euphemism for any accidental cause of death, being employed 518,629 times between 1700 and 2020 in the British Newspaper Archives. It has now become rather out of use.

glass of sulphuric acid, saying, 'Drink it down love – it will warm you'. Her patient found it undrinkable and spat the contents of the glass onto the bedclothes, which soon became a cobweb. Her barrister, Montagu Williams QC (1835–1892), succeeded in having her acquitted: 'The defence was the usual one; that the doctor was out when the prisoner called, and that the lad of fifteen in temporary charge had given the wrong medicine'. However, the police had been busy meanwhile, and no sooner had the foreman of the jury pronounced 'Not Guilty!' than she was rearrested for the murder of a Maria Soames, with six other murders waiting in the wings. It turned out that these victims had all been told they suffered from gout, and their deathbed symptoms were considered to have been due to poisoning with their Colchicum. Wilson had persuaded them all to leave her money in their wills and then killed them before they could change their minds. She was hung on circumstantial evidence at Newgate Gaol on 20 October 1862 in front of a crowd of over 20,000 onlookers, making her the last woman to be publicly executed in London.[83]

We end the chapter having come a long way down the path from the forgotten *Hermodactyl* of the Byzantine physicians via a commercial feeding frenzy over a French proprietary medicine to nineteenth-century tinctures of *Colchicum*. There was now a sea change in attitudes towards attacks of gout, as, despite all the pessimism, they could now be treated effectively and prevented. However, the *Colchicum* extracts were crude, unregulated and far from safe. Furthermore, the actual active chemical ingredient was unclear and how it worked was a mystery. The story unfolds further in Chapter 10.

Chapter 6

The Discovery of Uric Acid

In 1854, the Medical and Chirurgical Society of London[a] heard about an ingenious invention. Alfred Garrod (1819–1907) (see Figure 6.1(a)), aged 35, described how he had taken a blood sample from a patient with gout, allowed it to settle and then removed the clot. He had then dipped a simple linen thread into the clear blood serum remaining and added acetic acid.[b] Minute rhomboidal crystals then formed on the thread over the course of days, and he found these to be made of uric acid (see Figure 6.1(b)).[1] So what is uric acid anyway, and what was the background behind this simple procedure showing promise as a clinical test for gout?

Acidum Concretum

Winding the clock back to 50 years earlier, the rediscovery of *Colchicum* had been a breakthrough for the treatment of gout but had not set any boundaries to the definition of gout as a disease or helped understand the nature of Thomas Sydenham's 'morbific matter'. It was the emerging chemistry that changed the game, although, as we will see, only very slowly. The air, previously an amorphous emptiness, had become a mixture of oxygen, carbon dioxide, hydrogen and nitrogen through the work of Joseph Priestley (1733–1804) and Henry Cavendish (1731–1818) in

---

[a] Now, the Royal Society of Medicine.
[b] Acetic acid is vinegar.

121

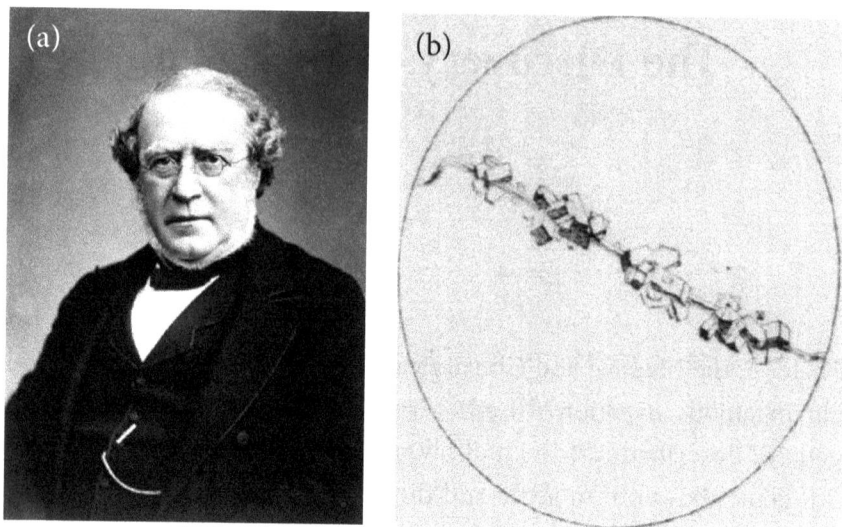

Figure 6.1.

(a) Alfred Baring Garrod later on in his career. Photograph by Elliott & Fry.

(b) Rhomboidal uric acid crystals deposited on a thread placed in acidified blood serum in Garrod's 'thread test'. From Garrod's *The Nature and Treatment of Gout and Rheumatic Gout* (1859).

Source: Both courtesy of the Wellcome Collection, public domain.

England, Joseph Black (1728–1799) and his student Daniel Rutherford (1749–1819) in Scotland, the Swedish Pomeranian Carl Scheele (1742–1786) and Antoine-Laurent de Lavoisier (1743–1794) in France. In addition, Lavoisier, Antoine de Fourcroy (1755–1809) and colleagues provided the basis for a new chemical nomenclature. It was time to apply these insights to medicine.

The story of uric acid begins with urinary stones, which, as mentioned earlier, were considered part of the 'Gouty Diathesis'. George Cheyne (see Chapter 3) had written:

that the Chalk Stones voided by the joints of Gouty Persons, and the Gravel Stones found in the bladder, are to all their essential Qualities, the same. They have both the same Colour, Taste and

Smell, yield both the same Principles, when chymically treated, they have both the same Texture of Parts, as far as can be known, and, even, the same outward Shape, when unbroken and unconfin'd by hard Substances, and they generally happen to one and the same Person. And this shows that they are both due to the same Conformation of Parts, and other general causes.[2]

This was insightful, although by no means all urinary stones have turned out to be related to gout.[3] The story of the chemical responsible for gout, therefore, begins with Carl Scheele identifying in a bladder stone and in normal urine a previously unknown substance that he called '*Acidum Concretum*' (see Figure 6.2(a)).[4] Sadly, Scheele did not live to

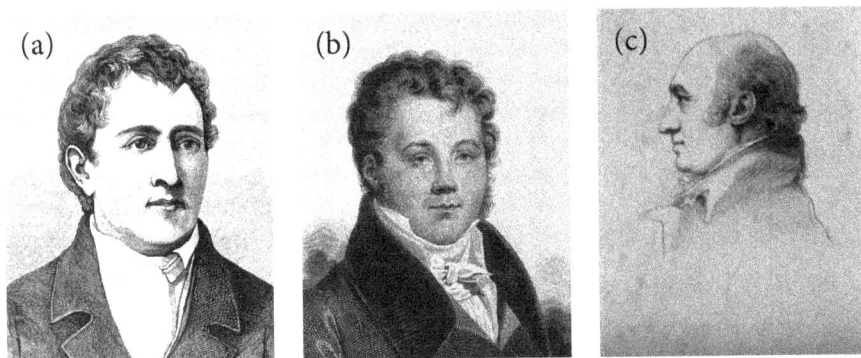

Figure 6.2.

Three chemists linked to the discovery of uric acid:

(a) Carl Scheele found a new chemical in a bladder stone and named it *acidum concretum*, from *Popular Science Monthly* (1887).

(b) The Parisian Antoine de Fourcroy, who renamed Scheele's substance lithic acid. Etching by Z. Belliard after A. C. G. Lemonnier.

(c) William Hyde Wollaston, who found the sodium salt of the same acid in a gouty tophus whilst still a physician. He subsequently gave up medicine to pursue science professionally. Etching by R. Lane after F. Chantrey.

Source: (a) Via Wikimedia Commons, public domain; (b) and (c) courtesy of the Wellcome Collection, public domain.

explore the discovery, as he died young at the age of only 43, probably poisoned by his chemicals. He would have worked without a fume hood, and it was common practice among chemists to evaluate compounds by applying the appearance, taste and smell test (see Chapter 5). He was by no means the only chemist, before or after, to be sickened or killed by laboratory work, as chemistry is a risky occupation. As we have seen, King Charles II probably poisoned himself with heavy metals in his alchemy workshop, and other chemists mentioned in this book also probably helped themselves on their way. These include Thomas Beddoes (aged 48), Humphry Davy and Philipp Geiger (both aged 50), Smithson Tennant (aged 53), Pierre-Joseph Pelletier and Antoine de Fourcroy (both aged 54). Lavoisier also died young, aged 50, but from political, not laboratory, toxicity: he was guillotined in Paris in 1794 during the Revolutionary Reign of Terror (see Chapter 14). Nowadays, laboratory workers tend to find modern health and safety regulations tiresome, but the premature deaths of these early chemists remind us that there can be a price to pay without them.

Detour to Thomas Beddoes and His Medical Pneumatic Institution

It took time for Scheele's work to impact the English-speaking world. His introduction to Britain was posthumous and is attributable largely to Thomas Beddoes (see Figure 6.3(a)), who converted Scheele's *Chemical Essays* from two existing German translations of the original Swedish into English and published them in 1786, soon after he died.[5] Beddoes was a man of many talents.[6] Born in the Shropshire market town of Shifnal in 1760, he was the son of a tanner. He was sent at the age of 16 to study medicine at Pembroke College, Oxford. He used his time there sensibly and gained access to new scientific developments abroad by learning French, Italian and German in his spare time. He subsequently spent three years studying anatomy in London and then moved to Edinburgh, where he learnt chemistry with Joseph Black. He then returned to Oxford to graduate as

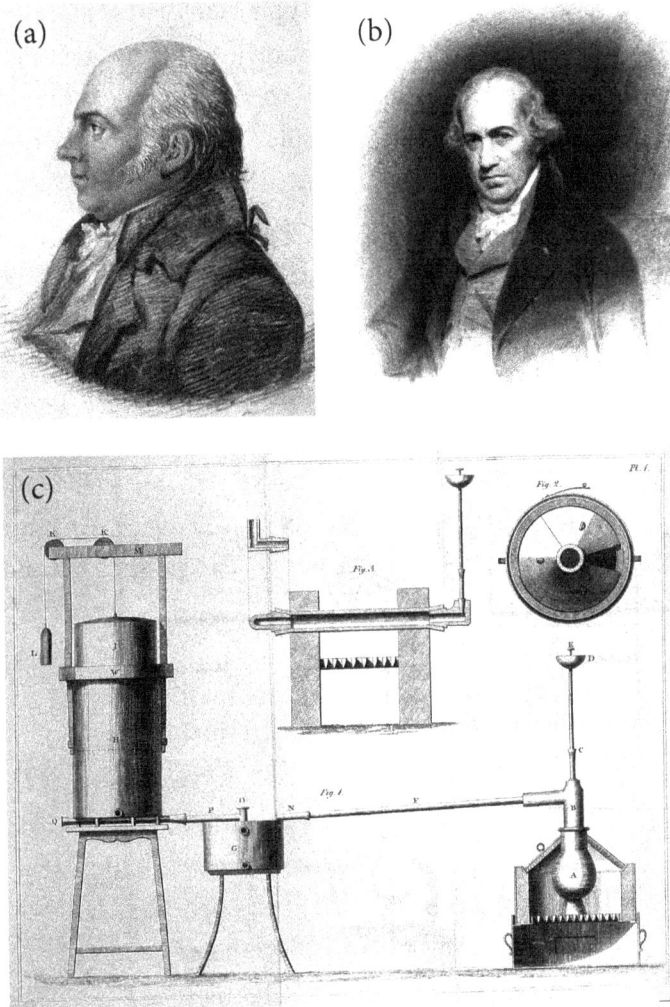

Figure 6.3.

(a) Pencil drawing of Thomas Beddoes by Edward Bird (1772–1819).

(b) James Watt. Stipple engraving by C. Picart, after W. Evans after Sir W. Beechey.

(c) Apparatus for generating gases at Beddoes' Pneumatic Institution designed by Watt. From *Considerations on the Medicinal Use of Factitious Airs and on the Manner of Obtaining Them in Large Quantities* by Beddoes and Watt.

Source: (a) Via Wikimedia Commons, CC BY 4.0; (b) and (c) courtesy of the Wellcome Collection, public domain.

a doctor of medicine and, in 1788, took up a faculty post teaching chemistry.[7] He was a keen geologist, participating in contemporary debates on the formation of the Earth, and in 1791, he sent a paper, 'Observations on the affinity between basaltes and granite', to the Royal Society, where it was communicated by Joseph Banks.[8] A cordial relationship with Banks was not going to last.

Despite the popularity of his lectures and a growing national reputation as a chemist, Beddoes left Oxford in 1792, jumping before he was pushed as his application for a new regius chair in chemistry was rejected.[9] This was not due to poor chemistry, but rather to his outspoken views deploring British colonial policy and lauding the French Revolution. These were well out of kilter with conservative Oxford and, indeed, had led to him being put under Government Home Office surveillance.[10] An anonymous contemporary verse attested Beddoes' republican politics in the wake of the French Revolution:

> Boast of proud Shropshire, Oxford's lasting shame,
> Whom none but Coxcombs scorn, but Fools defame,
> Eternal war with dulness born to wage,
> Thou Paracelsus of this wondrous age;
> BEDDOES, the philosophic Chymist's Guide,
> The Bigot's Scourge, of Democrats the Pride;
> Accept this lay; and to thy Brother, Friend,
> Or name more dear, a Sans Culotte attend[c,11]

In need of an occupation, he moved in 1793 to the fashionable Bristol suburb of Clifton, where he became the centre of a social set of political radicals, and over the next few years published a series of activist pamphlets, such as *Alternatives Compared: or What Shall the Rich Do to be Safe?* – the title speaking for itself.[12] He practised as a physician down the hill in

---

[c] 'Sans Cullote' literally means 'without silk knee breeches' but was a term used for the most radical French revolutionaries.

Hope Square at Hotwells, so named after a natural thermal water outlet on the bank of the River Avon. Hotwells had, years before, built itself up as a fashionable commercial spa but had failed to match the allure of Bath and, by this time, was in deep decline.[13] In many ways, Beddoes was to the end of the eighteenth century what George Cheyne had been at its start. Both were physicians on the fringe, and both were prolific authors of books on health for public consumption. However, whereas Cheyne's interests moved gradually towards metaphysics, Beddoes' driver was straight politics. Cheyne treated the better off in fashionable Bath, while Beddoes took on all comers in downmarket Hotwells. Physically and socially, the gargantuan and entertaining Cheyne would have eclipsed the short and stout Beddoes, who was described by the poet Robert Southey (1774–1843) as fitting the old medical literature by being by nature cold and dry.[14] What Cheyne and Beddoes would have agreed on was that gout was a punishment for the indulgencies of civilisation, a theme developed in parallel with Beddoes by the Scottish naval physician Thomas Trotter (1760–1832) in his *View of the Nervous Temperament*.[15]

In early 1794, Beddoes accepted an invitation to edit a benefit edition of *Elements of Medicine*[d] by the Scottish physician John Brown (1735–1788), who had died six years earlier, leaving his family destitute. Brown was a controversial character who had originally been William Cullen's protégé. The two had fallen out spectacularly, to the point of Brown being *persona non grata* in Edinburgh. He had migrated down to London to seek his fortune but died there in poverty. Central to Brown's exile from Edinburgh was his rejection of current medical theory (especially Cullen's) and his distillation of diseases into a simple scheme that emerged from his own experience of gout.[16] He came up with what became known as the 'Bruno-nian system', having found that his attacks were made worse rather than better by avoiding alcohol, to which he was much attached. His classification of diseases was based on imbalances between internal and external stimulation ('excitement') and capacity to be stimulated ('excitability').

---

[d] Originally published in 1780 as *Elementa Medicinae* in Latin.

The system is almost incomprehensible today but had strong adherents at the time, in part because its unconventional nature bucked the medical *status quo*. Brown placed gout as a disease in need of excitement, and this could be supplied by opium or alcohol:

> the diffusible stimuli are so powerful in removing the inflammation of the gout, that, sometimes, strong drink, undiluted, as wine, and spirits, or the latter diluted with water, as warm as can be borne, have in a few hours removed the most violent fit, and restored the use of the affected foot.[17]

This was certainly not how most people saw alcohol (see Chapter 12).

The Brunonian system appealed to the radical in Beddoes, but he pitied Brown's abrasive nature.[18] The point of labouring Beddoes' connection to Brown's system is that it played into his plans for using gases to treat consumption.[e] According to Brown, consumption was due to overstimulation, and Beddoes narrowed this down to over-oxygenation. Beddoes had kept in touch with Joseph Black after leaving Edinburgh and was aware through him that physicians around the country were testing the inhalation of 'fixed air'.[f].[19] He was also friends with Joseph Priestley, who clearly saw the medical potential of that and other purified gases.[20] These were competitive times for doctors, and most physicians did not share their clinical experience with each other. Beddoes bemoaned this and set up a correspondence with doctors around the country, garnering pilot experience with gases.[21] Later, in 1808, he published a public letter to Joseph Banks supporting Edward Harrison's campaign 'on the ineffective practice of medicine in Great Britain' (see Chapter 5).[22]

Although treatment with gases had already become quite fashionable, Beddoes takes the credit for trying to study the effects on

---

[e] Consumption was a catch-all term for chronic respiratory diseases, a high proportion of which would have been pulmonary tuberculosis. This was a death sentence at the time.

[f] i.e. carbon dioxide.

consumption systematically.[23] He set up a collaboration with Joseph Black's friend, James Watt (see Figure 6.3(b)), better known for developing a steam engine and kick-starting the industrial revolution.[24] Watt was interested, as consumption had recently claimed his daughter Jessie.[25] He engineered the equipment that allowed more reliable gas production and delivery (see Figure 6.3(c)) and also helped with fundraising for a treatment centre at Hotwells to be run by Beddoes. This opened in March 1799 as the Medical Pneumatic Institution and was the first ever dedicated medical research institute to be established in Britain, with facilities for 10 inpatients and 80 outpatients.[26] The venture was initially widely supported by the philanthropic contributions of Beddoes' friends. Beddoes' patroness, the socialite activist Georgiana Cavendish Duchess of Devonshire, attempted to obtain financial support from the Royal Society, but Joseph Banks turned her request down twice.[27] Banks initially did not wish to support a man 'who has openly avowed opinions utterly inimical to the present arrangement of the order of society in this country'. Although the Duchess won Banks round on that point, he remained negative on account of justified ethical concerns that the participants of the experiments in such uncharted waters faced unknown perils.

While it lasted, the Pneumatic Institution was something of a collecting point for emerging celebrities. First and foremost was the young Humphry Davy, introduced to Beddoes from Cornwall by James Watt's son, Gregory. Gregory had moved to Penzance on account of his failing health and was lodging with Davy's mother.[28] Davy was 19 and an apprentice apothecary surgeon with a bent for chemistry and an ambition to become a physician. He recognised the untapped potential of the new chemistry, writing before he met Beddoes: 'If we except the theories of a celebrated medical philosopher, Dr. Beddoes, it will be found that chemistry has as yet afforded but little assistance in the cure of diseases or in the explanation of organic functions'. Beddoes was thus pushing on an open door persuading Davy to move from Cornwall to join his venture as superintendent in a step up the medical ladder.[29] Another of Beddoes' assistants was Peter Roget (1779–1869), who went on to become a successful physician and, years later, compiled his well-known *Thesaurus of English Words and Phrases* (1852). Then, there were the young romantic literati Samuel Taylor Coleridge (1772–1834) (*The Rime of the Ancient Mariner*), Robert Southey (*The Story of the Three Bears*, the original Goldilocks), Thomas De Quincey (1785–1859) (*Confessions of an English Opium-Eater*) and Thomas Wedgwood (1771–1805) (a father of photography).

The central hypothesis being tested was that consumption was due to excessive oxygenation, and this could be corrected by lowering oxygen exposure through breathing different concentrations of hydrogen, carbon dioxide or nitrogen.[30] One presumes that these all failed as Beddoes left no record of the results. There was just one success, but not in the direction intended. Having succeeded in obtaining a pure preparation of nitrous oxide, Davy tested it initially on himself. Discovering its pleasurable effects, he went on to perform his famous 'laughing gas' tests on the social circle.[31] It would be a mistake to reduce these experiments to being merely entertainment, as nitrous oxide established beyond doubt that gases could have major physical and psychological effects and that inhalation could be used as a way to administer treatment. However, according to the theory being tested, nitrous oxide as a 'stimulant' was not predicted to cure consumption, nor did it do so. On the plus side, Davy found, instead, that it relieved his toothache and had the insight to realise its anaesthetic potential: 'As nitrous oxide in its extensive operation appears capable of destroying physical pain, it may probably be used with advantage during surgical operations in which no great effusion of blood takes place.'[32] However, Davy did not take this any further as he moved in March 1801 to other projects at the new Royal Institution in London, poached away by Benjamin Thompson (Count Rumford) (1753–1814) and Joseph Banks. It took another 44 years for nitrous oxide to be used for inhalation anaesthesia by the American dentist Horace Wells in 1844.[33] Ether vapour, as an anaesthetic, also derived from the Pneumatic Institution, as Beddoes had temporarily lost consciousness after inhaling it.[34]

By the summer of 1802, Beddoes had run out of money for more work on gases. He rebranded the establishment the Prevention Institution and then renamed it again in 1804 to the 'Medical Institution for benefit of the Sick and Drooping Poor'.[35] The latter name would not resonate well today, despite Beddoes' left-wing intentions.

As mentioned, John Brown placed gout as exemplary of the effects of under-stimulation and thus best treated with alcohol or opium. Beddoes may have seen nitrous oxide as a shorter-acting stimulant to achieve the same end; however, this probably went untested, as gout was rare among the low-income demographic of his clientele.[36] That does not mean that he had no experience of gout, as he later published a summary of some 17 gouty patients who he had treated with a promising but probably never-to-be-known medication.[37] He would have agreed with William Cadogan in seeing the gout and other chronic diseases as due to lifestyle, and his stance on it being a sign of sedentary under-stimulated lassitude and luxury had a political edge.[38] A worker with a decent manual job was protected: 'As to labour, it doubtless exempts multitudes from the Gout, and has been known to remove it. Among four thousand poor chronic invalids, scarce two instances occur of gout in this part of England.'[39] Beddoes also joined with William Heberden (see Chapter 3) in rocking the boat over gout's supposed salutary benefits:

> ... in attempting to speak of this disorder, one feels as if on *tabooed* ground. The public has unlearned an infinity of false opinions with regard to other disorders, but the prejudices of the darkest ages cling as fast as ever to the idea of gout... can it really deserve to be regarded in the favourable light it usually is? Is it reasonable to desire, and wise to cherish such a complaint? Or is it eagerness, with which we hear it sometimes invoked, to be placed among the most egregious examples of the *vanity of human wishes*?... But perhaps it is imagined that the dreadful disorders which follow in the trains of gout, are kept off by its occasional recurrence. There is nothing on the face of the facts to persuade a person, who reasons with the smallest degree of caution, that is more just than the opinion directly opposite – namely – that such and such person become

dropsical because they have suffered so much from the gout. Certainly, the gout seems to possess every qualification for rendering either the lymphatics or the nerves incapable of their function.[40]

From *Acidum Concretum* to Uric Acid

Being an Edinburgh Medical School alumnus, Beddoes had also picked up William Cullen's prejudice against gouty morbific matter and seems not to have realised from translating Carl Scheele's work that the *Acidum Concretum* of urinary stones was relevant to gout. A London surgeon, Murray Forbes, is often credited as being the first person to make the connection in print, publishing this view, unsupported by any chemical analysis, in his *Treatise Upon Gravel and Upon Gout* of 1787, initially for some reason anonymously and then under his own name in a further edition in 1793.[41]

Meanwhile, in Paris, Antoine de Fourcroy took up the challenge of examining the composition of bladder stones in more detail (see Figure 6.2(b)). Fourcroy was a major figure in the late-eighteenth-century 'chemical revolution' in France and was a father of clinical chemistry, believing that laboratory tests were needed to move medicine beyond anecdotes and case reports.[42] He was responsible for the introduction of chemical laboratory analyses into the routine activity of French hospitals. Like Beddoes, Fourcroy was a political radical, and he was a senior member of the National Convention, the elected government that devised the new constitution after the removal of the French monarchy. Fourcroy has been blamed historically for not using his influence to prevent Lavoisier from being guillotined during 'the Terror'. However, it seems more probable that he did try to intervene but had to back down when threatened with his own life.[43] Fourcroy published his massive *Élémens d'histoire naturelle et de chimie*[g] in 1789, and this provided further thoughts on *Acidum Concretum*, which Fourcroy renamed *Acide Lithique*.[h] He emphasised the insolubility of the substance in water and its propensity

---

[g] In English, *Elements of Natural History and Chemistry*.
[h] In English, lithic acid, from λιθοσ (*lithos*), the Greek word for stone.

to form salts with soda, potash and other factors.[i] He also touched on the question of whether gouty tophi and urinary calculi were of similar composition but considered that only future experiments could determine the issue.[44] In 1793, Fourcroy published an account of his large collection of urinary concretions, concluding correctly that his *Acide Lithique* was mainly composed of carbon and nitrogen, with a little oxygen and hydrogen.[45]

The chemical link between *Acidum Concretum* and gout was finally settled by the brilliant William Hyde Wollaston (1766–1828) (see Figure 6.2(c)). Wallaston was born into a prominent intellectual family, his great-grandfather William Wollaston (1659–1724) having written the bestselling *The Religion of Nature Delineated* and his grandfather, father and two uncles all being fellows of the Royal Society.[46] Groomed by his family to be a successful physician, Wollaston had been mentored by his uncle by marriage – none other than William Heberden (see Chapter 3).[47] In 1783, he entered Gonville and Caius College in Cambridge, which had a tradition of supporting medical studies. While there, he became friends with his future business partner, Smithson Tennant (1761–1815), who had met Scheele whilst travelling in Sweden. It was probably Tennant who brought Scheele's work, as translated by Beddoes, to Wollaston's attention. After graduating as MD in 1793, Wollaston moved to Bury St. Edmunds in Suffolk, where he built up a provincial medical practice. He had time to continue his amateur interest in chemistry and conducted an analysis of gouty tophaceous deposits and urinary stones. He moved back to London four years later and presented the results of his analyses to the Royal Society on 22 June 1797.

Wollaston began his subsequent publication, *On Gout and Urinary Concretions*, with a predictive statement on the importance of chemistry for medicine in general and for gout in particular:

> If in any case a chemical knowledge of the effects of diseases will assist us in the cure of them, in none does it seem more likely to be of service than in the removal of the several concretions that are formed in various parts of the body.[48]

---

i Soda and potash were early terms covering what are now known to be sodium and potassium salts.

He then went on to describe the chemical analyses he had performed on gouty tophi, which led him to conclude that they are neutral rather than acidic, and composed of lithiated soda, the sodium salt of lithic acid. This finding flew in the face of the widely held opinion that tophi emerged from underlying bones and consisted of common chalk, which in truth they do resemble to the naked eye. Wollaston was thus the first person to bring an evidence-based chemical footing to gouty tophi. Later on, he chemically characterised various other forms of urinary stones and, in the process, discovered cystine.[49] As we will see in Chapter 11, the proclivity to form cystine stones was to be at the forefront of medical genetics one hundred years later in the hands of Archibald Garrod (1857–1936).[50]

Wollaston moved back to London and practised as a physician for three years, performing dull College of Physicians duties, such as inspecting apothecaries and their premises. He then brought his medical career to an abrupt end, having been passed over for a prestigious staff post at St. George's Hospital. The other candidate, Charles Nevinson, was a well-liked clinician cut from the old cloth: 'Few physicians have ever more thoroughly and extensively secured the confidence of the aristocratic class of patients than Dr. Nevinson … it would be difficult to point out for the imitation of his brethren a more perfect model of the finished gentleman and profoundly skilled physician.'[51] The outcome was not close, with Nevinson gaining 111 votes against Wollaston's 78.[52] It is widely believed that Wollaston abandoning medicine was from a fit of pique over this, which may be partly true.[53] However, he disliked working with patients and yearned instead to devote his life to science. As touched on in Chapter 3, the Royal Society was at a low ebb in the mid-late eighteenth century, and fellowship could be obtained for the right sort by merely showing interest in natural philosophy plus having the right education and social connections.[54] Wollaston was elected a fellow at the age of 26 before even publishing a single scientific paper. However, some of the best appointments are made based on potential rather than achievement, and Wollaston went on to become Royal Society President in 1820, caretaking between the death in his 42nd year of office of Joseph Banks and the turning of a new leaf with the election to the presidency of Humphry Davy.[55] Wollaston's scientific achievements were diverse and remarkable; they included discovering ultraviolet radiation and dark gaps in the solar spectrum, identifying the elements palladium and rhodium, working out the mechanism of fungal circles ('fairy-rings') and inventing the camera lucida.[56]

The problem Wollaston initially faced when he gave up medicine was that being a scientist was not a 'proper job' with a reliable income, and it was not clear what he would live on. Wollaston took the risk of going into partnership with Smithson Tennant in a speculative business venture involving buying up much of the world supply of crude platinum and working out how to convert it into a malleable metal. This Wollaston succeeded in doing in a workroom at the back of his house. He did not publish his methods, as there was nothing obviously patentable in the procedures. Instead, he decided with Tennant to keep them secret, like a proprietary medicine, and to market anonymously the workable platinum they could now make at will. Initially, the problem was that there was no market for it, although the metal's very high melting point (1768°C) made it ideal for chemical laboratory crucibles. Later, Justus Liebig (1803–1873) (see Chapter 8) gave a platinum crucible as a prize to any students in his organic chemistry school in Giessen that mastered his chemical 'alphabet'[j].[57] However, the application for platinum which made Wollaston and Tennant wealthy was its use lining the touch-holes of flintlock guns.[58] Although these were obsolete by 1820 with improved firearms technology, they were standard fixtures through the later stages of the Napoleonic Wars. Wollaston only released the methodology for making platinum malleable towards the end of his life and then only after getting into trouble with Banks, who dictated that progress in science required knowledge to be open to all.

Soon after Wollaston published his analyses of gouty tophi, George Pearson (see Figure 6.4(a)) presented a similar but more comprehensive study.[59] Pearson was 15 years senior to Wollaston and was working as a

---

[j] Liebig's chemical alphabet challenge was to identify correctly the solids or solutions in 100 separate bottles.

physician at St. George's Hospital, where he set up the teaching of chemistry to the medical students.[60] Like Beddoes, he had studied under Joseph Black in Edinburgh. Surprisingly, Pearson failed to acknowledge Wollaston's prior communication, and he may have viewed Wollaston as an upstart rival. While one interpretation of why Wollaston was not appointed to the staff at St. George's is that Charles Nevinson was seen as a better fit socially, another is that Pearson undermined Wollaston's chances to protect his own patch. In any event, Wollaston did not apply when another vacancy for a staff physician came up at St. George's one month afterwards.

Although Pearson's paper was published after Wollaston's, it has its merits. Pearson had analysed many more urinary calculi and realised the great variability in their composition. As Scheele's substance was to be found in normal urine, Pearson argued that the generic name 'lithic' (i.e. 'from stone') was 'a gross solecism' and inappropriate and that 'uric' was better. Pearson also concluded, erroneously, that the substance was not an acid and proposed changing the name further to uric oxide. This infuriated Fourcroy, who then went to very great lengths to repeat

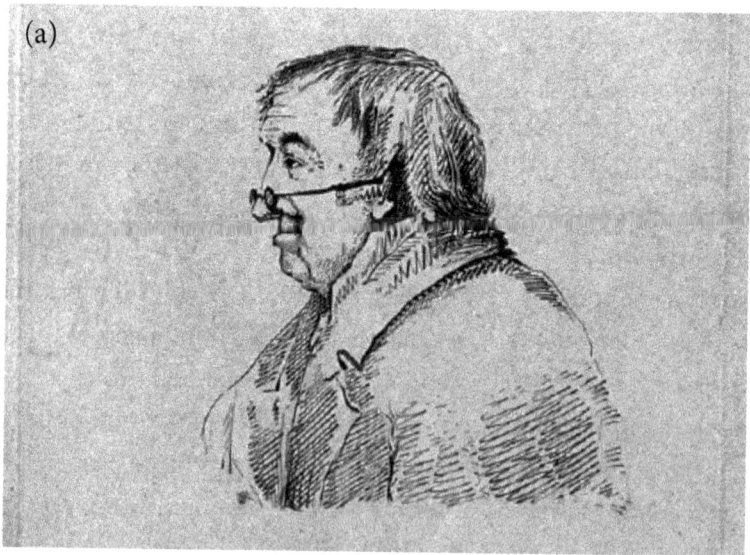

Figure 6.4.

(a) Drawing of George Pearson by an unknown artist.

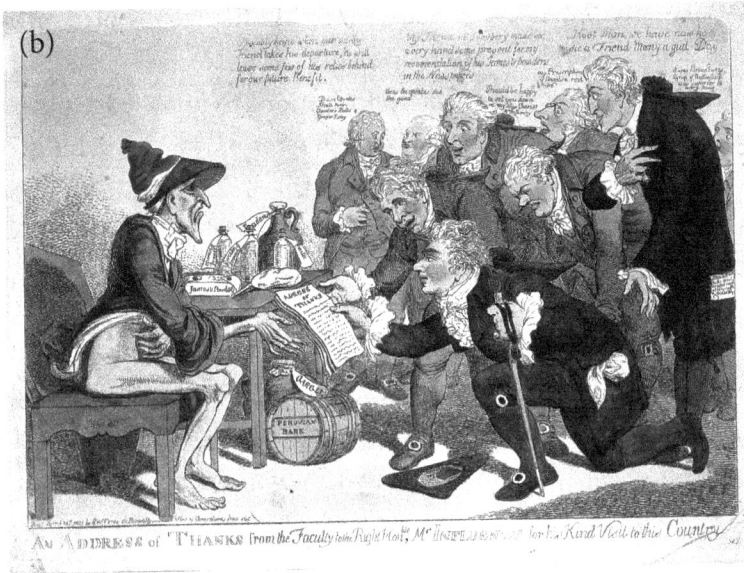

Figure 6.4. (*Continued*)

(b) 'An address of thanks from the faculty to the right honorable, Mr. Influenzy for his kind visit to this country' attributed to Temple West, published by S. W. Fores on 20 April 1803. A group of prominent physicians thank the visitor from France (identified as a revolutionary by his tricolour headdress) for bringing them work. George Pearson had earlier communicated his analysis of *Dr. James's Powder* to the Royal Society, with him, placed middle back, saying that 'My friend Mr. Newbery made me a very handsome present for my recommendation of his James's Powders in the Newspapers'. A packet of *Dr. James' Powder* rests on the table. It has been suggested that the man standing at the back on the left may be Thomas Beddoes, but Beddoes would not have approved of profiteering ill health.

Source: Both images courtesy of the Wellcome Collection: (a) public domain; (b) CC BY 4.0.

Pearson's experiments and ended up agreeing with Scheele as well as his own previous work that the substance was indeed an acid. Fourcroy did, however, accept Pearson's point on not calling it 'lithic', and so the lasting name became '*Acid Urique*', or uric acid in English.[61] It is intriguing that Fourcroy also did not acknowledge Wollaston's publication in his long-winded rebuttal of Pearson's work. Bearing in mind what he had already suggested in 1789, perhaps he found the results of Wollaston's chemical analyses obvious and not worthy of note.

Pearson made several other contributions to knowledge, including an analysis of *Dr. James' Powder* (see Chapter 4). James had described only vaguely in his patent how to prepare this by making an amalgam of mercury, antimony and silver in nitric acid, and it became well known that this description was wholly inadequate. In 1791, Joseph Banks communicated to the Royal Society Pearson's exhaustive effort to identify the exact composition. Pearson concluded that it was probably made by blending antimony with the calcium and phosphate in bone ashes.[62] Later on, a satirical cartoon by Temple West showed a group of acquisitive physicians thanking 'Mr. Influenzy' for coming from France to give them lucrative work and featured Pearson thanking Mr. Newbery for a 'handsome present' in return for providing free publicity for the powder (see Figure 6.4(b)).[63]

Robert Kinglake and James Parkinson

The physician Robert Kinglake had worked with Beddoes at the Pneumatic Institution and was the medical supervisor for the laughing gas experiments. After Hotwells, he went into practice in nearby Taunton. In 1804, he published his *Dissertation on Gout*, explaining that he offered 'a new view of the nature and cure of gouty affection'.[64] Like Beddoes, Kinglake stridently derided traditional opinions and adopted Cullen's dismissal of the humours and the importance of morbific matter. The notion that gout is due to whole-body dysfunction was wrong, and gout 'differs in no essential circumstance from common inflammation', being a local problem of tendinous and ligamentous structures. Many causes were possible, and the effects would always be the same. What made the book unpopular among doctors was not so much this theoretical view of the causes of gouty inflammation but more his practical recommendation that inflammation in affected joints should be treated by cooling. The idea probably came to Kinglake via Beddoes from a gouty William Harvey: 'The great Harvey, as I have heard from his relations, was accustomed to remove the pain by immersing his foot in cold water, as soon as he felt the pain approaching.'[65] However, cooling was still heresy to those who still thought that gouty inflammation should not be thwarted for fear of extending inwards. Even Beddoes felt it was too risky.[66]

A frontrunner in the charge against Kinglake was James Parkinson, who published his *Observations on the Nature and Cure of Gout* the following year in 1805 in protest.[67] Besides attacking Kinglake, Parkinson devoted some 12 pages to a detailed chronology of his own gout.[68] The work is remarkable in another way, in that it provided an early insight into the physiology and pathology related to uric acid, in which Wollaston had shown cursory interest and Kinglake none at all. Parkinson realised that uric acid in the urine is part of everyday physiological 'waste disposal' but that it was liable to crystallise in the urinary tract and form stones due to its limited solubility in water. Referring to Wollaston, he suggested that a similar argument applied to crystallisation of the sodium salt in gouty concretions. It is worth quoting at length Parkinson's remarkable intuition:

> The uric acid is, however, well known to be almost a constant ingredient in urine, and the quantity in which it exists, in that fluid, makes it evident that its removal, in an excrementitious state, is intended to be accomplished by such excretion.... It appears by Dr. Wollaston's experiments that uric acid, as well as that compound of it with soda, which forms the gouty concretions, requires a very large quantity of fluid to hold it in solution. Whenever, therefore, it exists in a morbid proportion in the human system, a strong disposition to its crystallization must prevail; and its separation in a solid form is reasonably to be expected. The part where this separation will take place, will necessarily depend on certain particularities in the diathesis, not, perhaps, to be explained. In some habits, the kidnies will prove to be the organs destined to effect this morbid separation; in which cases the saline concentration will be found either in the urine, bearing the appearance of a red sand, or forming one species of urinary calculus. In other habits,

the ligaments and tendons will be the parts on which the morbid excess of this acid will be deposited. In this case, gouty inflammation will be induced, and after every attack a thickening, with a considerable degree of stiffness, of the ligaments, and hindrance of motion, will be occasioned in consequence of the deposition of the gouty matter.[69]

No portrait of James Parkinson is known to exist. His memory lives on with his name, as he is of course best known for his *Essay on the Shaking Palsy*, published 12 years after his book on gout (see Figure 6.5(a)).[70] This was based on three of his patients, as well as on a further three

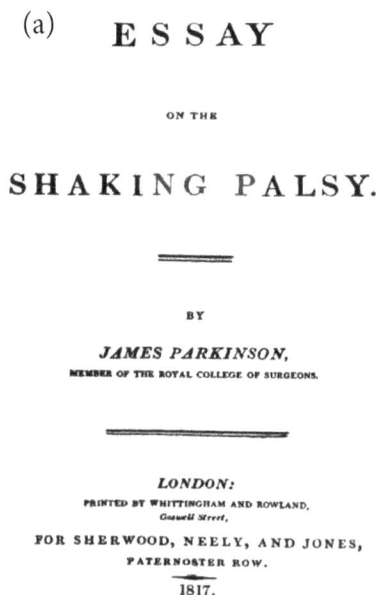

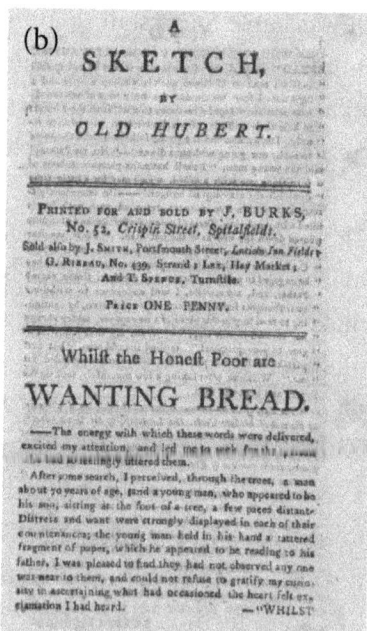

(a)

ESSAY

ON THE

SHAKING PALSY.

BY

JAMES PARKINSON,
MEMBER OF THE ROYAL COLLEGE OF SURGEONS.

LONDON:
PRINTED BY WHITTINGHAM AND ROWLAND,
Goswell Street,

FOR SHERWOOD, NEELY, AND JONES,
PATERNOSTER ROW.

1817.

(b)

A
SKETCH,
BY
OLD HUBERT.

PRINTED FOR AND SOLD BY J. BURKS,
No. 52, *Crispin Street, Spitalfields.*
Sold also by J. SMITH, Portfmouth Street, Lataiols Inn Fields;
G. RIEBAU, No. 439, Strand; LAX, Hay Market;
And T. SPENCE, Turnftile.

PRICE ONE PENNY.

Whilst the Honest Poor are

WANTING BREAD.

Figure 6.5.

(a) Title page of James Parkinson's *Essay on the Shaking Palsy*, the first report of what has become known as Parkinson's disease.

(b) Title page of Parkinson's *A Sketch by Old Hubert - Whilst the Honest Poor Are Wanting Bread*. This was a protest pamphlet on the food crisis in around 1795, and Old Hubert was a politically cautious pseudonym (Chapter 14).

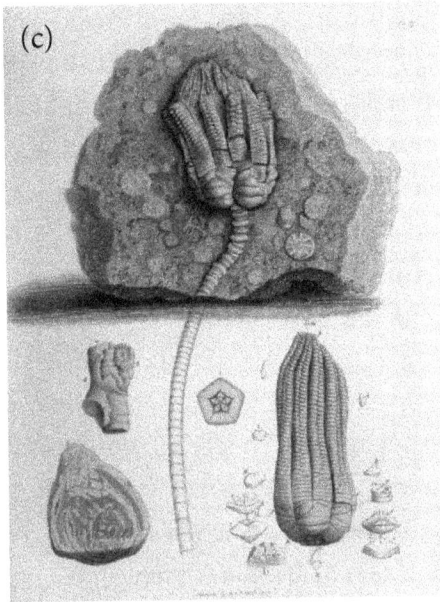

Figure 6.5. (*Continued*)

(c) Parkinson's drawing of fossilised 'lily encrinite', taken from the second edition (1833) of *Organic Remains of a Former World. An Examination of the Mineralized Remains of the Vegetables and Animals of the Antediluvian World*, tinted by his daughter Emma. Parkinson was the first person to use the word 'fossil' to refer to a vestige of living matter rather than just any old stone. He realised that different geological strata had distinct fossil signatures but drew short of rocking belief in Biblical creation.

Source: All courtesy of the Wellcome Collection, public domain.

individuals he observed walking ever so slowly in the streets around his home in Hoxton Square in the East End of London. Thus, Parkinson was the first to describe *Paralysis Agitans*, now known as Parkinson's disease, as a distinct medical entity. However, this was just a very small part of his achievements.[71] While working hard as an apothecary surgeon and being 'obliged to submit to the performance of the most laborious part of a harassing profession', this remarkable polymath also found time to write a compendium of chemistry as a pocketbook, a guide to parents aiming to send an offspring into medicine, household medicine books for ordinary families, a cautionary tale for children on dangerous sports and, as we will see further in Chapter 14, left-wing activist pamphlets on the hunger of the poor (see, for example, Figure 6.5(b)). His radical political views were similar to those of Beddoes, but with travel not being as easy or as frequent as it is today, the two probably never met.

As if all these achievements were not enough, Parkinson was a passionate fossil collector. He had been so impressed by the subject while attending the surgical lecture course of John Hunter[k] (see Chapter 9) that he decided to build up his own collection. He mostly purchased his specimens, one source being the vast collection of Ashton Lever auctioned off in 1806 by his namesake, another James Parkinson, after Joseph Banks had vetoed the purchase of the collection by the government. Parkinson brilliantly catalogued his collection in *Organic Remains of a Former World*, published over seven years (1804–1811) in three volumes, and was the first to apply the word 'fossil' specifically to the vestiges of living matter rather than to anything retrieved from the earth.[72] This giant work consisted of 1,198 pages of print and 50 multi-panelled plates with his own detailed line drawings coloured by his daughter Emma (see Figure 6.5(c)). His book on gout came out in 1805 during an interlude from this palaeontological *magnum opus*. Parkinson's geological publications were landmarks in the study of British fossils and greatly increased public interest in geology.[73] His efforts did not go unrecognised – he was a founding member of the Geological Society of London in 1807, along with Humphry Davy. His name survives in the *Parkinsoniidae* family of mid-Jurassic ammonites and in several other fossilised species. One can only marvel at Parkinson's fine illustrations and the definite hard graft, but his work on fossils still comes over somewhat similar to Christopher Merrett's *Pinax* (see Chapter 2) as a disconnected catalogue illustrating 'traces of the vast changes which this

---

[k] As the texts of Hunter's 68 lectures were burnt, Parkinson's meticulous shorthand notes are their sole surviving record. They were edited and published later by his son J. W. K. Parkinson.

planet has sustained'. Parkinson was aware of the contemporaneous seminal work of William Smith (1769–1839), showing that distinct fossils are present in different geological strata and indeed independently concluded that the same strata extend from England to France.[74] Nevertheless, he hesitated to cross swords with religious beliefs and interpreted geological age within a stretched-out timeline of Biblical creation recently proposed by Jean-André De Luc (1727–1817). Thus, he wrote:

> Circumstances will be observed, apparently contradictory to the Mosaic account, but which, it is presumed, serve to establish it as the revealed history of creation.... The discordance appears to be removed by the assumption of indefinite periods for the days of creation: an interpretation adopted by many learned and pious men.[75]

Alfred Garrod and Urate in the Blood

The big question was whether or not urate was in the blood as well as in tophi, as that might counter the ongoing erosion of the humoral basis to gout by the likes of Cullen, Beddoes and Kinglake. While analysing tophi was relatively easy, measuring substances in the blood was quite another matter. Parkinson was pessimistic and thought that uric acid was probably made locally in gouty tissues:

> No evidence indeed is likely to be adduced, to shew in what state, or in what state of combination, the principles of this peculiar acid exist in the blood. To have the least chance of success in such an inquiry, a series of experiments would be required on the healthy, as well as on that of the gouty; and were these experiments even to be performed, with all due accuracy, yet positive information would hardly be obtained.... It is most probable that the uric acid would not be found to exist, formally, in the blood.[76]

Forty more years therefore passed before there was anything new. A breakthrough, and really the breakthrough on which the history of gout pivots from concept to disease, then came with the work of Alfred Garrod. In 1848, six years before the Medical and Chirurgical Society meeting mentioned at the start of the chapter, Garrod announced that he had succeeded in detecting uric acid in the blood of patients with gout. If Fourcroy started clinical chemistry on urine, Garrod started chemical blood tests.

Garrod had been born in 1819, his father Robert being a successful estate agent and auctioneer in Ipswich.[77] Following schooling at Ipswich Grammar School, Garrod took up an apprenticeship at the East Suffolk and Ipswich Hospital and Dispensary, which is now a private nursing home. He then came to London to study medicine at University College. Garrod realised the importance of chemistry for medicine early on and gained practical experience as a student, presumably under the supervision of Thomas Graham (1805–1869), professor of chemistry. He won the University Gold Medal upon graduating as Batchelor of Medicine in 1842, as well as the Galen Medal for Botany of the Society of Apothecaries. The next year, he obtained his MD, again with the University of London Gold Medal. Not long after, he was appointed clinical assistant at University College Hospital, where his job description specified that he occupy himself chiefly with the analysis of morbid fluids and other substances occurring in hospital cases and sent to him by the medical officer.[78] Garrod's first paper from this appointment was read to the Medical and Chirurgical Society of London in February 1848 by his boss, the physician Charles Williams (1805–1889).[79] Williams had studied in Paris under René Laennec (1781–1826) and helped introduce Laennec's stethoscope into British medical practice.[80]

Uric acid is known to be formed by two positively charged hydrogen (H^+) cations combining with a negatively charged divalent urate anion. If the concentration of H^+ ions is somewhat exceeded by that of sodium (Na^+) ions, one of the two H^+ ions is displaced by a Na^+ ion to give monosodium urate, which is more soluble than uric acid

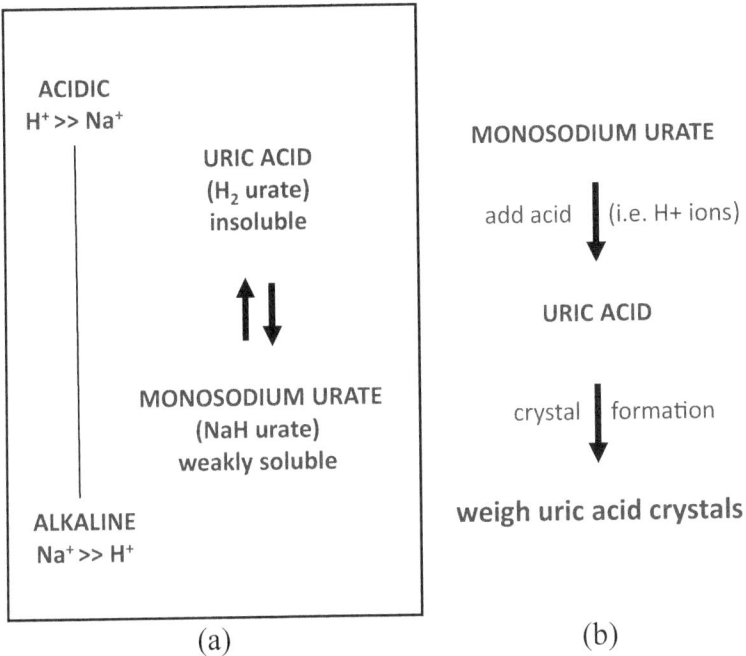

ACIDIC
$H^+ \gg Na^+$

URIC ACID
(H_2 urate)
insoluble

MONOSODIUM URATE
(NaH urate)
weakly soluble

ALKALINE
$Na^+ \gg H^+$

(a)

MONOSODIUM URATE

add acid (i.e. H+ ions)

URIC ACID

crystal formation

weigh uric acid crystals

(b)

Figure 6.6.

(a) The figure shows the effect of varying the hydrogen/sodium ion ratio on the formation of uric acid *versus* monosodium urate.

(b) Garrod found that raising the hydrogen ion concentration by adding an acid into blood serum from gouty subjects led to the conversion of weakly soluble monosodium urate to insoluble uric acid, which then formed crystals that could be weighted. This was the first clinical chemistry blood test.

(Figure 6.6(a)). As the blood is rich in sodium, Garrod hypothesised that it contains uric acid in the form of 'urate of soda' and that adding acid would result in the replacement of sodium by hydrogen ions and the precipitation of insoluble uric acid as crystals. Sure enough, this is just what Garrod found when he tested the blood of gouty patients (Figure 6.6(b)). At face value, this was a test for gout, as only trace amounts of crystals formed when blood samples from healthy individuals or from those with 'acute rheumatism'[1] were tested instead.[81]

Garrod realised that the chemical methods involved in his test were too cumbersome for routine use by practicing doctors, and so in 1854, he introduced a simpler version in the form of the 'uric acid thread' method with which this chapter opened (Figure 6.1(b)).[82] Although clearly an advance as far as the practicing physician was concerned, there were still significant problems diagnosing gout from a positive thread test, as, with more experience, it became clear to Garrod that some people had a raised level of urate in the blood without obviously having gout. A negative test seemed more useful, as the premise that everyone with gout has a readily detectable uric acid in the blood allowed Garrod to redefine so-called 'rheumatic gout'.[83] This was the diagnosis previously given to patients with features of both acute rheumatism and arthritis. Having found that such patients showed no evidence of a raised blood urate, Garrod coined the term 'rheumatoid arthritis', a condition intimated 50 years earlier by William Heberden (see Chapter 3).[84] All this was seminal stuff, but, as we will see in Chapter 9, we now know that categorically distinguishing gout from not gout simply on the basis of either a high or a low blood urate level does not hold true.

Apart from being a talented chemist, Garrod was a remarkable pathologist. He examined in depth a variety of gouty tissues with respect to the presence of urate and published his consolidated observations and views in his classic *The Nature and Treatment of Gout and Rheumatic Gout* (1859).[85] In this, he made 10 propositions on gout, many of which we will come across in later chapters, as they have turned out to be true. Paraphrasing, the propositions that have mostly stood the test of time in the absence of effective treatment are as follows: (#1) sodium urate is invariably present in the blood in abnormal quantities in true gout;

---

[1] 'Acute rheumatism' would have included a number of today's diagnostic entities that cause acute arthritis, but a majority probably had rheumatic fever.

(#2) true gouty inflammation is always associated with a deposition of sodium urate at the inflamed site; (#3) sodium urate deposits in cartilages and ligamentous structures and remains there indefinitely; (#4) sodium urate is the cause, and not the effect, of gouty inflammation; (#6) the kidneys are implicated, probably functionally in the early stages and certainly structurally in the chronic stages of gout; (#8) the precondition for gout is either increased formation of uric acid or increased retention of uric acid in the blood; and (#10) the deposition of sodium urate only occurs in true gout and not other diseases.

Garrod was appointed full physician and professor of material medica and therapeutics at University College in 1851 at the age of just 32. He resigned in 1863 and travelled south just over a mile to take up the chair of professor of material medica and therapeutics at King's College Hospital Medical School, then located at Lincoln Inn Fields. Reminiscent of Wollaston being turned down by St. George's, the move was probably triggered by not having been selected by University College for the chair of the principles and practice of medicine. Instead, the committee appointed William Jenner (1715–1798), a general physician who had made a name for himself drawing a distinction between typhoid and typhus fever.[86] Selection panels have to be wary of the consequences of passing over a good candidate. Apparently, the feedback to Garrod was that his lectures had an overemphasis on botany and chemistry and lacked sufficient attention to treatment. Garrod was knighted Sir Alfred in 1887 in the Queen's Golden Jubilee Honours List. That year, a medical banquet was hosted in his honour in his hometown, Ipswich. In the toast, a local physician concluded that Garrod had done for gout and rheumatic gout what William Jenner had done for typhus.[87] However, the role of uric acid in gout was by no means all sown up, as, although Garrod had demonstrated that those with gout have a raised urate level in the blood and had provided a wealth of pathological observations showing urate deposition in gouty tissues, experimental evidence supporting his contention that urate causes gout was still entirely lacking. In the same vein, as we will see, the actual diagnostic significance of finding a high urate level in the blood remained far from clear. Nevertheless, this did not stop the medicine trade equating uric acid with disease and spinning it into a poison badly requiring new and expensive proprietary treatments.

Chapter 7

More Pills and Potions

*C*olchicum (or colchicine; see Chapter 10) does not affect uric acid levels, and while it is effective in treating gouty inflammation, it does not prevent urate accumulation and tophus formation. Attempts to control uric acid by other means date back to the early 1800s. The *Lancaster Gazette* of June 1813 reported a presentation to the Royal Society by William Brande (1788–1866) on what he considered to be the successful use of magnesium powder for treating urinary stones.[1] Magnesium had originally been suggested as a treatment by Everard Home (see Chapter 6), on the basis that it is insoluble in water and might combine with uric acid in the gut, preventing it from entering the circulation from food.[2] However, the powder tended to aggregate and obstruct the bowels, so there was plenty of opportunity for improvement. One notable early magnesium solution was the surgeon James Murray's *Patent Aperient*.[3] This was renamed *Surgeon Murray's Antibilious Aperient or Portable Condensed Solution of Magnesia for Health or Pleasure* and specifically recommended for dissolving the uric acid in gravel or gout – and for many other indications related to neutralising stomach acidity and relieving the effects of intemperance.[4] Murray was knighted in 1833 for his services as a physician to the Lord Lieutenant of Ireland, after which the brand became *Sir James Murray's Fluid Magnesia*.[5] It was quite widely advertised in England and Ireland for over 30 years, but rivals sprang up. These included *Dinneford's Pure Fluid Magnesia*, which was offered all the same benefits but additionally advertised for partnering with *Colchicum* 'as a vehicle for the preparations of Colchicum for cases of Gout, its great utility must be evident to every medical man'.[6] Murray's preparation still lives on as *Milk of Magnesia*, although manufacturers have long since abandoned the fancy of it curing gout or urinary gravel and stones.

Uric Acid Poisoning

An unintended consequence of replacing candles with oil during the nineteenth century was an increase in household fires, and Hulbert Warner made his fortune in the United States dealing in fire-proof safes to protect people's valuables. He extended his commercial activity into healthcare with his *Warner's Safe Cure* (note the pun), each bottle being imprinted with an image of his safe door. His numerous advertisements carrying the heading *The Microscope: the many puzzling secrets revealed by this wonderful instrument* informed readers in 1887 that:

> Uric acid, which is a rank poison, is one of the substances which arise from destructive waste of our body, and must be thrown off daily, or we die. Now, before we understood the microscope it was impossible by any means at our command to know what was being passed out of our body, or from whence it came; and one great benefit this instrument has conferred upon humanity is in the relief of headaches, malaise, indigestion and other diseases, which are known to be caused by the retention of uric acid in the body. When an analysis of this fluid is made by a microchemical examination this substance can be traced in its proper quantity, and when the proper remedy is applied as soon secured, the cure being effected almost immediately.[7]

The need for the microscope is unclear but may have been to count uric acid crystals. However, all the public needed to know was that removing the 'rank poison' required a bottle of *Safe Cure*. In the old proprietary tradition of rags to riches, this turns out to have been simply a mix of senna, rhubarb, wintergreen (see the following), glycerine and potassium nitrate in alcohol.[8]

The focus on uric acid retention as a general cause of illness had its origins in the 'Gouty diathesis', which embraced both 'regular' and 'irregular' gout (see Chapter 1). Once Garrod found urate in the blood, the 'Gouty diathesis' was modernised by some to the equally vague 'uric acid diathesis'. This flourished particularly under the championship of the North London physician Alexander Haig (1853–1924), a cousin of the World Ward I Field Marshall Douglas Haig. Educated at Harrow and Oxford, Haig wrote his MD thesis on uric acid. He then came to London and worked as a casualty officer at St. Bartholomew's Hospital before obtaining a physician post at the Metropolitan Free Hospital in London. His duties would have been clinical rather than teaching or research. His interest in uric acid was at first personal, as he had worked out that a meat- and alcohol-free diet greatly reduced his incapacitating recurrent migraines. Convinced that his headaches had a dietary cause, he made detailed correlations of their incidence in relation to the uric acid content of his urine.[a] He concluded that uric acid was responsible for his headaches and then extended this reasoning to the point that it became a universal toxin, responsible for a long list of other complaints, including not only gout but also high blood pressure, epilepsy, depression, anaemia, diabetes and kidney disease:

> The fact which will appear when the whole of my researches have been published is that uric acid controls so completely the circulation of the blood that any accurate measurement of that circulation is a measure also of the quantity of uric acid in the blood and urine and corresponds in every way to this.[9]

---

[a] Methods for measuring urate in blood had not moved past Garrod's thread test and were too insensitive and cumbersome for Haig's experimental purposes.

Haig popularised what became a uric acid fetish in *Uric Acid as a Factor in the Causation of Disease* (1892), which was a bestseller among the health anxious.[10] He sent a deluge of open letters over 25 years or so to the *British Medical Journal* and *The Lancet*, mostly serving to remind colleagues about his book. However, even at the peak of his popularity, Haig's advocacy of the need to treat uric acid toxicity was by no means generally accepted by the profession, at home or abroad.[11] At a practical level, some laboratory studies failed to replicate Haig's analyses of urine.[12] Nevertheless, in his day, Haig was sufficiently mainstream to be invited to give a plenary lecture on the treatment of headaches at the Annual Meeting of the British Medical Association (BMA) in Portsmouth in 1899.[13] Two years later, James Goodhart (1845–1916), a consultant physician at Guy's Hospital in London, addressed the BMA's annual meeting in Cheltenham with:

> I find that the British public knows far more about uric acid and how to deal with it than I do with all my pains, and what men think they know in this respect, I fear that we, in the first place, and vulgar advertisement in the second place, have taught them.[14]

The vulgar advertisements to which Goodhart was referring were not only for *Warner's Safe Cure* but for a whole new generation of proprietary medicines.

Alkalis

Winding the clock back, doctors had been prescribing alkalis to try to clear urinary stones long before Scheele discovered uric acid. Some justification for the practice in the case of uric acid calculi came in late nineteenth century with the work of Lionel Beale (1828–1906) (see Figure 7.1(a)). Beale was nine years younger than Alfred Garrod and had been appointed to the chair of physiology at King's College Hospital in 1853, well before Garrod arrived there. Lacking any laboratory facilities, he set up his own private laboratory for research and for teaching students chemistry and

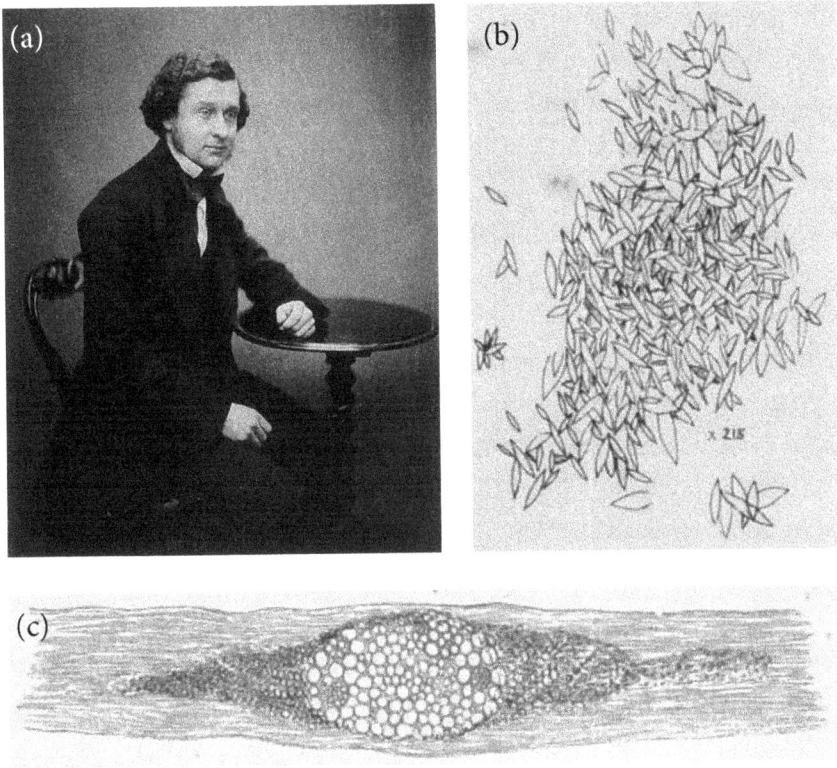

Figure 7.1.

(a) Lionel Smith Beale, photograph by Maull & Polyblank.

(b) Beale's drawing of uric acid crystals precipitated from an acid urine and connected together to form plates. Figure 17 of *Illustrations of the Constituents of Urine, Urinary Deposits, and Calculi* (1878).

(c) Beale later became a leading force in the vitalism movement, challenging the idea that evolution could be determined by simple biochemical rules, and was an ardent critic of Charles Darwin's theories. He used his undoubted microscopy skills to search for, and in his eyes find, evidence of vital forces (bioplasm) contained in tissues. The image is entitled 'Bioplasm and formed material from ordinary tendon' from *Protoplasm: Or, Matter and Life* (1874).

Source: All courtesy of the Wellcome Collection: (a) CC BY 4.0; (b) and (c) public domain.

microscopy. Testifying to the importance of urine as the window to the patient's chemical world in an era before routine blood tests, the *British Medical Journal* published Beale's lectures on the composition of urine in no less than 32 sequential articles over 1859–1860.[15] His research showed that the urate in the urine was in the form of monosodium urate, just as in blood. However, rhomboidal uric acid crystals can precipitate spontaneously when the urine becomes acidic, just as they did when Garrod added acid to blood serum (see Figure 7.1(b)).[16] Pure uric acid stones may thus form in the urinary tract, as do stones formed of uric acid mixed with calcium salts.[17] More modern analyses of urinary stones have borne out Beale's conclusions. He is now more remembered as a nineteenth-century champion of vitalism (Figure 7.1(c)), a belief that started unravelling with the work of Friedrich Wöhler (1800–1882) and Justus Liebig (1803–1873) and the birth of organic chemistry (see Chapter 8).

Between 5% and 20% of urinary stones are made mostly of uric acid, and many other urinary stones are complex assemblies around a uric acid nucleus.[18] Calcium citrate and other alkalis have survived as effective treatments for radiolucent urinary stones, or, in other words, those stones not showing opaque calcium on X-rays and assumed to contain uric acid.[19] The scientific basis for the therapeutic use, or rather non-use, of alkalis for gout is quite different. In the eighteenth century, William Cullen used to prescribe 'an alkali in various forms, such as the fixed alkali, both mild and caustic, lime-water, soap, and absorbent earths' to his gouty patients. He found the strategy effective in reducing acute attacks but was reluctant to pursue the treatment for long, being 'apprehensive that the long-continued use of them might produce a hurtful change in the state of the fluids'.[20] This was an entirely sensible approach, necessitated by a rudimentary understanding of disease mechanisms. Moving to the nineteenth century, alkalis became widely prescribed for gout on the assumption that gout was caused by uric acid or sodium urate precipitating in tissues when they were acidic, just as uric acid became known to do from acid urine.

It was not until the late 1890s that alkali treatment for gout was debunked by Arthur Luff, who found no evidence that blood becomes sufficiently acidic for uric acid or urate precipitation, not even during an acute gout attack.[21] Luff was a practising physician at St. Mary's Hospital in London and an early rheumatologist. He was an accomplished chemist and is remembered as one of the fathers of forensic medicine, with his seminal *Textbook of Forensic Medicine and Toxicology*, which was published in 1895 (see Figure 7.2(a)).[22] Luff's most famous case was the 'O. J. Simpson trial' of the early 1900s – that of 'Doctor' Hawley Harvey Crippen. Crippen was an American proprietary medicine distributor, and his wife Cora was a dressy, aspiring and talentless music hall singer with the stage name Belle Elmore (see Figure 7.2(b)). After Cora disappeared, Crippen told her friends that she had gone urgently to California, where she had died in the mountains. Soon after, Crippen and his mistress Ethel Le Neve were

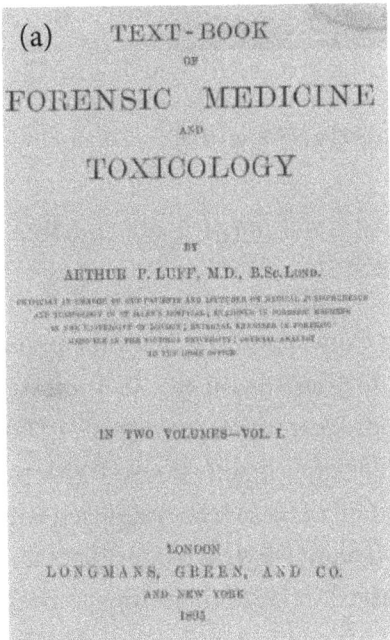

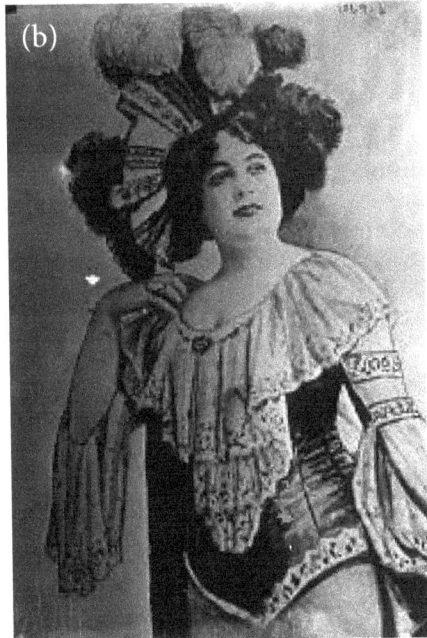

Figure 7.2.

(a) Title page to Arthur Luff's seminal *Textbook of Forensic Medicine and Toxicology.*

(b) Cora Crippen (*aka* Belle Elmore) dressed for the stage in 1910.

(Continued)

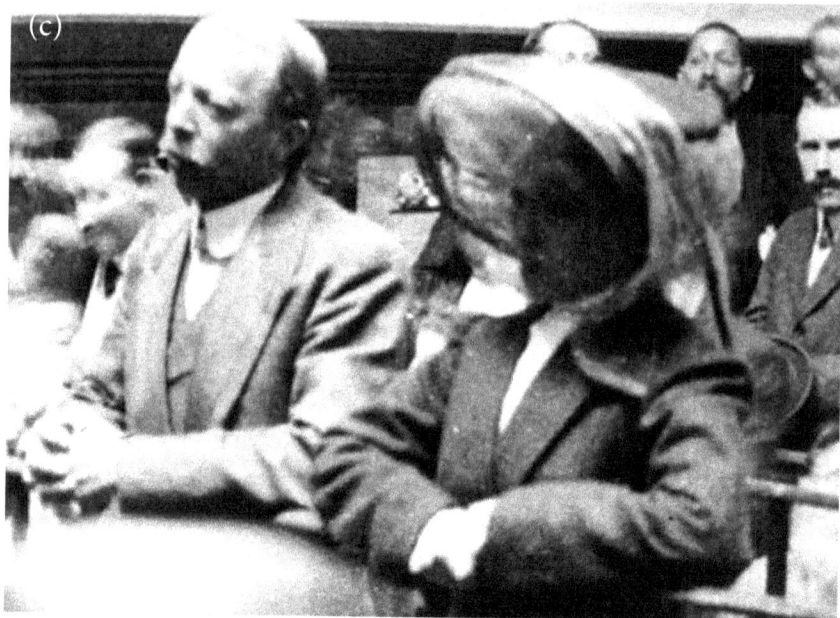

Figure 7.2. (*Continued*)

(c) Hawley Harvey Crippen and his mistress, Ethel Le Neve, on trial for Cora's murder in 1910.

Source: (a) Courtesy of the Wellcome Collection, public domain; (b) and (c) Bain News Service publisher via Wikimedia Commons, public domain.

seen out walking, with Le Neve wearing Cora's jewellery. With the police showing interest, the two fled London for Canada on the *SS Montrose*, disguised as Mister and Master Robinson. Meanwhile, an Inspector Dew found human remains buried in the cellar of Crippen's house. With the case now a newspaper sensation, the captain of *SS Montrose* realised who the Robinsons were and used his new Marconi wireless to alert Scotland Yard. Dew boarded a faster boat and arrived in Quebec in time to arrest the fugitive couple as they disembarked. Luff's toxicological analysis of the buried remains revealed a plant alkaloid (see Chapter 10) that dilated the pupil of a cat's eye. It turned out that Crippen had recently purchased a known pupil-dilator, hyoscine, from a local chemist, and further analysis supported this being the poison employed.[23] Crippen and Le Neve were duly tried (see Figure 7.2(c)), and Crippen was found guilty and hung in Pentonville Prison at 9 am on 23 November 1910. Le Neve was found to be an accessory after the fact and was acquitted. The remaining doubt as to whether the remains in Crippen's basement really were Cora's is doubt no more, as comparison of chromosomes and DNA sequences in archived tissue from the find with those of Cora's living relatives has shown that they were not – and also that they were those of a man.[23] However, the presence of any torso buried in Crippen's cellar does not speak well for his total innocence. We do not know what happened to Cora, nor, if she was alive, why she did not come forward to save her husband. For that matter, why did Crippen and Le Neve flee the country in such a furtive manner?

By 1900, the German physician Carl von Noorden (1858–1944) was lecturing to the British Medical Association that 'Alkalis in every form are utterly useless. They act excellently in nephrolithiasis[b], but in true gout they cause a diminution, that is, an actual retention of uric acid'.[24] Since then, a better understanding of acid–alkali balance has shown that the blood has a robust buffering system that maintains a slightly alkalinity at pH 7.4[c] and becomes acid only when the buffering system is overwhelmed during major life-threatening illnesses. The urine is not similarly buffered, explaining the precipitation of uric acid in an acid urine, as above. Simple alkalis to prevent uric acid stone formation are rational for urinary stones, but for gout they are pointless.

The Lithium Fad

A spin-off from the misguided use of alkalis for gout was the use of lithium. It is prescribed nowadays as a mood stabiliser for bipolar disorders, and it has rather been forgotten that it was introduced to medicine as a uric acid solvent. To set the background, the Swedish chemists Johan Arfwedson (1792–1841) and Jöns Jacob Berzelius (1779–1848) discovered the element

---

[b] i.e. kidney stones.

[c] pH is an index of acidity. The lower the pH, the more hydrogen ions and the more acidic, with pH 7 being neutral, below 7 acidic and above 7 alkaline.

within the mineral petalite in 1817. They named it from the Greek word λιθειοσ (*lithios*; stone-like), which is somewhat confusing for us in view of lithic acid being an early name for uric acid (see Chapter 6) and the term 'lithaemia' being used for years afterwards to describe a high blood urate level. A small quantity of pure lithium was isolated by Humphry Davy soon after it was discovered, and then larger amounts by his successor at the Royal Institution, William Brande.[25] Lithium's properties were explored in greater detail by the German chemist Alexander Lipowitz (1810–1873), who found that it had the remarkable ability to dissolve uric acid.[26] This is because lithium combines with the urate anion to form lithium urate, which is 36 times more soluble in water than uric acid and five times more soluble than monosodium urate. Subsequently. the English surgeon and chemist Alexander Ure (1808–1866) found that lithium carbonate could dissolve uric acid stones in a dish and suggested it might be effective if injected directly into the bladder. Unfortunately for Ure, but fortunately for his patients, lithium supplies were initially very limited, and he did not have enough to test his idea at the time.[27] When lithium became more readily available 20 years later, Ure published a report in *The Lancet* in 1860 of a patient with urinary stones whom he had treated with repeated installation of lithium carbonate into the bladder. It was not a success, as the patient soon developed a further stone and died.[28]

Advertisements for lithiated water started appearing in British news-papers as early as 1855.[29] By 1858, Garrod was telling the world how he was prescribing lithium salts to his gout patients, partly for their alkaline prop erties and partly to dissolve uric acid.[30] Following this, lithium citrate and lithium carbonate were featured as therapeutic agents for gout in the first edition of the *British Pharmacopoeia*, published in 1864.[31] Garrod was firmly convinced of their ability to prevent attacks of acute gout and clear tophaceous deposits, and he stuck to his guns for over 25 years, staunchly defending lithium in his Lumlean Lectures to the Royal College of Physicians in 1883.[32] He saw it as a natural supplement since it was present in animal and plant tissues: 'Lithia must therefore now be regarded, not as a drug foreign to the economy, but as a normal constituent of the body, and essential to its well-being'.[33] He considered chronic lithium therapy to be reasonably safe but acknowledged it could sometimes cause trembling hands and adversely affect the kidneys, both of which transpired to be all too true.

The spa resorts and mineral water companies jumped on the band-wagon once lithium chloride was detected in the thermal springs at Baden-Baden (Germany). Suppliers pushed on an open commercial door, helped by the uric acid phobia, into which the public was being guided. *Buffalo Springs Lithia Water* from Virginia was marketed as 'the best natural remedy for excess uric acid in the blood', while imbibers of *Londonderry Springs Lithia Water* from New Hampshire were instructed to 'drink six to ten glasses of Londonderry Lithia, the best known neutraliser of uric acid, which causes the trouble'.[34] Eventually, critical analyses both in England and in the United States found that these and similar bottled waters contained just trace levels of lithium at best.[35] Henry Jeffmann, chemical pathologist at Jefferson Medical College in Philadelphia, concluded his analytical report in 1910 with 'the time is now at hand to overthrow the lithia water fetish, the only use of which is to extract thousands of dollars from the pockets of real and imaginary suffers in this country'.[36] The suppliers adjusted their sales pitches by stating that 'lithia' was just part of the company name or that the low levels of lithium had powerful homoeopathic potency. *Buffalo Springs Lithia Water* survived as a brand name in the United States until 1917, when the company lost a prolonged misinformation legal wrangle that ended up in the US Supreme Court. In the opinion of the court, someone would have to drink over 150,000 gallons of the product to obtain a 'therapeutic dose' of lithium.[37] The company duly rebranded the water *Buffalo Mineral Springs Water*, which sold well in the US and Europe into the 1950s.[38] Some companies pivoted on the problem of natural lithia waters lacking lithium by adding lithium to their products, with Merck's Index of 1907 listing a staggering 43 different tablets and powders containing it.[39]

Garrod's views on lithium were endorsed by the gout author Dyce Duckworth (1840–1928), but other practitioners were not so sure.[40]

Certainly, William Roberts (1830–1899), otherwise one of Garrod's staunchest supporters, was far from convinced, and Arthur Luff warned against lithium on the basis that it depressed the heart.[41] Furthermore, subsequent studies by Luff and others failed to support lithium as an effective urate solvent in blood or as a means to stimulate urate excretion.[42] Actually, Alastair Haig, the high priest of uric acid phobia, did not support the use of lithium either, being aware that Garrod had paid little attention to whether the concentrations achieved by prescription were sufficient to dissolve uric acid in the body. This was because most lithium ingested could be expected to combine instead with other, more plentiful substances, such as phosphate.[43] Needless to say, the liberal and unregulated marketing of lithium led to increasing appreciation of its untoward effects on the nervous system and kidneys, and sales tailed off. However, the sale of commercial lithium tonics continued well into the twentieth century, albeit perhaps more as pick-me-ups than antidotes to uric acid. The most enduring beverage that once contained lithium is *Bib-Label Lithiated Lemon-Lime Soda Water*, introduced by the St. Louis-based Howdy Corporation in 1926. Now known as *7Up*, this contained lithium until 1948. There are various theories on the origin of the name, but the one that suits this story is that seven is the atomic mass of lithium. The irony is that although a 330 ml can of modern regular *7Up* sold in the UK has no lithium, it has 15 grams of sugar, which will help raise rather than lower the blood urate level (see Chapter 13).

Piperazine and Other Supposed Uric Acid Solvents

There were other 'uric acid solvents'. The neurologist Charles-Édouard Brown-Séquard (1817–1894) is remembered for describing a neurological consequence of spinal cord injury (Brown-Séquard syndrome). Having clocked up 72 years, he perhaps reasonably became interested in ageing and experimented with injecting extracts of monkey testicles in the hope of rejuvenating sexual prowess. His work led to Philipp Schreiner (1846–1914) isolating a supposed anti-ageing testicular derivative, named spermine.[44] In fact, Anton van Leeuwenhoek (see Chapter 9) had unknowingly previously observed spermine crystals in seminal fluid in the 1600s while making the first sighting of spermatozoa.[45] The obvious commercial potential of spermine led to many synthetic analogues, and out of this effort came the Schering Company's piperazine.

Advertisements started appearing around 1892 lauding piperazine as the solvent for use in gout and urinary stones. One in *The Morning Post* informed readers that:

> The greatest discovery since the introduction of quinine into medical practice is the ammonia derivate piperazine. Its peculiar affinity for uric acid gives it a capacity of dissolving all urinary and other concretions in the body, and goutie, stone and so-called old-aged patients may be considered to have at last found a remedy which is certain to give relief. Piperazine is pronounced by numerous medical authorities to be non-poisonous, non-irritant, and not to interfere with the circulation of the blood or the action of the heart.[46]

The august *Journal of the American Medical Association* carried an editorial the same year, telling readers that 'the popular knowledge in regard to the new "gout-water" containing piperazine is spreading, and laymen in the horse-cars have been overheard discussing the merits of the water' and that it was also available as tablets or more palatable effervescent powders.[47] The editorial also mentioned that the German physician Ernst Schweninger (ca. 1686–ca. 1744) had prescribed piperazine to over a hundred patients and had stated that 'no remedial substance has done so much good for gouty patients, in many years of trial of many remedies, as has this new product.' Schweninger was the unconventional professor of dermatology at the Charité Hospital in Berlin, having been placed there against strong academic opposition by his patron, the German Chancellor Otto von Bismarck, whom he was treating for gout and obesity.[48]

A *British Medical Journal* report in 1894 from doctors in Aberdeen, showing that piperazine was more effective than lithium in dissolving uric acid stones in a dish, was considered important enough to be announced by the local newspaper.[49] Two months later, 'Doctor's Corner' in the *Newcastle Weekly Chronicle* was telling readers that piperazine was the best treatment for the many mental and physical conditions of ill health linked to that 'insidious form of blood poisoning – uric acid in the blood'. The article then gently introduced the subsidiary matter of a sensible diet.[50]

Sadly, for piperazine, urate dissolution was not observed at concentrations achievable in urine, and William Roberts taught that it was as useless as lithium.[51] Moreover, the anti-vivisection correspondent of *The Courier* picked up on it having been tested on animals, and derided it as a 'delusion and a sham' in being no better than cheap sodium bicarbonate, and it gloated at 'another medical bubble burst'.[52] Despite the mounting evidence on its lack of efficacy, a *British Medical Journal* book review in 1906 castigated the work in question for not including piperazine 'among the drugs selected as serviceable for the relief of Gout'.[53] The *Sporting Times* adapted a Christmas carol: 'Hark the Herald, angel's sing, "Piperazine's the only thing".'[54] Piperazine's career thus lasted for a few more years – drug companies kept it alive, doctors continued to prescribe it and patients swore by it. Indeed, the supposed role of uric acid as a general poison led to the recommendations for piperazine being extended, for example by Dr. Reynold Webb, professor of medicine and therapeutics in New York, for use by those with insomnia 'should the patient be afflicted with Goutiness'.[55] Keen to extend further the unmet need, the Pipérazine Midi Company produced a series of promotional booklets with broad claims: 'It constitutes without contradiction the medication of choice for acute gout and gravel. In addition, it gives the most remarkable results in chronic gout and in other manifestations of the uric acid diathesis: skin disease, neuralgia, sciatica, sore throat, atherosclerosis etc.'[d,56]

---

[d] Originally in French: '*Dans la goutte aiguë et la gravelle, elle constitute sans contredit le medicament de choix. Enfin elle donne les plus remarquables résultats dans la goutte chronique et dans les autres manigestaions de la diathèse urique : dermatoses, névralgies, sciatique, angine granuleuse (Fauvel), artériosclérose, etc.*'.

Other agents that were introduced in the 1890s with claims to dissolve uric acid even better included piperidine, urotropine,[e] and lysidine.[57] Faced with evidence that individual drugs were insufficiently effective, manufacturers moved on to combinations that were advertised as improvements. The formulation from Willcock's in Datchet mixed piperazine with phenocoll[f] and added lithium for good measure.[58] Lithium was combined with quinate by Zimmer and Co. of Frankfurt in their Urosine, the inclusion of quinate deriving from this being held to be the ingredient responsible for the supposed ability of eating large quantities of cherries (see Chapter 12), strawberries or grapes to reduce uric acid levels.[59] The combination of quinate with piperazine in Schering's Sidonal was so expensive that the manufacturers then introduced the marketing strategy of issuing New Sidonal. This was sold at less than half the price but was still costly, being the equivalent of £12 per tablet in today's money.[60]

The combination of Sidonal, lysidine and urotropine was patented in 1907 by the urologist Lucien Graux and marketed as Urodonal, with an imaginative promotional campaign making claims of renewing the system and providing second youth. One revealing advertisement stated:

> There are, at any rate, a few points which have been agreed upon, among which is the fact that nine times out of ten the rheumatic diathesis is characterised by excess of uric acid in the system.... It no longer matters much to know exactly what rheumatism is when we possess such an unrivalled means to relieve it. It is possible that in studying the effects of URODONAL the problem will finally be solved.[61]

This and similar advertisements for Urodonal ran for 297 successive weeks in the upmarket *Illustrated London News*, placed there presumably

---

[e] The early urinary anti-septic hexamethylenetetramine.

[f] Phenocoll was used to relieve pain and fever.

to reach a gouty readership (see Figures 7.3(a) and (b)). The version of 1 July 1916 had the title 'Urodonal maintains youth of the heart and arteries'. [62] Sadly, the drug could not maintain the youth of the 318,700 soldiers who died at the Battle of the Somme, which opened that same day. Urodonal's inventor, Lucein Graux, became a popular novelist and publisher and also the founder of a successful perfume company. He was

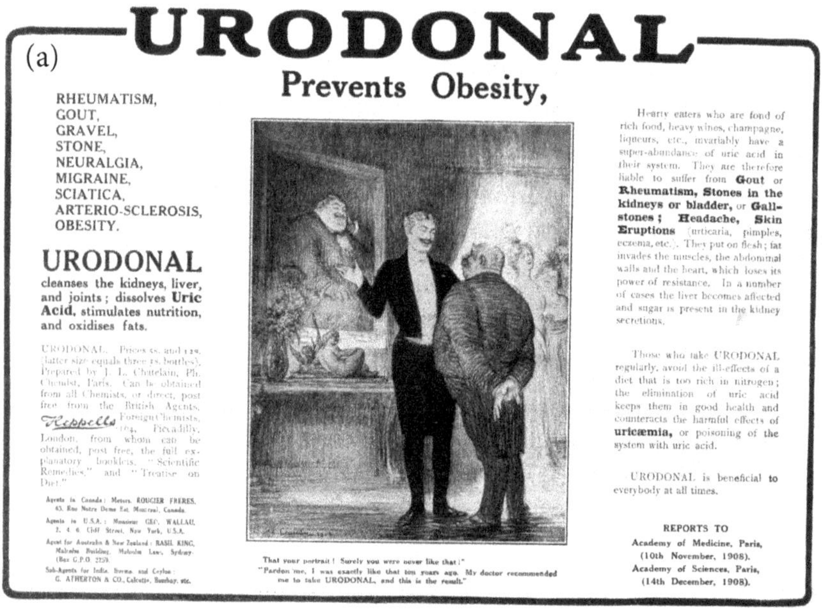

Figure 7.3.

Two advertisements for Urodonal that appeared in 1916 in the *Illustrated London News*, an upmarket magazine likely to have been read in private member's clubs. These and many similar advertisements kept uric acid alive in the public mind as a poison responsible for a variety of conditions. None of these links had been scientifically established, nor had the ability of Urodonal to cure them. Hence, they were no different from advertisements for any other medication at the time.

(a) Highlights a link with obesity that will be addressed in Chapter 14. The caption reads: 'That's your portrait! Surely you were never like that!', followed by 'Pardon me, I was exactly like that ten years ago. My doctor recommended me to take URODONAL and this is the result.' (2 September 1916).

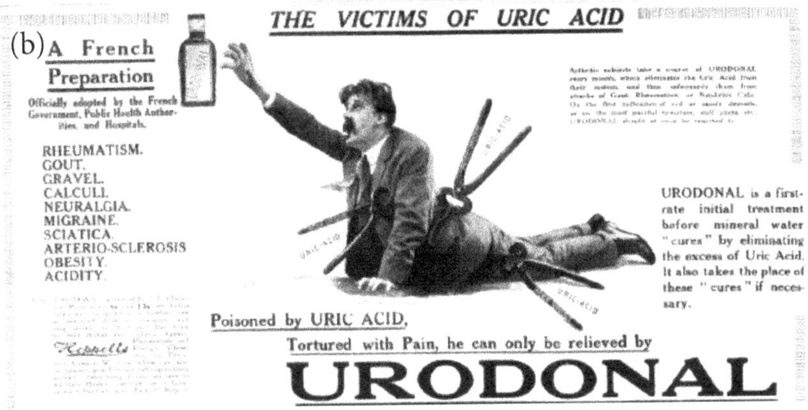

Figure 7.3. (*Continued*)

(b) Focuses on Urodonal for treating pain (29 April 1916).

Source: Under licence @ Illustrated London News/Mary Evans.

arrested by the Germans for French resistance activity during World War II and subsequently died in the Dachau concentration camp in 1944.

The last advertisement for Urodonal accessible via the British Newspaper Archive appeared in 1932, but it remains an over-the-counter product in some countries. However, its use for lowering uric acid has been dropped, and it is now promoted to help with mental problems. Use of lithium, piperazine and other supposed uric acid solvents also dwindled away, and by the 1930s, medical interest had all but vanished.[63] Piperazine has subsequently re-entered medicine as a treatment for worms and has since become a lead compound for many derivative drugs still in use today. Closing the loop on Brown-Séquard's quest for rejuvenation, one of these is sildenafil (Viagra).[g]

Salicylates

By the 1880s, an alternative to the supposed solvents had emerged in the form of salicylic acid and its derivatives. James Goodhart had this to say at

---

[g] Viagra is commonly used nowadays to correct erectile dysfunction.

his 1901 BMA address: 'I suppose there is not a single case of gout in the whole world that has not had sodium salicylate and other easily enumerated drugs, and had them freely; and why? Because they are supposed to eliminate the cause of the disease'.[64]

The bark and leaves of the common willow (*Salix alba*) had been used in ancient times to treat inflammation, pain and fever but had largely been forgotten.[65] Their ability to quench fevers was rediscovered by the Reverend Edmund Stone,[h] a chaplain near Chipping Norton in Oxfordshire, and communicated by letter to the Royal Society in 1763.[66] Johann Buchner (1783–1852), working at the University of Munich, later isolated an active extract and called it salicin.[67] Ten years after that, the Neopolitan chemist Raffaele Piria (1815–1865) (see Figure 7.4(a)) isolated the salicylate radical

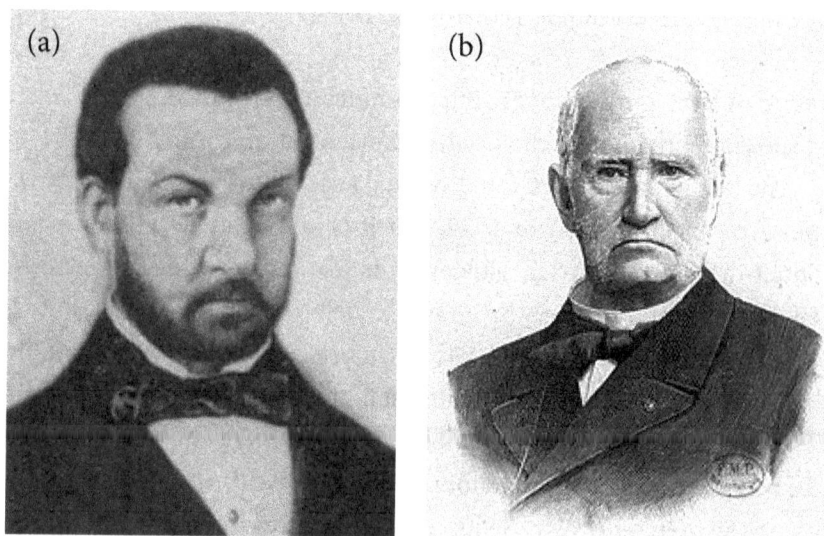

Figure 7.4.

(a) Raffaele Piria, who in 1838 isolated the salicylate anion.

(b) Germain Sée, professor of clinical medicine at Hôtel-Dieu in Paris. Sée was the first to advocate the use of salicylates for treating gouty arthritis and also appreciated their ability to increase urinary loss of urate.

---

[h] Stone's first name may have been Edward, not Edmund.

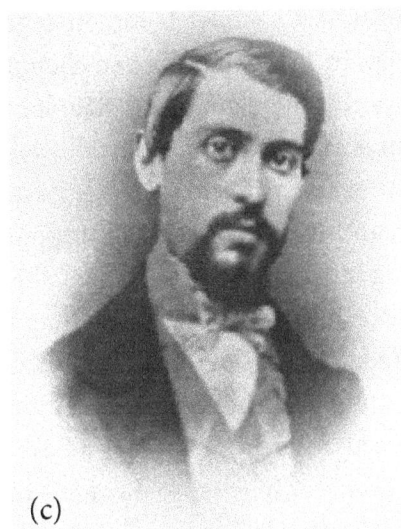

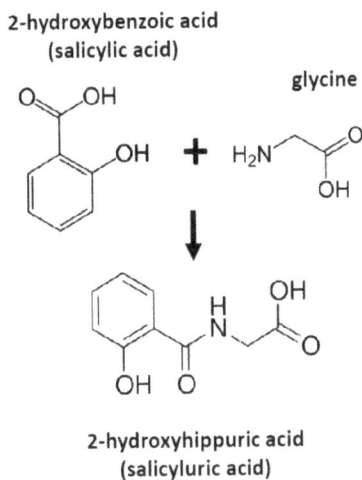

2-hydroxybenzoic acid
(salicylic acid)

glycine

2-hydroxyhippuric acid
(salicyluric acid)

(c)

(d)

Figure 7.4. (*Continued*)

(c) Piria's former student, Cesare Bertagnini. He analysed urine passed following salicylic acid ingestion and realised that salicylate appeared as *acido salicilurico*, a novel compound composed of salicylate conjugated to an unidentified nitrogenous substance. The latter was later identified as the amino acid glycine.

(d) This was the first insight into how foreign chemical compounds are detoxified in the body. The involvement of glycine in the process led to an erroneous speculation that the deviation of glycine from uric acid synthesis might be responsible for urate lowering effects of salicylates.

Source: (a)–(c) Via Wikimedia Commons: (a) and (c) public domain, (b) Bibliothèque interuniversitaire de Santé, Licence Ouverte.

from salicin, thereby discovering salicylic acid.[68] Although the words salicin and salicylic come from *Salix* (i.e. willow), salicylates have been extracted from many other plants, including the flowers of Meadowsweet (*Filipendula ulmaria*) and Wintergreens (genus *Gaultheria*). Like many other plant chemicals that have been adopted for medicinal purposes (including colchicine, see Chapter 10), salicylates play an important role in plant defence against herbivores and pathogens.[69]

Although fêted as providing an improvement on quinine, initial clinical experience with salicin and then salicylic acid was not encouraging, and over the next few years, they were almost completely forgotten, just as willow bark had been before.[70] Then, in 1860, the German chemists Hermann Kolbe (1818–1884) and Edward Lautemann (1836–868) found that they could create salicylic acid from phenol and carbon dioxide. Kolbe refined the technique so that, by the 1870s, salicylic acid was widely available. At first, it was mainly used as an antiseptic, being added to wound dressings, and was also used for treating infections such as cholera, diphtheria, and typhoid. In veterinary practice, it was used as a disinfectant for cattle with foot-and-mouth disease.[71] Trade was not slow on the uptake, and salicylic acid rapidly became an anti-septic household panacea. Tidman and Sons of Finsbury, London, advertised 'Salicylic Soap – for a healthy skin and a clear complexion', and the *Thanet Advertiser* told readers that a salicylic acid tooth powder and mouth wash 'deodorises, decomposes, and removes all the carious and depository substances forming upon or attaching themselves to the teeth, and in all cases keeps the gums in a healthy state'.[72] It became widely used as a household disinfectant and was added as a preservative to fish, meat, fruits, beer and wine by food and beverage manufacturers.[73]

The use of salicylic acid for general anti-inflammatory purposes originates with Germain Sée, professor of clinical medicine at the Hôtel-Dieu in Paris (see Figure 7.4(b)), who found that it reduced the fever and inflammation occurring in 'acute rheumatism'.[i] Sée also found that salicylic acid attenuated acute attacks of gout and tested the combination of salicylate with lithium, 'which has undeniable advantages in the treatment of this disease'[j] but could not convince himself that this was better than sodium salicylate alone.[74] By the 1880s, salicylates were being widely used as a safer alternative to *Colchicum* extracts for settling the inflammation of acute attacks of gout. However, salicylic acid was not popular, as it has a bitter taste and causes nausea and abdominal discomfort. A particular

---

[i] This would have mainly been streptococcus-related rheumatic fever.

[j] Originally in French, '*qui a des avantages incontestables dans le traitement de cette maladie*'.

problem was its insolubility, and aggregates caused ulcers by adhering to the lining of the throat, oesophagus and stomach.[75] It was to circumvent these issues that the Bayer Company tinkered with the salicylate anion.[76] Of several variants, acetyl salicylic acid stood out as the most soluble, and the company developed this as aspirin, so called because the starting material for its synthesis was *Spirea ulmaria,* an obsolete Latin name for Meadowsweet.[k] Aspirin was introduced to British doctors at the trade 'museum' of the BMA Annual Meeting in 1899.[77] It is a 'prodrug' as it is inert until deacetylated into salicylic acid once within the body.

How salicylates work in general was still a mystery. One view stemmed from research in the 1850s of an Italian chemist, Cesare Bertagnini (1827–1857) (see Figure 7.4(c)), who had tested enough salicylate on himself to cause ringing in the ears and then looked for it in his urine. What he found was a new compound that he called '*acide salicylurique*'[l] and which he deduced was salicylic acid linked chemically to a nitrogen-containing substance.[78] This was the first evidence that drugs are metabolised internally and set in motion a large and still active research field looking into the biochemical mechanisms that have evolved to enable the body to detoxify foreign chemicals. The nitrogenous factor was later identified as glycine (see Figure 7.4(d)). This amino acid was already in the limelight, with the Austrian chemist Ivan Horbachevsky (1854–1942) having succeeded in combining it with urea to make uric acid (see Chapter 11), and the success of Peter Latham (1832–1923) in reproducing the work was considered sufficiently important to justify an article in *The Lancet.*[79] Latham was Downing Professor of Medicine at Cambridge and a proponent of the uric acid diathesis. He wrongly proposed that the clinical effectiveness of salicylate was due to it stealing the glycine needed for uric acid synthesis and hence lowering uric acid levels.[80] On reading the text of his Croonian Lecture on the subject, one marvels not only at

---

[k] *Filipendula ulmaria.*
[l] i.e. salicyluric acid.

the sophisticated level of chemistry he conducted but also at his capacity to draw the wrong conclusion.

Germain Sée had recorded that salicylic acid led in his hands to an increase in the amount of uric acid in the urine.[81] Many agreed that salicylates sometimes increased uric acid excretion and, indeed, once the blood urate level could be measured accurately, sometimes also lowered urate in the blood.[82] However, there was a problem, as others found the opposite.[83] The paradox was solved in 1907 by the French zoologist Pierre Fauvel (1866–1958) of the Catholic University in Anges, who demonstrated that it had to do with dosage: low doses of salicylate reduced uric acid excretion, while high doses (5–6 grams daily) increased it.[84] The important point for gout was that this, as well as that coming from a parallel work on cinchophen (see the following), was the first good evidence that drugs could deplete the body of uric acid by enhancing its urinary excretion (see Chapter 8). Nevertheless, continued use of high-dose salicylate was not practicable. I should emphasise, however, that the suppressive effects of salicylates on inflammation, in general, or on gouty inflammation, in particular, are not related to altering uric acid levels. John Vane shared the 1982 Nobel Prize for Physiology or Medicine for discovering that the immediate anti-inflammatory action of salicylates is due to inhibition of cyclooxygenases that make prostaglandins.[m]

Cinchophen

Cinchophen[n] owes its discovery to the links that the emerging pharmaceutical industry in Germany had with dye manufacturers. Dyes were commonly used as starting points for the synthesis of novel compounds with possible medical applications. The compound was first synthesised at the E. Schering Company in 1887, being the result of boiling aniline dye, pyruvic acid and benzaldehyde in absolute alcohol.[85] It was first tested for

---

[m] Prostaglandins are lipid-derived chemical mediators of inflammation unconnected to uric acid.

[n] 2-phenyl-quinoline-4-carboxylic acid.

its effects as a drug by the physician Arthur Nicolaier (1862–1942), who had already made his name as a medical student by isolating the toxin that causes tetanus. For many years afterwards, the bacteria responsible for releasing the toxin, *Clostridium tetani*, was known as 'Nicolaier's Bacillus'.

Nicolaier was well acquainted with uric acid and gout, having worked with Wilhelm Ebstein (1836–1912) (see Chapter 9) in Göttingen in the mid-1890s on an inconclusive project, which involved injecting uric acid into rabbits and dogs to explore its effects on their kidneys and on stone formation.[86] Having moved to Berlin, he made use of his training by testing the pharmacological effects of new compounds. He gave cinchophen to rabbits, dogs, pigs and a rooster, after which he decided it was safe enough to test on himself and finally studied its effects on some other healthy volunteers. He found that urine became unexpectedly cloudy about 45 minutes following ingestion of the compound as long as the urine was acidic, and this was due to precipitation of uric acid crystals. Nicolaier then established that the compound led to a rapid increase in urinary urate excretion that was greater than seen with high-dose salicylates.[87]

Cinchophen was first tested in patients by Wilhelm Weintraud (1866–1920), director of internal medicine at the municipal hospital in Wiesbaden. Weintraud substantiated that the observations that Nicolaier and several others had made on healthy volunteers held true for patients with gout. In addition, the increased urinary excretion of urate was paralleled by attenuation of inflammation, so much so that Weintraud suggested cinchophen might replace colchicine in being as effective and with fewer side effects.[88] A new drug to enhance urate excretion and also treat inflammation had considerable commercial potential, and the Schering Company expectantly came up with the trade name Atophan.° It was launched to the public in Berlin in 1911 and quickly achieved fad status. The drug was introduced to British doctors as an 'exceptionally powerful eliminant of uric acid' at the trade exhibition of the BMA's annual meeting in Birmingham in September 1911.[89] With the outbreak of World War I in 1914, Atophan could no longer

---

° i.e. no tophi.

be imported from Germany, but demand was such that British chemists produced an equivalent named Phenoquin. As time went on, cinchophen was such a success that it was further mimicked, with various minor chemical modifications to evade the patent, by over 20 other drug houses, each obviously with a different brand name.[90] Schering also introduced an esterified[p] version, named Novatophan, with a less unpleasant taste. It is estimated that over 43,000 kilos of Atophan alone were manufactured in a year, leaving aside the many derivatives. Bearing in mind the maximum daily dose was 3 grams per day, that translates to over 14 million doses per year. As far as gout is concerned, it was viewed as effective in treating and preventing acute attacks but not useful for clearing tophi, probably because the increase in urate excretion was only temporary.[91]

Sadly, things did not go as well for Nicolaier himself, as, like Lucien Graux, he became a victim of the Nazis. In 1933, the newly enforced racial laws meant that, as a Jew, he had to give up his position at the Charité Hospital in Berlin. Having decided not to emigrate, he received a letter in August 1942 informing him that he was scheduled for the next 'Alterstransport'[q] to the Theresienstadt ghetto, now known to have been a waystation to the extermination camps. He settled his affairs and the next day injected himself with a fatal dose of morphine. He left one sentence as farewell, which, translated into English, read, 'I depart voluntarily from this life'. The letter was later found to contain a hidden watermark: 'INVICTUS', Latin for unconquered.

In occasional individuals, cinchophen led to a serious and frequently fatal liver reaction that was first recorded in 1923. Nothing was done to prevent its over-the-counter sales, such that nine years later, a medical review article had found 191 cases of what had become known as acute liver atrophy, and 88 of these were fatal.[92] An adverse coroner's report in Birmingham in 1934 then led to a question being asked in the House of Commons by Alec Cunningham Reid, a former World War I Royal Flying Corps ace and Conservative Member for St. Marylebone. He asked why

---

[p] i.e. an alkyl group of atoms replaced a hydrogen.
[q] Translates as 'age transport'.

cinchophen was not branded a poison.[93] The Home Secretary, John Gilmore, responded with true parliamentary deference to the aviator: 'I am bringing the case to which my hon. and gallant Friend refers to the notice of the Lord President of the Council and the Council of the Pharmaceutical Society, who are the authorities at present responsible for additions to the Schedule of Poisons'.[94] The status of the drug in Britain was changed in 1936 to prescription-only, but a chemist shop owner in Grimsby was still prosecuted in 1938 for selling it over the counter.[95]

Requiring a doctor's prescription did not make cinchophen any safer, and in 1954, thirty years after the problem first surfaced, the *West London Observer* reported the death of a woman being treated with it for gout, who had gone to her doctor because she was turning yellow. At the inquest, her doctor said that 'he had heard of toxic symptoms developing after the use of this drug but had never come across a case himself'. The coroner, showing due respect to the medical profession, deliberated 'that this particular drug was a recognised drug and had been properly prescribed by the doctor' and recorded a verdict of misadventure.[96] Two years later, *Price's Textbook of Medicine* advised that cinchophen was best avoided because of its toxicity; however, in the absence of regulations, it was still an option.[97] Cinchophen is no longer available for use in humans in Britain or the US, but it had had a great run, and as with *Colchicum*, a racehorse was named after it in 1947.[98] It can still be prescribed to dogs for their osteoarthritis. As for inquests, a recent survey found that coroners in the UK do highlight the adverse effects of drugs, but often sufficient notice is still not taken of serious reports and not enough learned.[99]

Reflections on the Monitoring of Drug Efficacy and Safety

The common denominator of all the commercial and non-commercial medicinal preparations mentioned in this chapter, as well as in Chapters 4 and 5, is that none had been tested in formal clinical trials for efficacy and safety. Many were almost certainly ineffective, other than as placebos, and many were unsafe, sometimes fatally, through poor labelling, impurity,

contamination and idiosyncratic adverse effects. It took two further trag-
edies to change the ways governments regulate the licensing of new drugs
and survey their post-marketing safety.

The first was the Elixir Sulfanilamide scandal. The S. E. Massengill
Company of Bristol, Tennessee, already had a tarnished reputation, having been fined in 1934 for selling a *Colchicum* extract that exceeded the
United States Pharmacopoeia standard in drug activity. Three years later,
the company distributed a new formulation of the antimicrobial sulphanil-
amide without having conducted any safety testing. Two hundred and forty
gallons were manufactured, but the drug had to be withdrawn rapidly
after eleven gallons and six pints had been prescribed and dispensed and
over a hundred recipients had died. The toxic component turned out to be
diethylene glycol, in which the drug was dissolved, and which the company
should have known from published work to be poisonous.[100]

The second and better-known disaster was the birth of babies with
limb malformations when women took thalidomide during pregnancy,
with the thalidomide having been marketed in the early 1960s as a safe
sedative to take when having a baby.[101]

These incidents were the watershed that led to national drug policies
in the twentieth and twenty-first centuries, which have placed potentially
dangerous drugs in the hands of suitably licensed medical practitioners
and which require rigorous preclinical and clinical testing of efficacy and
safety. The unintended consequence is, of course, the enormous expense
nowadays of developing new drugs, especially when large numbers
of patients are needed to establish statistical superiority over existing
standard treatments. The research and development of a new agent that
passes through the very tight testing process now requires as much as a
billion US dollars, and most fail along the way. The immense cost of new
drugs is now partly due to pharmaceutical companies recovering outlays
on research and development, partly due to huge marketing budgets and
partly due to recouping the expense of previous costly failures, not to mention the need to make a profit for shareholders.[102] The price we have to pay
for drugs that really work and are safe is a major factor in the escalating
cost of healthcare, with all its political ramifications.

Chapter 8

Controlling Uric Acid

Winding the clock forward from the various expensive failures discussed in Chapter 7, uric acid no longer held quite the same status as a universal poison by the 1940s, and gout had rather fallen out of fashion. Moreover, how, or even if, uric acid caused gout was still far from clear. Consequently, uric acid and gout were low priorities for the drug discovery programmes of the booming pharmaceutical corporations. The big breakthroughs in regulating uric acid levels, and showing scientifically that these mattered, thus came by serendipity.

The Discovery of Probenecid

The problem for penicillin

The story is well known of how Alexander Fleming (1881–1955) noticed that a fungal colony had killed the bacteria surrounding it on a culture plate (see Figure 8.1(a)).[1] Fleming realised the therapeutic potential of the factor released by the *Penicillium rubrum* mould, which he named 'penicillin'; however, working in the bacteriology laboratory at St. Mary's Hospital in London, he was not equipped to develop it as a drug. That was left to Howard Florey (1898–1968) and his colleagues at the Dunn School of Pathology in Oxford. Florey came to England from Australia and was appointed professor at the Dunn School in 1935. He teamed up with Ernst Cheyne (1906–1979), a biochemist trained in the German organic chemistry tradition who, by then, had relocated to Oxford as a refugee from the Nazis. At the outbreak of World War II, Florey, Cheyne and colleagues established a makeshift *Penicillium* culture system in their laboratory using bespoke ceramic flasks sourced from Staffordshire potteries. These flasks were glazed only on the inside to reduce costs and made flat to enable stacking. The first patient to receive their lab-brewed penicillin isolate showed a good early response but succumbed once the small stock of the drug was used up. It soon became clear that a serious limitation was the very rapid loss of penicillin in the urine, which greatly increased the amount needed to maintain its level in blood and overcome serious infections.[2] Ingeniously, the Oxford team (see Figure 8.1(b)) collected the urine from the first patient, extracted the penicillin and used it to boost the dose for the next patient. This was a boy with a bone infection, whose survival from what had previously been an untreatable problem became a medical landmark. Subsequent mass production by pharmaceutical companies in the United States then greatly improved outcomes for military and civilian casualties during the war (see Figure 8.1(c)).[3]

By the end of the war, some bacterial strains had become resistant to penicillin, necessitating increasingly high doses. The Sharpe & Dohme Company's drug discovery team, led by Karl Beyer Jr. (1914–1996) at West Point, Pennsylvania (see Figure 8.2), wondered whether higher and more prolonged blood levels might result from preventing the very rapid urinary loss. Beyer had graduated from the University of Wisconsin with dual training in medicine and physiology. He realised that universities and hospitals lacked the resources needed for developing new drugs and was one of a new cadre of scientifically trained physicians electing to work in the industry. In 1942, he joined Sharpe & Dohme, where he built up an elite team of renal pharmacologists. He championed a new philosophy of synthesising chemical compounds to modify measurable physiological processes as intermediate stepping stones to treating disease rather than heading straight into treatment.[4]

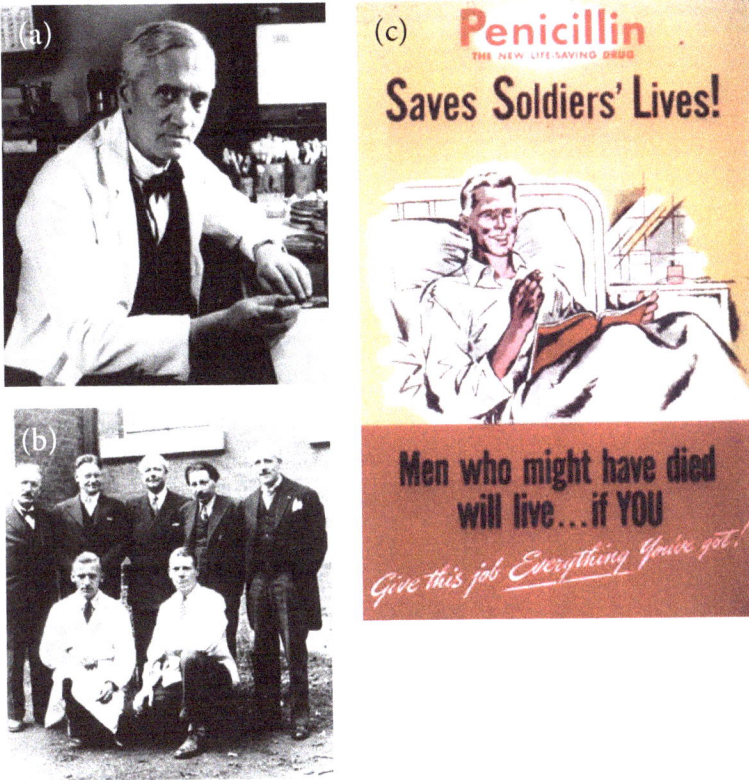

Figure 8.1.

(a) Photograph of Alexander Fleming, who realised the therapeutic significance of a culture plate in which *Staphylococcus* bacterial colonies failed to grow around a colony of *Penicillium* mould; Fleming gave the name 'penicillin' to the presumed substance that prevented bacterial proliferation.

(b) Oxford researchers working on the purification of penicillin during World War II: (back row, left to right) S. Waksman, H. Florey, J. Trefouel, E. Chain and A. Gratia; (front row, left to right) P. Fredericq and Maurice Welsch. Photographer unknown.

(c) Penicillin – THE NEW LIFE-SAVING DRUG, a United States Federal Government World War II propaganda poster; note the cigarette. By the end of the war, supplies were insufficient to keep up with the ever-increasing requirement for higher doses due to the emergence of bacterial resistance.

Source: (a) Via Wikimedia Commons: Calibuon at English Wikibooks, cropped by User: AlanM1, CC0. 1.0 Deed; (b) courtesy of the Wellcome Collection. Attribution 4.0 International (CC BY 4.0); (c) Science History Institute, via Wikimedia Commons, public domain.

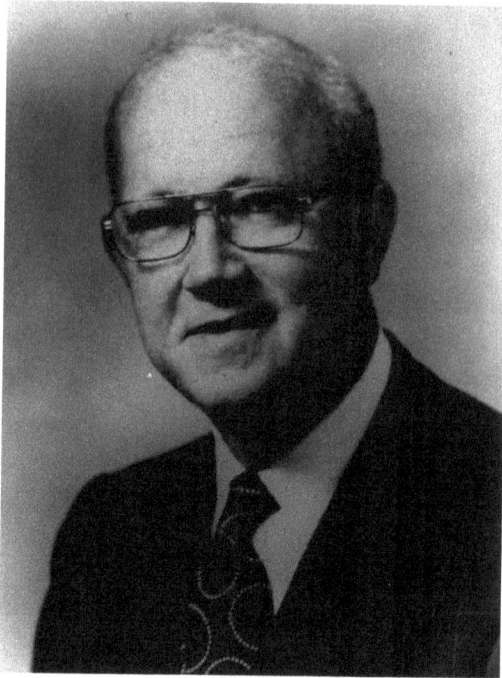

Figure 8.2.

Karl Beyer Jr., whose team at Sharpe & Dohme Company worked out how to prevent the loss of penicillin into urine and, in so doing, discovered probenecid as a treatment for gout. Beyer and his team then continued the research programme, linking medicinal chemistry with renal physiology, and in 1975, he received a special Lasker award for discovering thiazide diuretics as a new class of drugs for the treatment of high blood pressure and heart failure.

Source: Courtesy of the US Library of Medicine, Public Domain Mark 1.0 Universal.

Introduction to renal physiology

To understand how Beyer and his team achieved their aim of reducing penicillin excretion, we need to take a brief look at what was known about the workings of the kidney. We start with Marcello Malpighi (1628–1694), an early microscopist who described numerous small bodies[a] in the

---

[a] Now known as Malpighian bodies.

kidney, each containing a network of blood capillaries called a glomerulus. Malpighi found that these readily filled with dye once injected into the artery supplying the kidney and proposed that they were the origin of urine. This common-sense conclusion was critically challenged ~250 years later by William Bowman (1816–1892), a surgeon at King's College Hospital in London (Figure 8.3(a)). Bowman was also a meticulous microscopist[b] and saw how blood flows into each glomerulus via an afferent small artery and leaves via an efferent small artery.[c] He described a capsule, now known as 'Bowman's capsule', which surrounds each glomerulus and acts as the origin of what he called 'uriniferous tubes' (see Figure 8.3(b)). These tubules, as they are now called, then pass the fluid filtered through the glomeruli into collecting ducts for the ureter that leads to the urinary bladder. Bowman noticed that the small efferent arteries, taking blood out of the glomeruli, lead on to a previously unobserved network of capillaries that wraps around the tubules. He concluded that glomerular filtration was not the whole story of urine formation and that:

> ... there are in the kidney *two perfectly distinct systems of capillary vessels*, through both of which blood passes in its course from the arteries into the veins: the 1st, that inserted into the dilated extremities of the uriniferous tubes, and in immediate connection with the arteries; the 2nd, that enveloping the convolutions of the tubes, and communicating directly with the veins. ...To these distinct capillary systems, I am inclined to attribute distinct parts of the function of the organ.[5]

On the basis of the passage of injected dyes through the kidney, Bowman further proposed that salts can enter the urine via the blood capillaries around the tubules and that the filtrate of the glomeruli serves to wash

---

[b] Bowman also described "Bowman's glands" in the nose and "Bowman's membrane" on the outer surface of the cornea of the eye.

[c] Afferent and efferent mean entry and exit, respectively.

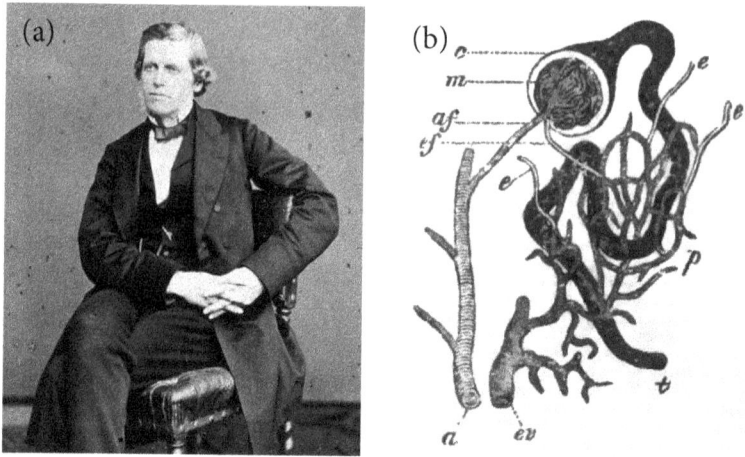

Figure 8.3.

(a) William Bowman in 1867. Photograph by Ernest Edwards, 1867.

(b) Drawing by Bowman of the relationships between the blood supply, the glomerulus and the proximal renal tubule. An afferent arteriole (*af*) supplies the capillaries of the glomerulus ('Malpighian corpuscle') (*m*). The glomerulus is surrounded by a capsule (*c*) that drains into a convoluted tubule (*t*). An efferent blood vessel takes the blood from the glomerular capillary plexus into a capillary plexus (*p*) that surrounds the tubule before passing into efferent venules (*e*), and thence to an efferent vein (*ev*). Bowman realised that many salts may move from blood to urine via the capillary plexus that surrounds the tubules rather than just by glomerular filtration. From Todd and Bowman (1856).

Source: (a) Courtesy of the Wellcome Collection, public domain; (b) courtesy of the US National Library of Medicine. CC0 1.0 Universal Public Domain Dedication.

them towards the bladder. The consequence of both the glomeruli and tubules being involved in producing urine is that either one or both may fail in disease. This explains the clinical pitch of Alfred Garrod's seminal 1848 paper, in which he gave the first account of measuring urate in the blood (see Chapter 6). Garrod actually centred that paper as much on a comparison of the kidney in gout *versus* Bright's disease[d] as on his new

---

[d] Bright's disease is an old term for inflammation of glomeruli and was named after the English physician Richard Bright, who, in 1827, described patients with protein in the urine accompanied by tissue oedema.

measuring system. He found an excess of urea[e] in the blood in Bright's disease and a varying amount of urate, whereas in gout it was the opposite. With remarkable insight, he concluded:

> the excreting functions of the kidney, with respect to the solid portions of the urine, are not simple, but that the urea and uric acid are separately eliminated; also that one of these functions may be impaired or destroyed, the other remaining entire. With regard to the solid and fluid portions of the urine, Mr. Bowman has already shown the probability that different structures in the kidneys being concerned in their secretions. ...Gout would thus appear partly to depend on a loss of power (temporary or permanent) of the 'uric-acid-excreting function' of the kidneys.[6]

Bowman's proposal that the kidney possesses a dual excretory system was not generally accepted, and Garrod's supporting observations appear to have been ignored. However, Bowman was championed later by the professor of physiology at Breslau, Rudolph Heidenhain (1834–1897), who showed that dyes injected into rabbits can still be detected coming into tubules after the blood pressure had been reduced to the point where filtration through glomeruli ceases.[7] Subsequently, the concept of passage of salts and other solutes directly via the renal tubules into the developing urine became known as the Bowman–Heidenhain theory.[8] The principle of tubular secretion was finally established once John Geraghty (1876–1940) and Leonard Rowntree (1883–1959) at Johns Hopkins University School of Medicine introduced the use of phenol red dye[f] for measuring renal blood flow and excretory function.[9] This allowed Eli Kennerly Marshall (1889–1966), the professor of physiology at Johns Hopkins, to provide definitive proof that solutes are actively secreted into urine by the epithelial

---

[e] Urea and urate are the most important compounds for excreting waste nitrogen, and their distinction is discussed in more detail in Chapter 13. Urea is $CO(NH_2)_2$, and the urate anion is $C_5H_2N_4O_3^{2-}$.

[f] Phenolsulphone phthalein.

cells lining the tubules.[10] Using the same experimental approach as Heidenhain of lowering the blood pressure to stop glomerular filtration, he measured the amount of dye accumulating in the kidneys of anaesthetised dogs and found that this was up to 12 times that in their blood plasma. As the dye had to travel against a concentration gradient, the implication was that active transport must have occurred across the cell walls of the tubules.[11] In a follow-up paper, Marshall showed that the efficiency of phenol red secretion from the tubules drops when plasma levels increase, implying that the tubular transport system could be saturated.[12]

One drug to complement the effects of another

It soon became clear that many other compounds are secreted into the urine via the tubular route, including *p*-aminohippurate (PAH) and two X-ray contrast agents: diodrast[g] and hippuran.[h,13] Consistent with the saturability of the secretory channels in the tubules, these agents were found to compete with one another for passage.[14] If penicillin were to pass into the urine in the same way, a drug might be found to compete with it and thereby prevent its loss through urination and extend therapeutic blood levels. Diodrast and PAH were both found to do so, and towards the end of World War II, PAH was tested on a few patients with serious heart valve infections, with some success in raising penicillin levels.[15] However, as PAH is also secreted by the tubules, several grams at a time needed to be administered intravenously, which proved to be both inconvenient and poorly tolerated. Beyer's team, therefore, set about chemically engineering a compound to prevent penicillin tubular transport without itself being secreted.[16]

Beyer published the new concept of designing a drug to reduce the urinary excretion of another drug in an article in *Science*. In the same article, he announced the discovery of caronamide,[i,17] which significantly

---

[g] 3,5-diiodo-4-pyridone-*N*-acetic acid diethanolamine.
[h] Iodohippuric acid.
[i] 4'-carboxyphenylmethanesulfonanilide.

reduced penicillin loss in urine and raised its blood levels, but again was only effective if 18–24 grams were taken daily.[18] However, a related compound increased penicillin levels at a much lower dose.[19] Given the name probenecid,[j] this was first marketed as an adjunct to penicillin treatment in 1951 under the trade name 'Benemid'. However, it was not a commercial success for this purpose, as alternative antibiotics to penicillin had already become available. Its main achievement in fighting infections was when it was combined with penicillin as a single 'hit-and-run' cure for gonorrhoea. This strategy remains in use today and is also currently being investigated for boosting blood concentrations of other microbial agents and combatting the development of resistant bacterial strains.[20]

Increasing urate in the urine

With a better understanding of the complex mechanisms of urine formation, it became clear that Garrod's 'uric acid excreting function' depends on the tubules rather than the glomeruli. To cut a very long story short, once blood is filtered, urate is reabsorbed from the filtrate across the walls of the proximal renal tubules[k] before it is secreted in the distal tubules[l] back into the urine. After this, some of the secreted urate is then once again reabsorbed. The net flux is such that, in humans, only around 10% of urate that is filtered through glomeruli ends up in final urine, with the remainder eventually passing back into the blood.[21] This understanding opened up the possibility of pharmacologically preventing urate reabsorption by the tubules, thereby depleting the body of uric acid by augmenting its urinary loss – the opposite of what was intended for penicillin. Diodrast was found to partially achieve this, and similar effects also explained the uric acid excretory effects of high-dose salicylate and cinchophen (see Chapter 7).[22] Beyer had already observed that caronamide increased urate excretion and predicted this would hold true for probenecid.[23] This turned out to be the

---

[j] p-[di-*n*-propylsulfamyl]-benzoic acid.
[k] i.e. immediately downstream of the glomeruli.
[l] i.e. further downstream.

case. Probenecid was first mentioned in the medical literature as a drug for accelerating urinary urate loss in gout in a report from a 1950 hospital staff round by Alexander Gutman (1902–1973), professor of medicine at Columbia University.[24] More formal evidence that probenecid enhances urate excretion and lowers blood levels emerged the following year in a paper by John Talbott (1902–1990) and colleagues from the University of Buffalo School of Medicine.[25] Even more importantly, it soon became clear that it was possible to take probenecid for much longer durations than high-dose salicylates, and that prolonged treatment led to the clearance of gouty tophi.[26]

Gout, therefore, proved to be the silver lining to the Benemid cloud, leading Sharpe & Dohme to repurpose the drug. However, this did not receive the fanfare it would have garnered a century earlier, and there was minimal interest from medical journals or public newspapers. No doubt it was seen as an incremental advance after salicylates and cinchophen. Nevertheless, the long-standing question of whether tophi could be removed by anything other than surgery had been answered. Other 'uricosuric' agents soon followed, including sulfinpyrazone and benzbromarone.[27] However, a major limitation of all such drugs is that they depend on healthy kidneys, which many of those with gout do not have. Another is that increased excretion of urate comes with the risk of forming urinary stones, particularly as patients with gout are predisposed to developing them. As a class, these agents have largely been superseded by drugs that prevent uric acid production rather than accelerate its removal. To these we now turn our attention.

The Discovery of Allopurinol

If the level of uric acid can be reduced by increasing its loss in the urine, should it not also be possible to achieve the same result by reducing its synthesis in the body? It certainly is, and this was established through cancer research.

Introduction to purines

When William Hyde Wollaston announced in 1797 that he had detected urate in gouty tophi (see Chapter 6), he could not have known how it came to be there. Organic matter was once considered subject to separate vital rules from those of inert, inorganic chemicals. The German chemist Friedrich Wöhler (1800–1882) put the first dent into vitalism's armour when he discovered that urea can be synthesised from two inorganic compounds: potassium cyanate and ammonium sulphate.[28] Together with Justus Liebig, Wöhler then founded the field of organic chemistry, in which compounds are assembled and interconverted following inorganic rules. Much of the early organic chemistry research in medicine focused on urine and urinary stones, as they were so easy to come by and more straightforward to analyse compared to blood or other tissues.

Alexander Marcet (1770–1822) was a Swiss Huguenot who came to Britain as a political refugee from revolutionary Geneva. Like Thomas Beddoes and George Pearson (see Chapter 6), he trained in chemistry under Joseph Black in Edinburgh. He was an accomplished chemist, promoting the correct view that the main alkali metal in normal and diseased animal body fluids is sodium, crossing swords with the acrimonious Pearson, who believed it to be potassium.[29] In 1807, Marcet became a staff physician at Guy's Hospital in London.[30] Tasked with teaching urinary calculi to the students, he published his lectures as *An Essay on the Chemical History and Medical Treatment of Calculous Diseases* in 1817. He dedicated this to William Hyde Wollaston (see Chapter 6), writing that his work was 'little more than a sketch' of Wollaston's discoveries, particularly emulating Wollaston's technical innovations in small scale chemical analyses.[31] Just as Wollaston had first discovered cystine in a stone, Marcet found a stone made of a novel substance which was much more soluble than uric acid and gave a yellow colour when treated with nitric acid; hence, he named it xanthic oxide after Ξάνθος (*xanthos*, Greek for 'yellow').[32] Twenty years later, Wöhler and Liebig managed to obtain a piece of Marcet's stone and showed that 'xanthic oxide' was similar chemically to uric acid, except that it had one fewer oxygen residue.[33] They renamed the substance xanthine. It is likely that the stone originated from a patient suffering from the rare condition known as xanthinuria, caused by xanthine buildup due to a genetic deficiency in the enzyme xanthine oxidase (see the following).

Other substances with chemical similarities to uric acid that were isolated during the 1800s include guanine[m] and adenine.[n] It was the German biochemist Albrecht Kossel (1853–1927) who established that these, as well as the pyrimidines thymine, cytosine and uracil, are the major components of the nucleic acids deoxyribonucleic acid (DNA) and ribonucleic acid (RNA).[34] Kossel's findings were considered important at the time; consequently, he was awarded the Nobel Prize for Physiology or Medicine in 1910. However, nobody realised just how important they were. Nucleic acids were originally believed to play a merely structural role within cells, as in the organisation of chromosomes; of course, they are now known to be the molecular basis of the genetic code and the translation of genes into proteins. Chemical modifications of adenine and guanine also provide a general means for energising intracellular organic molecular reactions, such as those resulting from the interconversions between adenosine monophosphate (AMP), adenosine diphosphate (ADP) and adenosine triphosphate (ATP). We return to the genetic code in Chapter 13.

Emil Fischer (1852–1919) (see Figure 8.4(a)) collected uric acid, xanthine, guanine and adenine together into a chemical family that also included hypoxanthine and the plant compounds caffeine (trimethyl-xanthine) and theophylline (dimethyl-xanthine). Having shown experimentally that these were chemically interconnected, he named the family of compounds 'purines', after their theoretical common

---

[m] Guanine was so named by Julius Unger, who isolated it from guano in 1846 – see Chapters 11 and 14.

[n] Adenine was isolated in 1885 from pancreas by Albrecht Kossel and named after ἀδήν (aden, Greek for 'gland').

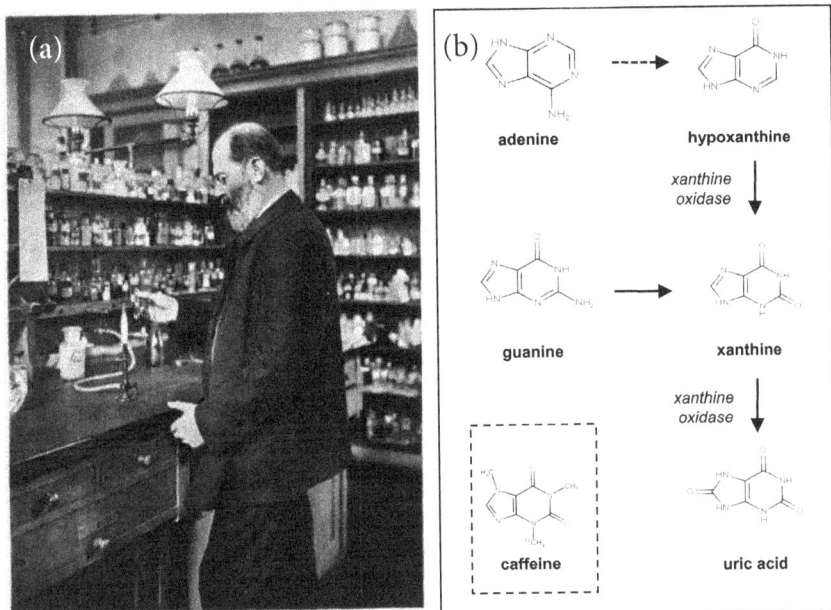

Figure 8.4.

(a) Emil Fischer in his laboratory circa 1912. He established purines as a family of nitrogen-rich organic compounds and charted their molecular similarities and differences. His 'purine' was a theoretical common denominator that is not known to exist in nature.

(b) Flow diagram of how the two purines, adenine and guanine, are converted to uric acid. Xanthine oxidase catalyses both the oxidation of hypoxanthine to xanthine and the oxidation of xanthine to uric acid. The insert shows how caffeine (trimethylxanthine) fits structurally into the purine family.

Source: (a) Via Wikimedia Commons, public domain.

denominator.[o,35] In his Nobel Prize acceptance lecture of 1902, Fischer declared that the era of discovering organic compounds was drawing to a close and that it was time to start understanding their functions in biology.[36]

---

[o] The word 'purine' comes from the Latin *purum uricum*, meaning 'pure urine'.

Discovery of xanthine oxidase

Given the links between the different purines, could uric acid be made within the body? The discovery of the enzyme that catalyses endogenous uric acid synthesis is credited to Austrian chemist and bacteriologist Franz Schardinger (1853–1920), whose interests were focused far away from gout. Schardinger studied carbohydrates, and, today, he is better known as a pioneer in the field of cyclodextrins.[p,37] He found an enzyme that stimulates the oxidation of aldehydes in fresh milk, and only later did it become clear that the same enzyme can convert xanthine to uric acid.[38] Indeed, the enzyme is now called xanthine oxidoreductase, or xanthine oxidase for short. As it is present at a high concentration in milk, it is relatively easy to obtain in large quantities for laboratory analysis. This led to it being one of the first enzymes to be purified, and the relationship between its molecular structure and its biochemical function has been particularly thoroughly studied.[39] By 1912, it was known that adenine and guanine are converted in the body, respectively, to hypoxanthine[q] and xanthine; and that xanthine oxidase converts hypoxanthine to xanthine and also xanthine to uric acid (see Figure 8.4(b)).[40]

Targeting leukaemia

We now skip ahead 30 years and go to the Burrows Wellcome Laboratories in Tuckahoe, a New York village some 16 miles north of Manhattan, and look at the work of George Hitchings (1905–1998) and Gertrude 'Trudi' Elion (1918–1999) (see Figure 8.5(a)).[41] Hitchings had obtained his PhD in 1933 by studying nucleic acids (i.e. DNA and RNA) with Otto Folin (1867–1934) in the Department of Biological Chemistry at Harvard (see Chapter 9). Jobs were hard to come by during the economic depression of the 1930s, so he had to make do with a series of part-time positions until he was hired in 1942 as a senior biochemist by the Burroughs

---

[p] Cyclodextrins are derived from the digestion of starch and are extensively used in chemical engineering.

[q] Hypoxanthine was discovered by Justus Liebig's student Johann Scherer in 1850.

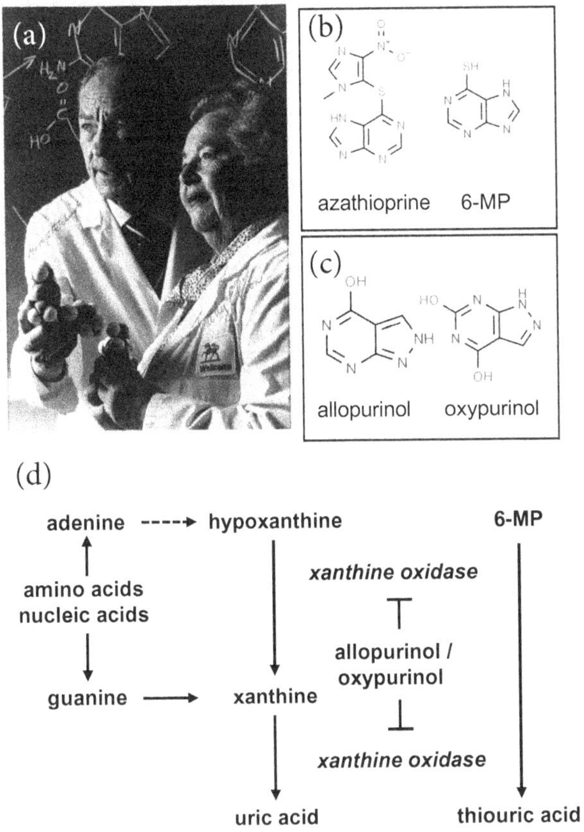

Figure 8.5.

(a) George Hitchings and Gertrude Elion, who together developed the first xanthine oxidase inhibitor allopurinol at the Burroughs Wellcome Laboratories in Tuckahoe, New York. Photograph by Will and Deni McIntyre.

(b) The prodrug azathioprine is cleaved in the body to give the active drug 6-mercaptopurine (6-MP).

(c) Allopurinol is a purine analogue that is oxidised in the body by xanthine oxidase to oxypurinol.

(d) 6-MP is inactivated by xanthine oxidase, which converts it to thiouric acid. Both allopurinol and oxypurinol prevent xanthine oxidase inactivating 6-MP and in so doing maintain 6-MP blood levels. At the same time, allopurinol and oxypurinol also block the normal conversion of hypoxanthine to xanthine and xanthine to uric acid, thus preventing uric acid synthesis and lowering blood urate levels.

Source: (a) Courtesy of the Wellcome Collection, CC BY 4.0.

Wellcome company. The company was undergoing a major reorganisation, and Hitchings was charged with building up a new research group, into which he recruited Elion two years later as an assistant. Elion was a New Yorker with immigrant parents: her dentist father coming from Lithuania and her mother from Russia.[42] She was largely self-trained, having worked as a technician in several small chemical laboratories, before joining Burroughs Wellcome. The group's goal was to develop new ways to treat cancer, specifically by developing drugs that prevent cancer cell division by interfering with the synthesis of nucleic acids.

It is worth first pointing out the novelty of their experimental approach. One hundred and fifty years earlier, *Colchicum* extracts were tested by John Want and others directly and rather crudely on a few hand-picked patients (see Chapter 5), and, as above, only 10 years prior, Karl Beyer and colleagues used mammals to test the effects of probenecid on urine formation. However, the Burrows Wellcome group was able to make use of purine biochemistry, which is incredibly ancient. Virtually all single and multicellular life-forms possess the complete, or nearly complete, set of enzymes required for purine synthesis and interconversion, with only occasional exceptions, such as a few archaea species, which must rob purines from other organisms.[43] In fact, adenine, guanine, hypoxanthine and xanthine have all been identified in extraterrestrial meteorites, and it is possible that purines from outer space could have contributed to the generation of the first single-cell organisms on Earth.[44] Because of this extreme conservation of purine biochemistry, the Burrows Wellcome drug discovery programme could be initiated cost-effectively and humanely in bacteria.

The basic idea was that purine-like analogues might mimic natural purines and act as 'anti-metabolites', interfering with DNA synthesis. Cancer cells should be more sensitive than normal cells to such agents, as they divide faster and have greater demands for fresh DNA.[45] One hundred or so purine variants were tested on the growth of *Lactobacillus casei*, a bacterial organism traditionally used for cheese production and nowadays used as a dietary probiotic.[46] Normally, bacteria release lactic acid when proliferating, and so a reduction of lactic acid in the culture broths was used as evidence of impaired bacterial growth. It became clear that guanine- or hypoxanthine-like compounds in which sulphur was substituted for oxygen were effective. Consequently, the agent 6-mercaptopurine (6-MP) was advanced for further testing and shown to suppress the growth of tumours in mice.[47] This was then tested by Joseph Burchenal (1912–2006) on patients attending the Sloane Kettering Institute in New York, under the leadership of cancer research pioneer Cornelius Rhoads (1898–1959).[48] The initial results were sufficiently promising for the drug to receive US Food and Drug Administration approval in 1953 for use in acute childhood leukaemia, just two years after the agent had first been synthesised. This was a stepping-stone for Burchenal's career, which eventually led to him receiving the 1972 Lasker Award for his work on the chemotherapy of Burkitt's lymphoma.

Improvement of leukaemia following 6-MP treatment proved to be a false dawn, as cancer cells rapidly became resistant to the drug. As a limiting factor was the amount of drug that could be administered without causing side effects, it was possible that treating patients with a prodrug, which cancer cells convert to 6-MP faster than normal cells, would allow a higher and more effective local concentration. This led to the development of azathioprine, which is metabolised into 6-MP once within the body (see Figure 8.5(b)).[49] Although azathioprine did not turn out to be an improvement over 6-MP for treating leukaemia, another use for the two compounds emerged. These were the early days of cellular immunology, and Robert S. Schwartz (1928–2017), working at Tuft's University in Boston with the haematologist William Dameshek (1900–1969), noticed visual similarities between lymphoblastic leukaemia cells and healthy lymphocytes that become activated during a normal immune response.[50] Schwartz's work showing that 6-MP and azathioprine suppressed antibody formation and skin graft rejection in rabbits led him to coin the term 'immunosuppression'.[51] This was a major milestone in organ transplantation and, subsequently, also in the treatment of autoimmune diseases, such as systemic lupus erythematosus and rheumatoid arthritis.

Meanwhile, Elion and Hitchings did not give up on 6-MP and aza-thioprine in their cancer programme. They found that as much as 25% of injected radiolabelled 6-MP appeared in the urine as inert 6-thiouric acid.[52] They worked out that xanthine oxidase was responsible for this conversion and investigated whether inhibiting the enzyme might make 6-MP last longer in the body, thereby increasing its effectiveness.[53] The idea was similar to probenecid raising penicillin levels but involved preventing the internal degradation of a drug rather than its urinary excretion. Of the purine analogues they tested for inhibiting the conversion of 6-MP to 6-thiouric acid, the one they took forward was a structural isomer of hypox-anthine,[r] which was originally synthesised by Roland Robins (1926–1992) at New Mexico Highlands University and which they named allopurinol.[s,54] Allopurinol is converted by xanthine oxidase to oxypurinol, which then inhibits the enzyme (see Figure 8.5(c)). Wayne Rundles (1911–1991), a haematologist at Duke University in Durham, North Carolina, tested allopurinol as an adjunct to 6-MP or azathioprine in a few leukemic patients; however, the results were disappointing. Although it reduced the dose of 6-MP needed to achieve therapeutic blood levels by around fourfold, it did not help treat leukaemia.[55]

Allopurinol lowers uric acid

Although allopurinol failed as an anti-cancer therapy adjunct, it was soon discovered that it could attenuate the 'tumour lysis syndrome'. This is the multiorgan failure that occurs when drug-induced cancer cell death and the release of purines from nucleic acids lead to a surge in uric acid synthesis and widespread precipitation of urate crystals (see Chapter 9) in tissues.[56] Allopurinol was found to not only prevent 6-MP conversion to 6-thiouric acid but also prevent the endogenous conversion of hypoxanthine and

---

[r] 4-hydroxypyrazolo (3,4-d) pyrimidine.
[s] Chosen from the combination of the Greek *allo* ('other') and *purinol* ('purine-like').

xanthine into uric acid (see Figure 8.5(d)).[57] As hypoxanthine and xanthine are more soluble than uric acid, they are safely excreted in the urine.

It was now a small step to see whether allopurinol could lower urate levels in the absence of cancer and help treat gout. This was put to the test by Wayne Rundles at Duke in collaboration with gout specialist James Wyngaarden (1924–2019), and at the American Rheumatism Association meeting in Atlantic City in June 1963, they reported positive preliminary results showing that allopurinol reduced urate levels in both blood and urine.[58] This was followed by seminal publications by the Duke group as well as from Alexander Gutman and his long-standing collaborator Ts'ai Fan Yu, the first female full professor of medicine at Mount Sinai School of Medicine in New York. Both papers showed the power of allopurinol in lowering urate levels.[59] It soon became clear, from observations reported by Charley Smyth in Denver, that allopurinol lowers blood urate levels enough to clear tophi (see Figure 8.6(a)).[60] The drug was approved by the United States Food and Drug Administration for the treatment of gout in 1966 (see Figure 8.6(b)). In recognition of the discovery of allopurinol, additional contributions to cancer chemotherapy and the development of acyclovir,[†] Hitchings and Elion were awarded the Nobel Prize for Physiology or Medicine in 1988, jointly with James Black (1924–2010) (who developed the beta blocker propranolol and the histamine H2 receptor antagonist cimetidine).

Allopurinol is the only drug listed in the World Health Organization Model List of Essential Medicines for the prevention of gout and protection from tumour lysis syndrome. It has long since been off-patent and is available cheaply in its generic formulation under a variety of trade names. It has been estimated that, in 2002–2003, as many as 200,000 people were on treatment with the drug in England alone.[61] However, although it has made a huge difference in the treatment of gout, it is not without some serious limitations, one of which is that it is excreted from the body via urination.

[†] The first antiviral drug.

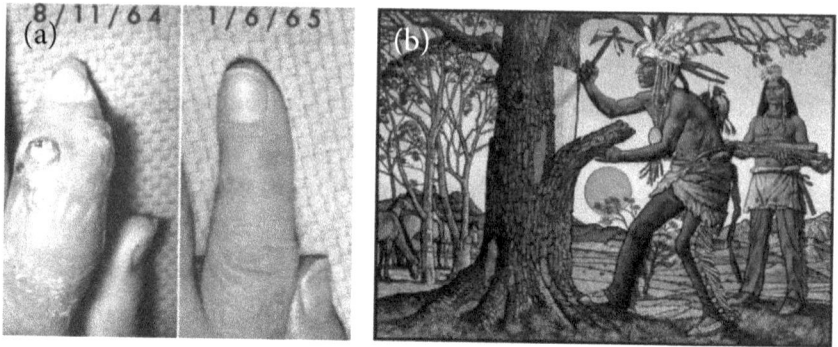

Figure 8.6.

(a) An example of the ability of allopurinol to clear gouty tophi, taken from Smyth (1965).

(b) 'Wherever gout strikes – Zyloric protects'. This 1971 Burroughs Wellcome marketing image for allopurinol tapped nostalgia for natural medicine with the following narrative: 'Collection of bark for medicinal purposes: Bark among the Cherokees was always taken from the east or sunny side of the tree. Roots and branches running towards the east were also used since this side was thought to absorb more of the sun's power.' Note that allopurinol is a synthetic agent and does not itself derive from a bark.

Source: (a) Used with kind permission of John Wiley & Sons, conveyed through Copyright Clearance Center, Inc.; (b) in copyright and courtesy of the Wellcome Collection.

Although it is unlike probenecid and other uricosuric agents, which require adequate renal function for their therapeutic effects, allopurinol must be used with great caution or not at all by those with reduced renal function to avoid the accumulation of its metabolite, oxypurinol, and subsequent side effects. Lowering the dose to avoid this often limits the reduction in uric acid levels that can be achieved, making it inadequate for preventing gout attacks. Furthermore, allopurinol is a purine mimic rather than a specific inhibitor of xanthine oxidase and has effects on other enzymes. It has a number of side effects, the most important of which is the occurrence of allergic reactions that were first reported in 1970 and can be very serious.[62] The effects of ethnicity and genetics on allopurinol sensitivity are touched on in Chapter 11.

Newer Urate-Lowering Agents

Recent years have seen additions to the repertoire of urate-lowering agents. For over two decades, allopurinol has been the only licensed xanthine oxidase inhibitor. With an awareness of the increasing frequency of gout and of allopurinol's shortcomings, Teijin Pharma in Japan instigated a drug discovery programme in 1988. The outcome was febuxostat, which is a novel compound rather than a purine mimic, with a thousand-fold greater potency and greater specificity than allopurinol for inhibiting xanthine oxidase. It is also less dependent, compared to allopurinol, on renal function for its elimination. In a head-to-head comparison, febuxostat was found to be superior to allopurinol (at a fixed dosage) in lowering urate levels.[63] Febuxostat is now marketed in over 60 countries, and US sales, via licencing to Takeda, amounted to US$1.9 million between 2012 and 2017 alone. However, it is relatively more expensive than allopurinol and is often reserved for cases of allopurinol 'failure'. There have been concerns that febuxostat treatment may predispose individuals to cardiovascular complications, which led to a US Food and Drug Administration warning regarding the drug.[64] However, a recent direct comparison of febuxostat with allopurinol has not revealed any difference in untoward cardiovascular effects.[65] A further non-purine xanthine oxidase inhibitor, topiroxostat, is under development.[66]

As mentioned, uricosuric agents have largely been superseded as first-line urate-lowering agents, and their use in gout is mainly as 'add-ons' for patients with healthy renal function who have not responded adequately to a xanthine oxidase inhibitor. At least in the UK, probenecid, benzbromarone and sulfinpyrazone are no longer readily available, but other uricosuric agents continue to be developed. Research on an antiviral drug for treating HIV-1 infection led to the observation that its metabolite, RDEA594, enhanced urate excretion. RDEA594 was redesignated as lesinurad and received approval from the United States Food and Drug Administration and the European Medicines Agency.[67] However, the manufacturers withdrew it from the market in 2018, reportedly due to the reluctance of physicians to risk causing urinary tract stone formation (see above), as well as a low demand relative to its relatively high cost.[68] Other uricosuric agents under development are dotinurad, verinurad and arhalofenate acid. Dotinurad is a chemically-engineered variant of benz-bromarone, designed to avoid the latter's occasional serious liver toxicity, and is approved for use in Japan.[69] Verinurad is an effective urate-lowering agent but is still under evaluation.[70] Arhalofenate acid is being developed for its combined uricosuric and anti-inflammatory activity (see the following).[71] These various new uricosuric agents all have in common with probenecid, sulphinpyrazone and benzbromarone the ability to prevent urate reabsorption from renal tubules via the URAT1 solute transporter channel (see Chapter 11). However, many, if not all, also block other solute transporter channels in the kidney and elsewhere; therefore, their effects could be potentially much broader than simply promoting urate excretion. Time will tell whether the newer uricosuric agents meet with commercial success.

In addition to drugs specifically developed to increase uric acid excretion, others have emerged that achieve the same as an 'added bonus'. The most topical are drugs collectively known as sodium glucose cotransporter 2 (SGLT2) inhibitors, such as canagliflozin, dapagliflozin and empagliflozin. These are used to treat type 2 diabetes and act on glucose transporter channels in the kidney to enhance glucose loss in the urine. A consequence of this increased glucose excretion is a parallel increase in urate excretion.[72] There is now evidence that SGLT2 inhibition not only modestly lowers serum urate levels but also helps prevent acute attacks of gout. As type 2 diabetes and gout are closely linked (see Chapter 14), an SGLT2 inhibitor may sometimes kill two birds with one stone.[73]

An innovation in recent years has been the use of uricase, the enzyme that digests uric acid (see Chapter 13). Uricase isolated from the fungus *Aspergillus flavus* was shown in 1968 to be capable of lowering urate levels in humans.[74] Pegloticase is a genetically engineered pig uricase that is highly effective in rapidly reducing urate levels and clearing tophi. It needs to be injected, and, as a foreign protein, it has the disadvantage of inducing an immune response that can result in allergic reactions to administration and loss of efficacy. To some extent, this is prevented by complexing the uricase in pegloticase with polyethylene glycol.[75] A further pharmaceutical strategy to reduce immunogenicity is to combine the administration of pegloticase with the immune-modulating agent methotrexate.[76] Use of uricase is mostly limited to chronic, refractory tophaceous gout in which other urate-lowering therapies have failed.

The Inflammation Paradox

For all the pessimism that Georgian physicians held regarding gout being untreatable, the chapter ends on a high with clear evidence that it is indeed manageable through long-term urate-lowering therapy. However, urate-lowering agents do not in themselves provide proof that uric acid directly causes gouty inflammation, and, right from the first use of probenecid, a paradox emerged that led to doubts that it does so. The paradox is that commencing urate-lowering treatment often actually triggers an acute gout attack.[77] I discuss the likely reason for this and how it can square with uric acid being responsible for inflammation in Chapter 12. It is only after urate deposits are depleted that acute attacks become less frequent, and that may take months or even years. The practical consequence of this is that adherence to urate-lowering drug treatment is notoriously low, and a clear understanding of the problem is essential to avoid discouragement.[78] Acute attacks during treatment initiation can be avoided by the coadministration of a non-steroidal anti-inflammatory agent or colchicine (see Chapter 10) for the early period. Arhalofenate acid, mentioned above, is being developed with this in mind, as its direct effects are both uricosuric and anti-inflammatory.[79] As the faster urate is lowered, the higher the chance of an acute gout flare, it makes sense to adopt a 'start-low and go-slow' strategy of escalating the drug dose gradually to achieve the target level. In the case of allopurinol, this may reduce drug-specific side effects.[80] However, unfortunately, this strategy does not substitute for the need for anti-inflammatory cover.[81]

Reflections on Urate-Lowering Therapy

Urate-lowering therapy has been transformational for gout, and there is no doubt that it can reduce the frequency of acute attacks and clear tophi, provided it is correctly adhered to.[82] However, it is not a substitute for life-style measures (see Chapter 12), and these may be sufficient. How far the blood urate should be reduced remains an open question, as uric acid has potentially beneficial roles, which will be discussed in Chapter 13. Several urate-lowering clinical trials have shown a trend towards higher cardiovascular mortality in those with the largest reductions in urate level.[83] It is as well to be cautious; the current British Society for Rheumatology Guidelines recommend treating to an initial target level of blood urate less than 0.30 mmol/l (5 mg/100 ml), reducing drug doses to bring the urate level up to between 0.30 and 0.36 mmol/l (6.1 mg/100 ml) once acute gout attacks have ceased and tophi have cleared. These levels are well below the theoretical solubility level of monosodium urate (0.41 mmol/l [6.89 mg/100 ml]; see Chapter 9), below which there is likely to be little further significant urate deposition.[84]

Chapter 9

Crystallising Inflammation

Acute gouty arthritis is a vigorous inflammatory response in and around a joint, with all the hallmarks of inflammation described by the Roman physician Aulus Celsus.[a] With the introduction of probenecid in the early 1950s, it became clear that enhancing the urinary excretion of uric acid could clear tophi (see Chapter 8); however, many people found that they suffered a return of acute gout soon after starting treatment.[1] Clearly, this ran in the face of Alfred Garrod's fourth proposition that 'the urate of soda is the cause, not the effect of inflammation' (see Chapter 6).[2] Referring to probenecid, the distinguished London rheumatologist and gout specialist Michael Mason went so far as to write in 1954:

It is evident that, whatever the changes in blood levels in a naturally occurring attack of gout, acute paroxysms can occur at a time when the level has been sharply brought to normal. This finding renders it difficult to believe that uric acid per se can be responsible for initiating the acute paroxysm of gout.[3]

In this chapter, I explain how, on this occasion, Mason was wrong and how uric acid, or more precisely, monosodium urate, is indeed the instigator of gouty inflammation.

---

[a] Celsus' hallmarks of inflammation were *ubor, tumor, calor* and *dolor*, which translate from Latin as redness, swelling, warmth and pain, respectively.

Inflammation in John Hunter's Day

First, some introduction to inflammation in general, starting when handed-down dogma was giving way to scientific enquiry. John Hunter (1818–1883) (see Figure 9.1(a)), who is widely regarded as the father of scientific surgery, provided the late-eighteenth-century *vade mecum* of inflammation.[4] His working life began in London, demonstrating at his brother William Hunter's School of Anatomy in Great Windmill Street, Soho. He put together his own bespoke medical education, as all would-be doctors had to do in the absence of state-regulated courses,

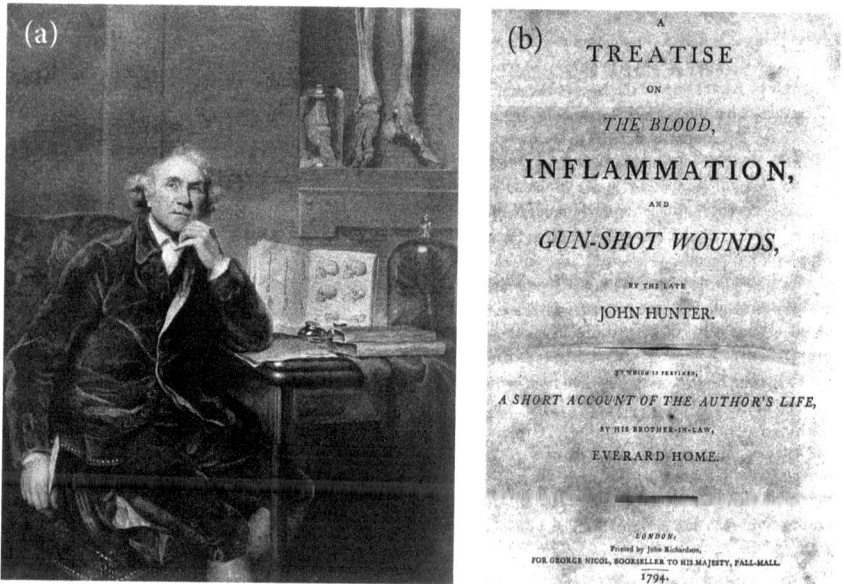

Figure 9.1.

(a) John Hunter by Joshua Reynolds. The spines of the two closed volumes on the table have the titles *Natural History of Fossils* and *Natural History of Vegetables*. These are pointers to Hunter's wide scientific interests rather than actual book titles.

(b) Title page of his *Treatise on the Blood, Inflammation, and Gun-Shot Wounds* (1794), containing a biography by his brother-in-law, Everard Home.

Source: Both images courtesy of the Wellcome Collection, public domain.

and in 1756, he secured a house surgeon post at St. George's Hospital. Burnout is not new among doctors; after six years of hard graft, he quit his job and enlisted as an army surgeon. This was during the Seven Years' War, and Hunter's first battle experience was with the force that captured Belle-Île[b] from France. He then went on to work alongside William Cadogan (see Chapter 3) in a military hospital behind the lines in Portugal. The war exposed him to a wide variety of battle wounds, with all their inflammatory consequences. He began lecturing on the subject in around 1770, but it was not until soon after he died in 1794 that his seminal *Treatise on the Blood, Inflammation, and Gun-Shot Wounds* (see Figure 9.1(b)) appeared in print, organised by his brother-in-law and mentee Everard Home (see Chapter 5).

   Hunter regarded inflammation as the body's natural way to repair physical injury:

> Inflammation is to be considered only as a disturbed state of parts, which requires an new but salutary mode of action to restore them to that state wherein a natural mode of action alone is necessary: from such a view of the subject, therefore, inflammation in itself is not to be considered as a disease, but as a salutary operation, consequent either to some violence or some disease.[5]

While inflammation was restorative in principle, weakness in the body led to suppuration with pus formation,[c] adhesions or ulceration. Which one occurred depended largely on where the problem was situated. Hunter saw acute gout, which he suffered from badly himself, as a special form of inflammation, differing from others in almost always resolving spontaneously without any of these consequences.[6] Note that, although Hunter used the word 'salutary', he meant it in a different way to Thomas Sydenham (see Chapter 2). Whereas Sydenham, as a physician, emphasised the

---

[b] A small island off the coast of Brittany.

[c] As in an abscess.

constitutional healthiness of acute gout, Hunter took a surgical view and saw it as a local corrective process.

On top of his contributions to surgery, Hunter is particularly remembered for his anatomical studies relating the physique of animals to their lifestyles. He purchased the bodies of dead circus animals and established his own animal menage in Earl's Court, London. He may well have been the inspiration for Hugh Lofting's *Dr. Dolittle* books.[7] Hunter realised that studying animals with relatively simple makeups can help understand general principles that can be brought to bear on the more complex human situation. Although his main interest was comparing anatomies, this was a fundamental approach to biology, and it is the same reasoning that has led to the modern emphasis on studying small plants, yeasts, fruit flies, worms, etc. We saw in the previous chapter how the conservation of purine biochemistry since life began allowed the Burroughs Wellcome group to use bacteria to discover 6-mercaptopurine.

It was because of Hunter that James Parkinson started collecting fossils (see Chapter 6). Hunter saw fossils as comparative anatomy's fourth dimension, a window to a bygone age. He corresponded for years with his student, the vaccinologist Edward Jenner (see Chapter 5), often asking him to send fossils from the West Country.[8] By the time he died, Hunter had assembled the fossils of 1,215 vertebrates, 2,202 invertebrates and 292 plants.[9] Tragically, most of his collection was destroyed in the London bombings of 1941. As Hunter's publications on fossils appeared posthumously, the importance he attached to the subject has tended to be underestimated. *Observations and Reflections on Geology* only turned up in 1859, years after Hunter died.[10] Hunter had intended this to be an introduction to the catalogue of his fossil collection, but the work goes beyond that by anticipating Charles Darwin's and Alfred Wallace's theories of natural selection. He suggested that fossils are indicators of gradual alterations in the Earth's surface and a demonstration that species come and go in response to changes in local geography. The implication was that fossils are not imprints of life destroyed by the Biblical deluge but instead evidence of a much older and episodic past. James Rennell (see Chapter 5), whom Hunter asked to review the book, was at pains to point out the heretical nature of the conclusions:

> ... you have used the term <u>many thousands of centuries</u>, which brings us almost to the *yogues* of the Hindoos. Now, although I have no quarrel with any opinions relating to the antiquity of the globe, yet there are ... persons very numerous and respectable in every point apart but their pardonable <u>superstitions</u>, who will dislike any mention of a specific period that ascends beyond 6000 years: I would, therefore, with submission, qualify the expression by many thousand YEARS, instead of CENTURIES.[11]

Hunter yielded and altered centuries to years but then never submitted the manuscript himself for publication.[12]

The Origin of the Cells in Inflammation

Hunter's understanding of inflammation was entirely clinical. The ability to explore further improved with the introduction of ever more powerful and visually faithful microscopes with which to observe the tissues. The focus was still on general principles rather than whatever might be specifically happening in gout. The big unknown was whether the many visible 'corpuscles[d]' that are present in inflamed tissues derive from the blood or are generated locally at the site of inflammation. By the 1840s, the general view was that these arose from hypothetical germinal structures in the tissues known as 'blastemas'. This was challenged by William Addison (1802–1881), who, using microscopy, focused his attention on the colourless corpuscles in the blood that are larger and more motile than the red cells, which now, of course, are known as white cells or leukocytes. By 1842, Addison had concluded that all the varieties of cells in inflamed tissues 'are more or less altered colorless blood corpuscles – altered either

---

[d] Corpuscle is an old word for cell.

by imbibing and growing larger, or by exhaling, shrivelling, and becoming less'.[13] Addison was a traditionalist and was keen to use his observations to justify therapeutic bleeding. Indeed, it is likely that it was through therapeutic bleeding that Addison obtained enough blood to conduct his extensive haematological studies. Fast-forwarding to the present, although bleeding has long been out of vogue, the physical removal of leukocytes from the blood is still taken seriously and has been explored as a treatment for inflammatory disease in this century.[14]

Addison met with some stiff resistance at the time. Although he noted that leukocytes adhered to the walls of blood vessels at sites of local irritation, he did not actually witness them moving into the tissues. Following Addison, the medical physiologist Augustus Waller (1816–1870) (Figure 9.2(a)) then devised a method that allowed him to visualise under the microscope the blood vessels in the outstretched tongues of frogs, and he actually observed leukocytes moving out of the blood into their surroundings (see Figures 9.2(b) and (c)). The nature of small blood vessels was still not known, and Waller probably conceived of them more as fibrous tubes than cellular structures. He proposed a digestive process whereby leukocytes move from the inner to the outer side of the blood vessel without rupturing the vessel and causing bleeding:

> It may be surmised either that the corpuscle, after remaining a certain time in contact with the vessel, gives off by exudation from within itself some substance possessing a solvent power over the vessel, or that the solution of the vessel takes place in virtue of some of those molecular actions which arise from the contact of two bodies; actions which are now known as exerting such extensive influence in digestion and are referred to what is termed the catalytic power.[15]

Waller went on to use the same frog tongue preparation to discover 'Wallerian degeneration' of nerves after injury, for which he is better known.[16]

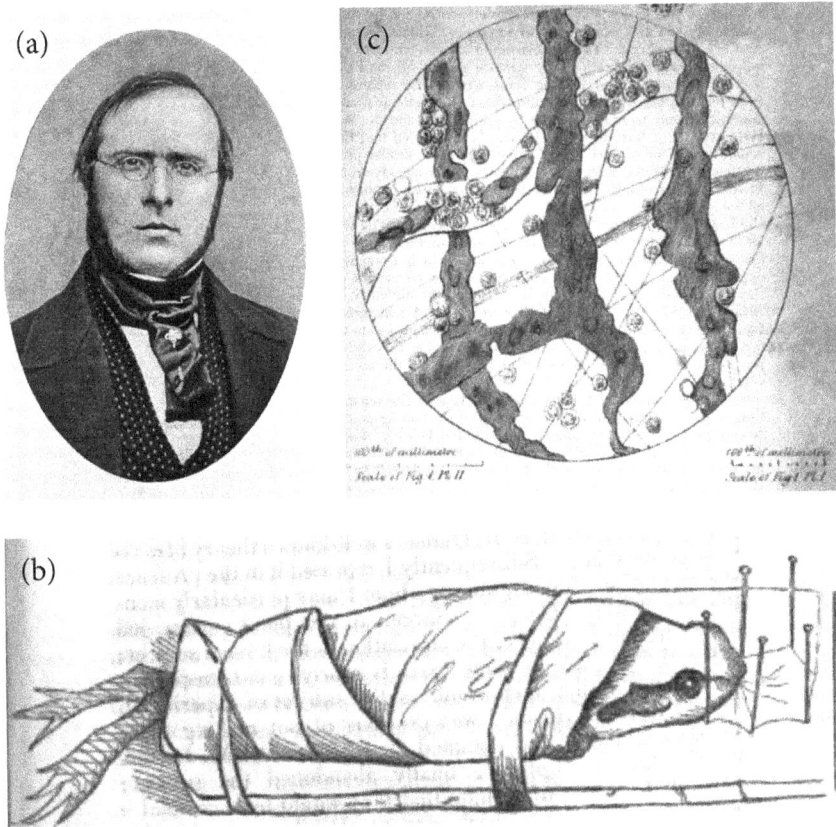

Figure 9.2.

(a) Augustus Waller by an unknown photographer.

(b) Diagram by Waller of how he exposed the tongue of frogs to study the small blood vessels under the microscope.

(c) Using this technique, Waller became the first to observe leukocytes emigrating out of blood vessels. In his words, the drawing 'represents vessels of the inferior surface of the tongue as they appear after the escape of the corpuscles, filled with stationary blood, deformed and indented at the points of escape, near which the corpuscles are generally found. A portion of a vessel with an internal current is likewise seen with discs, and internal and external corpuscles. No indentations are seen near these, probably from the force of the current, which directly restored the form of the vessel'.

Source: (a) Courtesy of the US National Library of Medicine, public domain; (b) and (c) are from Waller, 1846a and 1846b, respectively, and both courtesy of the Biodiversity Heritage Library, public domain.

The Cellular Basis of Disease

The works of Addison and Waller were somewhat marginalised once the centre of medical scientific gravity shifted to Germany in the 1850s, which is where most modern recollections of the inflammation story begin. Rudolf Virchow (1821–1902) transformed thinking about disease, publishing his seminal paper on its cellular basis in 1855.[17] He introduced his collection of 20 lectures as professor of pathology at the Charité Hospital in Berlin as follows:

> They were more particularly intended as an attempt to offer in a better arranged form than had hitherto been done, a view of the cellular nature of all vital processes, both physiological and pathological, animal and vegetable, so as distinctly to set forth what even the people have long been dimly conscious of, namely, the unity of life in all organized beings, in opposition to the one-sided humoral and neuristical (solidistic) tendencies which have been transmitted from the mythical days of antiquity to our own times, and at the same time to contrast with the equally one-sided interpretations of a grossly mechanical and chemical bias – the more delicate mechanism and chemistry of the cell.[18]

With this, Virchow threw the schools of traditional humours, iatrome-chanics and iatrochemistry all out of the same window and replaced them with his dictum *Omnis cellula e cellula.*[e] As far as inflammation was concerned, Virchow updated the old blastema theory with modern cells.

Besides being one of the most influential medical scientists of his generation, Virchow was also a champion of social justice, regarding medicine and politics as closely allied. He was heavily involved in the

---

[e] 'All cells are from cells'.

evolutionary controversies of the mid-late 1800s that followed the theories of natural selection. The issue for Virchow was not so much about whether biblical creation was true as about the social, moral and political implications of our being connected to apes. Although often considered an anti-evolutionist, Virchow's position was actually the danger of accepting theories as facts and teaching these as such.[19] In addressing a meeting of the German Association of Naturalists and Physicians in Munich in 1877, he warned, 'I may say that I look forward with real fear to the events which will happen among our neighbours in the course of the next years'. What he foresaw was natural selection thinking being applied to nations and justifying the spiral that started with Otto Bismarck's German Imperialism and led on to World Wars I and II, as well as of course the Holocaust. Virchow maintaining that the fossilised remains of a Neanderthal were probably those of a human crippled by rickets is now thought to have been an anti-racist rather than an anti-evolution stance and motivated, at least in part, by a reluctance to separate Germans from peoples of the world who others might have regarded at an 'intermediate' stage along an evolutionary pathway.[20]

Virchow encouraged his pupil, Julius Cohnheim (1839–1884), to take an interest in inflammation.[21] Like Hunter, Cohnheim had been an army surgeon and had gained clinical experience of inflammation in the Prussian forces during the second Schleswig–Holstein war. He performed painstaking microscopy on the living tissues of frogs and rabbits, aided by being able to stain tissues with new dyes, and determined, first, that small arteries are not usually occluded in inflammation and, second, that small veins are the portal through which leukocytes emigrate into the tissues. His conclusions were similar to those of Addison and Waller but were supported by much more thorough experimentation and more detail. Cohnheim did pay passing reference to Addison in his groundbreaking paper of 1867, but none to Waller, who should take the historical credit for being the first to visualise leukocytes emigrating from the blood into inflamed tissues.[22] No doubt Cohnheim was unaware of Waller's work at the time, as he did include a reference to it in the second edition of his *Lectures on General Pathology* of 1882.[23] Cohnheim would probably have gone from strength to strength had he not died aged only 45, supposedly from the effects of gout.[24]

While Waller had emphasised a likely enzymatic digestive mechanism whereby leukocytes penetrate blood vessel walls, Cohnheim proposed that the adhesion of leukocytes to the walls of small veins and their subsequent transmigration out of the vessel could be explained by chemical changes in the lining of the vessel: 'I believe I can prove strictly that it is only and solely the vessel wall which is responsible for the entire series of events'.[25] It took another hundred years for us to begin understanding the mechanisms that enable leukocytes to emigrate out of small blood vessels into sites of inflammation at a molecular level (see the following).

The Discovery of Phagocytosis

After Cohnheim, it was accepted that leukocytes pass into inflamed tissues from the blood; however, no one quite knew what they did once they got there. Twenty-five years later, Ilya Ilyich Metchnikoff (1845–1916) (see Figure 9.3(a)), a Russian zoologist and pupil of Louis Pasteur (1822–1895), described the phenomenon of phagocytosis,[f] whereby leukocytes become amoeba-like eater cells ('phagocytes') that ingest and degrade bacteria and other foreign bodies as well as dead tissue (Figure 9.3(b)).[26] This was groundbreaking and set the foundations for the field of innate cellular immunology.[27] In 1908, Metchnikoff was awarded the Nobel Prize for Medicine or Physiology, which he shared with the early humoral immunologist Paul Ehrlich (1854–1915).[g] Metchnikoff was heavily influenced by Charles Darwin and saw inflammation in an evolutionary context: a cellular protective strategy in the battle for species survival against bacteria and

---

[f] From Ancient Greek φαγεῖν (*phagein*, meaning 'to eat'), and κύτος (*kytos*, meaning 'cell').

[g] Humoral immunology is the science of antibodies and other soluble mediators of immunity.

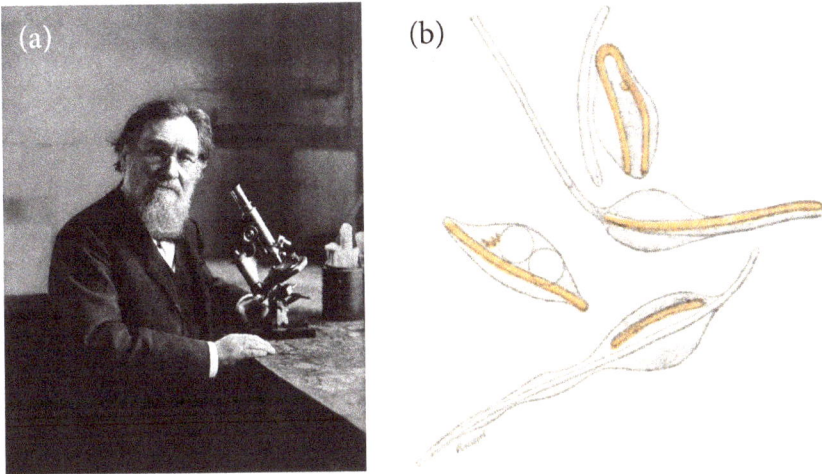

Figure 9.3.

(a) Metchnikoff in his laboratory. He discovered phagocytic cells and is considered the pioneer of macrophage biology and innate cellular immunology. Photogravure after Henri Manuel.

(b) Four frog phagocytes with live bacteria (white) and internal dead bacteria (brown) from Metchnikoff in 1892.

Source: Both images courtesy of the Wellcome Collection, public domain.

other microorganisms.[28] With the same scientific philosophy as Hunter, Metchnikoff looked for commonalities between species:

> Medicine has hitherto excluded all the pathological phenomena which occur in the lower animals. And yet the study of these animals, affording as they do infinitely simpler and more primitive conditions than those in man and vertebrata, really furnishes the key to the comprehension of the complex pathological phenomena which are of special interest in medical science.[29]

We now know that phagocytes recognise and engulf 'danger' in the form of bacteria or other unwanted entities. They then send chemical signals to local small blood vessels to make these dilate, increase blood flow and leak out defensive blood proteins into the local site of injury. This is responsible for inflammation's cardinal features of redness, warmth and swelling. The pain is due to the chemical signals stimulating local sensory nerve terminals. The protective system soon becomes self-propagating as the endothelial cells that form the inner lining of small veins also respond to messages from phagocytes by expressing adhesion proteins that capture more phagocytic leukocytes passing by in the blood, as proposed conceptually by Cohnheim. Further chemicals act as 'chemotactic' factors that attract the leukocytes captured from the blood to migrate towards the source of the problem, with their movement within the tissue being aided by enzymes on their cell surfaces, as proposed by Waller. Thus, the complementary hypotheses of Waller and Cohnheim were both upheld. In deference to the old blastema theory and to Virchow, we also now know that some local proliferation of resident phagocytic cells does also occur.

The Discovery of Urate Crystals in Gout

So, with the general principles of inflammation now in place, is there anything special about inflammation in gout? We saw in Chapter 6 how Robert Kinglake had proposed in 1804 that there was not, suggesting that gout was simply local inflammation and could have any number of causes.[30] Metchnikoff himself challenged this, putting his money mistakenly on gout being a disease due to an as yet undiscovered germ.[31]

We also saw in Chapter 6 how Alfred Garrod had championed in his propositions that gouty inflammation is a reaction to monosodium urate depositing in tissues.[32] Garrod was well aware that the urate deposition was in crystalline form, but he was not the first person to describe the presence of crystals in gout – for that, we need to go back 150 years earlier to Anton van Leeuwenhoek. Van Leeuwenhoek was a Dutch cloth merchant who developed his own microscopes to test the quality of his cloths and became obsessed with the new world that he saw through them. He wrote a series of letters to the Royal Society in London detailing many tiny entities, some of which he found moved with seemingly vital energies. Robert Hooke had described microscopic fungi a little earlier in 1665, but it was van Leeuwenhoek who made the first sightings of motile bacteria and spermatozoa.[33] No such minute life forces were thought possible, and claims to their existence were initially not well received. The Royal Society sent a site visit that substantiated van Leeuwenhoek's claims, and he was duly elected an international fellow in 1680. Robert Boyle sensitively described in his *Short Memoirs for the Experimental History of Mineral Waters* how he was won around:

> ... to convince these doubters, of whose number I was myself at first inclined to be, I devised the following experiment: having laid upon the magnifying glass a part of a drop of water, wherein I could see store of these little animals frisking up and down, we put to the liquor, with a bristle or some such very slender thing, part of a drop of spirit of salt, which, as was expected, presently killed these little tender creatures, and depriving them of their animal motion, left them to be carried so slowly to and fro in the liquor, as to make it visible, that they were then dead, and had been before alive.[34]

One of van Leeuwenhoek's letters to the Royal Society, sent in 1685, described the microscopic appearance of material scraped out from a gouty tophus (see Figure 9.4(a)):

> A relation of mine, much troubled with the Gout, has his heel spoyl't with the great quantity of Chalk, that breaks out of it; this matter I examined in my Method, and separated the same in 3 parts, the first was the driest, and whitest, made of small irregular parts, as if some small sands lay together; these thro' the Microscope appeared very dark bodies, and each of then consisted of a great number of long transparent figures; which I can liken to nothing better, than to cut Horse-hair, something sharp at both ends. These figures I judged so thin, that more than 1000 of them lying close together, would not make out, the thickness of a hair of our head.[35]

Van Leeuwenhoek may or may not have realised the significance of these structures for gout, but, anyway, it had little to no impact compared to many of his other discoveries. Hooke and Boyle were friends with Thomas Sydenham, and it seems very possible that he would have heard from them about van Leeuwenhoek's work. However, Sydenham was not a proponent

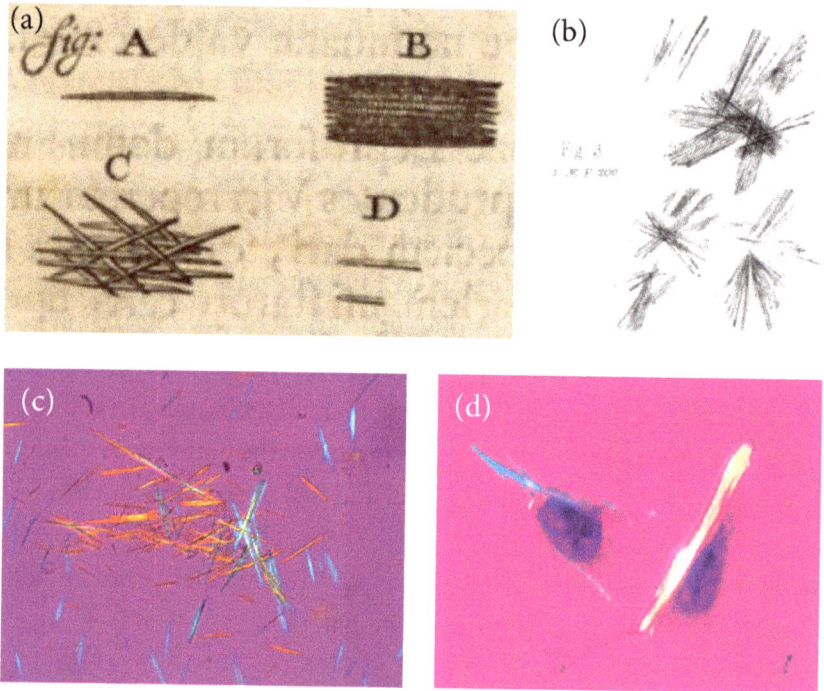

Figure 9.4.

(a) Anton van Leeuwenhoek's drawings of the needle-shaped structures he saw in the scrapings of a gouty tophus. From van Leewenhoek's *Opera Omnia* (1722–1730) Volume 1.

(b) Alfred Garrod's drawing of the needle-shaped crystals in a tophus, which he identified as monosodium urate. From Garrod (1859).

(c) Polarising microscopy of monosodium urate crystals, which are strongly negatively birefringent and either yellow or blue depending on the plane of the light.

(d) Polarising microscopy of monosodium urate crystals that have been internalised by monocytic phagocytes. From Yagnik *et al.* (2000).

(e)

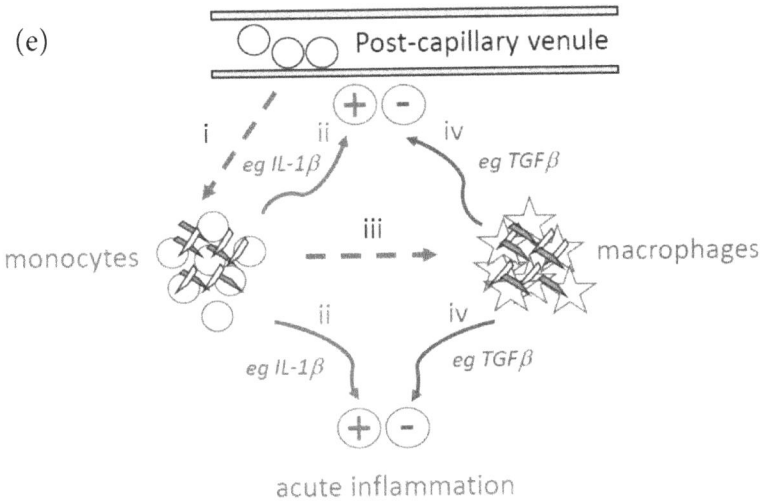

Figure 9.4. (*Continued*)

(e) Simple scheme of monosodium urate crystals triggering an inflammatory response that resolves spontaneously: (i) leukocytes adhere to the endothelial cells that line post-capillary venules and migrate into the local tissue containing naked monosodium urate crystals, attracted by chemokines, (ii) monocytes phagocytose crystals and release factors such as IL-1β that amplify inflammation through actions on vascular endothelial and other cells within the local environment, (iii) monocytes differentiate to anti-inflammatory macrophages that, (iv) release factors such as TGFβ that dampen the inflammatory response.

Source: (a) and (b) Courtesy of the Wellcome Collection, public domain; (c) Bobjgalindo, via Wikimedia Commons, CC BY-SA 4.0; (d) with permission from John Wiley and Sons.

of microscopy anyway (see Chapter 2), and if he knew about van Leeuwenhoek observing 'long transparent figures' in tophaceous conretions, he would not necessarily have considered it of any consequence. In the subsequent long period after van Leeuwenhoek, William Stukeley had proposed in 1834 that sharp, pointed particles triggered inflammation in gout; however, this was probably entirely theoretical and based on his mentor Richard Mead's work on snake venom (see Chapter 3).[36] However, by the early 1840s, it was well recognised by physicians that the crystallisation of uric acid or its sodium salt could be responsible for inflammation. For instance, William Robertson (1810–1897) wrote in his very considered and readable *The Nature and Treatment of Gout* (1845):

> It is not improbable, that the irritation of the capillaries of the part, resulting from the throwing down of crystalline particles of lithic acid or of its compounds with alkali, may be the true cause of gouty inflammation, and may help explain many of the phenomena and peculiarities of the disease.[37]

Fictitious quadriurate

By the late 1800s, most physicians who wrote about gout agreed that 'no uric acid, no gout'; however, the role of crystals was by no means settled. Garrod had been at pains mid-century to document the presence of monosodium urate crystals in gouty tissues (see Figure 9.4(b)) and was a strong advocate for their importance. Supporting him was his former student, William Roberts, who somewhat muddied the water with an excessively elaborate theory on urate crystal formation.[38] The notion that monosodium urate crystals form from the dispersal of soluble quadriurate (a supposed combination of monosodium urate with uric acid) had originally been proposed by Henry Bence Jones (1813–1873) (see Chapter 13) and was further developed by Roberts to the extent that he devoted all four of his Royal College of Physicians Croonian Lectures in 1892 to the topic.[39] Although chemically based on shaky ground, quadriurates entered the medical vocabulary and were featured in textbooks and monographs, not least that by the discerning Arthur Luff (see Chapter 7) in his excellent *Gout: Its Pathology and Treatment* of 1898.[40] Others were more sceptical, and the existence of quadriurate was finally debunked in 1900 as just a loose mixture of urates and uric acid rather than a bonded chemical entity.[41] Quadriurates then passed into oblivion.

Opposition to the importance of urate crystals

Among the many who challenged the importance of urate crystals, Dyce Duckworth rekindled the old neurological explanation of gout, extending the pre-uric-acid lines of William Cullen and, before him, Thomas Willis, with uric acid acting as a stimulus for the nervous system in causing acute inflammation without the need for crystals. [42] This thinking was encouraged by the discovery by the French neurologist Jean-Martin Charcot (1825–1893) of inflammatory arthritis due to syphilitic injury to the nerves[h].[43] 'Doctor's Corner' in the *Newcastle Weekly Chronicle* carried an update in 1894 on gout entitled 'An Insidious Poison', some 35 years after the first publication of Garrod's book. This briefed the public that 'it is more than probable that the symptoms observed to be present when uric acid exists in excess in the economy are due to its action on the nervous system' and made no mention of crystals.[44] In a facile way, the involvement of the nervous system is self-evident, given the local pain and tenderness along the path of adjacent nerves during acute gouty arthritis.[45] Moreover, although we no longer think that the nervous system has primacy of place, suggesting its involvement is by no means incorrect. We now know that small peripheral nerves play a major role in the progression of inflammation, in part through increasing the flow of blood through blood vessels and the accumulation of fluid and cells.

The many different countertheories to Garrod's mostly shared the view that uric acid was inert, largely because injecting urate in solution into animals did not elicit a gout-like inflammatory response. The crystalline urate in gouty tissues was seen as a consequence rather than a cause of inflammation. The Polish-German physician Wilhelm Ebstein (1836–1912) was particularly outspoken in his disagreement that urate crystals were important. Ebstein is now remembered more for describing the congenital

---

[h] An inflammatory arthritis caused by peripheral nerve injury is now referred to as a Charcot's joint.

malformation of the heart's tricuspid valve that has become known as Ebstein's anomaly.[46] As he detected dead matter but no urate crystals in some gouty tissues, he maintained that the inflammation was primarily due to the irritating effects of urate in solution, causing stasis of blood within the veins, and that this led to tissue breakdown and crystal formation. Ebstein attempted to support his theory with a number of animal experiments involving instilling a urate solution on the surface of rabbit eyes and raising urate levels in birds by occluding urine flow.[47] Although these were wholly futile and inconclusive, his theory was taken seriously well into the twentieth century.[48]

Urate crystals trigger inflammation

Experimental support for urate crystals being the key to gout eventually came from Leipzig. Cohnheim had built up pathology research there during the last six years of his life, and this must have established a conducive experimental climate. A dermatologist there, Gustav Riehl, published in 1897 a careful microscopic study of gouty tophi. He detected crystals in areas of tissue showing no evidence of necrosis and challenged the conclusions of Ebstein and others on the basis that they had missed seeing crystals by taking insufficient care to prevent them from dissolving while preparing their microscope slides.[49] Riehl's descriptive work was then extended experimentally in the laboratory of Wilhelm His Jr. (1863–1934). His' father, Wilhelm His Sr. (1831–1904), was a distinguished embryologist who had invented the microtome, a slicing device for preparing tissue sections for microscopic analysis, and who from 1872 to 1904 held the chair of anatomy in Leipzig. His son was primarily a physician but, soon after graduating, published a paper on the neuromuscular band that conducts electrical impulses and coordinates contractions in the heart – since known as the Bundle of His.[50] In 1895, His Jnr. was appointed assistant professor in clinical medicine in Leipzig, and subsequently, his interests shifted from the heart to the emerging speciality of rheumatology. He encouraged his student, Max Freudweiler, to experiment on uric acid and inflammation. Freudweiler injected urate crystals into the skin of rabbits, dogs, guinea pigs and chickens, as well as into his own upper arm. On all occasions, his microscopic analysis of the excised injected sites showed evidence of intense inflammation, whereas injection of a solution of monosodium urate without crystals had only a minor effect. He observed needle-shaped crystals within the phagocytic cells Metchnikoff had described, and these had the strong negative birefringence of monosodium urate under polarised light (see Figures 9.4(c) and (d)). Freudweiler's microscopic findings now provided a solid basis for the idea that crystals cause inflammation directly.[51]

Sadly, that was as far as Freudweiler's work went, as he left Leipzig in 1901 to become director of a new Institute of Physical Therapy in Zurich and died soon after. Wilhelm His Jnr. authored a subsequent similar report showing the effects of injecting urate into rabbits, but he moved in 1907 to Berlin, where his interests shifted to the use of radium in the treatment of gout and other rheumatic diseases. [52] The Leipzig papers appear to have had virtually no impact and were soon forgotten, if ever read. The relevance of urate crystals then remained up in the air, and indeed an adverse tide set in once it became clear that urate was commonly found at a high level in the blood of people without evidence of gout (see the following). In 1905, Clifford Allbutt (1836–1925)[i] placed William Roberts's chapter on gout, written for his much-used *Systems of Medicine*, in the section on 'General Diseases of Obscure Causation'.[53] The situation was no clearer by 1921, when the Bath physician Llewellyn Jones Llewellyn (1871–1934) wrote a detailed account of the various competing theories on the mechanisms of gout, putting forward his own idea that there may be an infective cause.[54] Notably, Llewellyn made no mention of urate crystals in his long and otherwise scholarly monograph. Likewise, Alexander Gutman failed to

---

[i] Clifford Allbutt was the inventor of the bedside mercury-in-glass thermometer.

mention crystals when asked as late as 1950 whether uric acid caused an acute attack of gouty arthritis. Gutman was the founding editor of the *American Journal of Medicine* and, himself a substantial gout expert, considered that acute gout could be an allergic phenomenon. He replied that 'there are, however, many reasons to doubt that uric acid *per se* is immediately concerned with the symptoms of acute gout. From all indications, uric acid is a physiologically inert substance'.[55]

The matter was not finally settled until the early 1960s, a decade after urate-lowering therapy with probenecid was introduced (Chapter 8). Two American research groups (James Faires and Daniel McCarty in Philadelphia; and Jay Seegmiller and colleagues at the National Institute for Health) separately performed similar experiments to Freudweiler's, with similar results. Seegmiller's group also elicited acute arthritis by injecting urate crystals into the knee joints of heroic human volunteers.[56] Neither group had been aware of Freudweiler's work, and McCarty, aided by Joseph Brill, gracefully republished the Freudweiler papers with commentaries once he discovered them in a literature search. They quoted George Santayana's saying that those who do not remember the past are condemned to repeat it.[57] On the one hand, the initial bypassing of Waller's work by the German school and then Freudweiler's by the Americans speaks to the fallibility of scientific research citation. On the other, it needs to be remembered that discovering forgotten papers was often a project in itself before the scientific literature was so widely accessible using modern information technology.

In attributing causation to an agent in disease, it is conventional to check 'Koch's postulates', a set of criteria for infective organisms used by the German microbiologist Robert Koch (1843–1910), who discovered the bacterial causes of tuberculosis, cholera and anthrax. The involvement of urate crystals in acute gouty inflammation now passed an adaptation of these postulates as follows: (i) urate crystals could be found in the tissues in all natural cases of acute gout; (ii) these urate crystals were identical to synthetic urate crystals; (iii) injecting the crystals reproduced the gouty inflammation; and (iv) crystals could be recovered and identified from the injected tissue lesions after inflammation was established.

A High Blood Urate Level Does Not Equal Gout

Thomas Beddoes bemoaned doctors in the early nineteenth century for not sharing clinical experience (see Chapter 6), but even when doctors do so, hospitals, clinics and private practices are not the best places to research the propensity to disease. Individuals who attend a clinic have either been referred there or have chosen to attend, and this introduces selection bias into the results. Modern epidemiology came into its own in the decades immediately after World War II, with the brief of discovering environmental and genetic influences and their interactions responsible for the maintenance and breakdown of health. The initial means to this end were local surveys of randomly selected participants living in defined communities, such as the Framlingham Heart Study, a highly influential community survey based in Massachusetts. These allowed the acquisition of detailed information on lifestyle as well as the collection of blood and other samples for laboratory analyses. By the early 1900s, biochemical techniques had become available for measuring urate in the blood quickly and more sensitively than Alfred Garrod could do, in large part through the work of Otto Folin and Willey Denis at Harvard.[58] These now allowed an exploration of how urate levels and gout vary at the population level, either at a single time point ('a cross-sectional study') or at sequential time points ('a longitudinal study'). The most informative longitudinal approach is prospective, meaning that clinical information and samples for laboratory tests are collected at the beginning of the study, and then participants are followed up over time for the emergence of disease. Because humans are so variable, such studies require large numbers of subjects and sophisticated statistical analyses to avoid the influence of extraneous confounding variables.

A study of hospital patients based at the National Institutes of Health in Bethesda showed, in 1959, not only that those with a high urate level do not have persistent gouty inflammation but that most do not get gout at all.[59] This lack of inevitability in those with a high urate level was found to apply at a population level by the Framlingham Heart Study.[60] A monosodium urate concentration in blood of 0.41 mmol/litre (6.9 mg/100 ml) can be considered the theoretical limit of its solubility in water.[61] In the Framlingham study, only 16.7% of participants found to have a slightly high urate level (0.42–0.47 mmol/l, or 7.0–7.9 mg/100 ml) at any time measured had experienced gouty inflammation, rising to 25% with a moderately high level (0.48–0.53 mmol/l, or 8.0–8.9 mg/100 ml) and 90% with a very high level (>0.53 mmol/l, or >9.0 mg/100 ml) (see Figure 9.5). [62] Then, in the 1980s, the Normative Aging Study conducted at the Massachusetts General Hospital in Boston published the results of a similar study, but

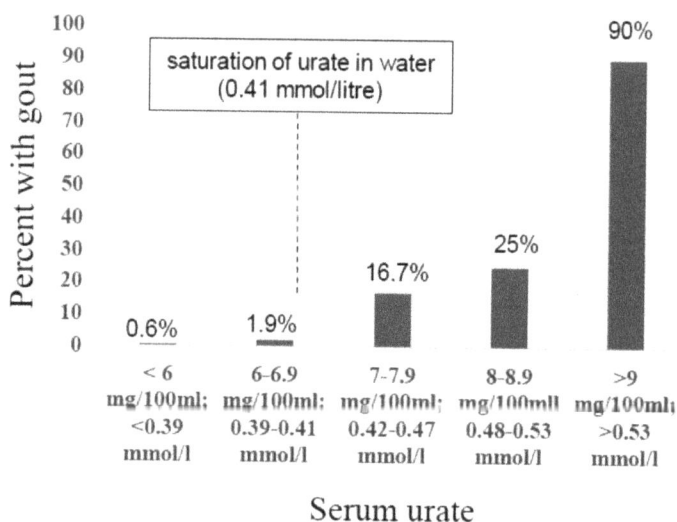

Figure 9.5.

Data extracted from the Framlingham study on the relationship between blood urate levels and gout. The study not only showed that the higher the urate level, the more risk of gout, but also that the majority of men with urate levels above the saturation point of monosodium urate in water (0.41 mmol/litre, or 6.9 mg/100 ml) have not experienced an acute gout attack.

Source: Graph generated from data in Hall *et al.* (1967).

this time forward-looking. They found that only 22% of individuals with very high urate levels (>0.54 mmol/l, or 9.08 mg/100 ml) at the initial sampling developed gout over five years. The proportions were much lower at 4.1% and just 2% in those with levels in the ranges 0.48–0.53 mmol/l (8.0–8.9 mg/100 ml) and 0.42–0.47 mmol/l (7.0–7.9 mg/100 ml), respectively.[63] More recently, dual-energy CT scanning has been shown to effectively identify deposits of monosodium urate in tissues non-invasively and provide a measurement of the total body solid urate load.[64] Using this technique, only around a quarter of those with blood serum urate levels above 0.41 mmol/l (6.9 mg/100 ml) were found to even have evidence of urate crystal deposition.[65]

Urate Crystal Formation

So, what protects individuals with hyperuricaemia[j] from urate precipitating as crystals in tissues and triggering inflammation? For reasons that are poorly understood, the amount of urate dissolved in blood plasma can be much greater than predicted by its solubility in water. At concentrations above 0.41 mmol/litre (6.89 mg/100 ml), plasma becomes supersaturated. In a test tube, crystals may not form spontaneously until the monosodium urate concentration is more than 10 times allowed by its theoretical solubility.[66] As with any supersaturated solution, whether or not a crystal forms is dependent on the interplay between factors that enhance solubility and factors that promote crystal nucleation. Once an initial crystal forms, further crystals can then precipitate around it in a secondary manner. The exact variables which affect urate crystal formation in the body are currently unknown, but there may be something about gouty individuals that makes them particularly prone.[67] It is also not known why urate crystal formation takes place preferentially at the typical sites susceptible to acute gout (i.e. the ball of the big toe) and tophus formation (i.e. the outer ear), as the whole body is exposed to a high urate level. A possible explanation is that this

---

[j] i.e. a high blood monosodium urate level.

may be related to the effect of a lower temperature in affected sites reducing urate solubility and disposing to crystallisation – a notion that would have been favoured by Abraham Buzaglo (see Chapter 4)! [68] Taking this line of thought further, maybe Thomas Sydenham's observation that the first fit of gout (in England) usually occurs in January or February was due to this being the coldest time of year, particularly in seventeenth-century houses without central heating.[69]

Freudweiler had attempted to address the issue of whether a small quantity of urate crystals in tissues might be able to 'seed' secondary crystal nucleation but was unable to find evidence for this with his animal injections.[70] This chain reaction concept was popularised later by Jay Seegmiller and colleagues, who suggested that the acidic microenvironment created by early gouty inflammation might lead to further crystal precipitation, with amplification and prolongation of the response; however, again, this was not supported by experimental evidence.[71] Moreover, recent studies have actually shown that monosodium urate is slightly more soluble in a mildly acidic environment, and so that could not be the whole story. A plausible hypothesis is that the local slightly acidic milieu of inflammation releases calcium ions from attachment to proteins, making them free to form calcium urate and trigger secondary monosodium urate crystallisation.[72] Along the same lines, lead cations can readily combine with urate anions to produce insoluble lead urate and be the seed for secondary crystal formation. I discuss in Chapter 12 the theory that lead pollution was a major player accounting for the assumed high prevalence of eighteenth-century gout.[73]

A final point to bring out is that mechanical shock can enhance urate crystal formation, at least in the laboratory.[74] This may help explain how an acute gout attack is commonly triggered by a knock or blow to a joint.

Urate Crystal Phagocytosis and Its Consequences

Once formed, urate crystals may be phagocytosed by leukocytes, just as Metchnikoff described for bacteria. This leads to the release of chemical mediators, such as interleukin-1 beta (IL-1β), which build up inflammation through the recruitment of white blood cells and their activation, as discussed above. That leukocytes are necessary for gouty inflammation seems obvious now, but this was experimentally shown to be the case by McCarty and colleagues in 1966. They found that gouty arthritis failed to occur in dog joints injected with urate crystals if blood leukocytes had previously been depleted from the bone marrow.[75]

Acute gouty inflammation is self-perpetuating as recruited leukocytes encounter fresh urate crystals. However, it is also self-limiting, whereas bacterial inflammation often results in abscess formation if left untreated by antibiotics. This failure of gouty inflammation to suppurate with pus formation was recognised as early as the 1600s and highlighted by Ben Welles in his *Treatise on the Gout or Joint-Evil* (1669).[76] As mentioned earlier, this was why John Hunter saw gouty arthritis as a 'true specific inflammation'.[77] Alfred Garrod, likewise, regarded the lack of suppuration as the hallmark of gouty inflammation:

> Gouty inflammation differs from common phlegmonous inflammation ... especially in not being followed by suppuration. If a medical man, by chance entirely ignorant of the nature of gout, were to see a toe affected with this disease in its full intensity, swollen, hot, red, and tender, he would probably think that the affection must of necessity terminate in suppuration; yet I believe this never happens as the result of simple gouty inflammation.[78]

Spontaneous Resolution

Gouty inflammation does not suppurate because it terminates by itself. Using a similar approach to Max Freudweiler, the team in my laboratory at the Hammersmith found in the 1990s that the phase of leukocyte recruitment from the blood is quite brief, peaking at about six hours after experimental injection of urate crystals.[79] Furthermore, inflammation subsides as phagocytic monocytes differentiate over time into a type of macrophage that ingests crystals without releasing proinflammatory factors but instead releases factors such as Transforming Growth Factor β (TGFβ),

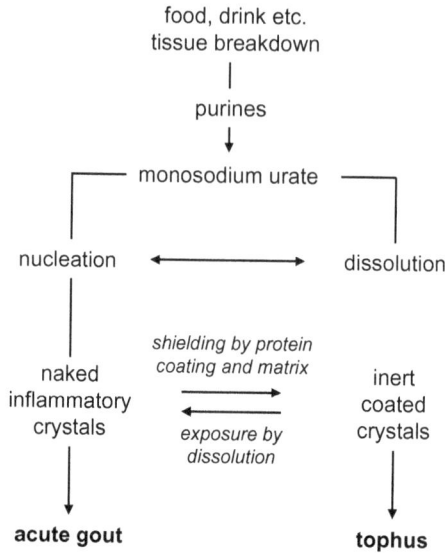

food, drink etc.
tissue breakdown

|

purines

↓

monosodium urate

nucleation ←——————→ dissolution

*shielding by protein
coating and matrix*

naked
inflammatory
crystals

inert
coated
crystals

*exposure by
dissolution*

acute gout   **tophus**

Figure 9.6.

Simple schematic diagram illustrating how monosodium urate crystals triggering of an acute inflammatory response depends (i) on the balance between crystal nucleation and solubilisation, and (ii) whether or not crystals are naked or shielded by protein coating and surrounding matrix.

which actively suppress inflammation (see Figure 9.4(e)).[80] Also, as will be discussed further in Chapter 12, urate crystals are much less inflammatory once they become coated with certain body fluid proteins and encased by a matrix within the tissues.[81] This chemical and physical protection most likely explains how urate crystals can be present in tophi without causing inflammation. A schematic diagram illustrating the role of urate crystals in gout is shown in Figure 9.6.

Crystals and the Diagnosis of Gout

There can be little doubt that the inflammation seen in James Gillray's *The Gout* (see Chapter 1) and so brilliantly documented in writing by

Sydenham (see Chapter 2) was what we call gout today. However, back in the day, some people saw gout and arthritis as much the same thing. Thomas Dover (see Chapter 4) wrote a chapter on 'Gout or Arthritis' in his popular *An Ancient Physician's Legacy to his Country* (1762) for general readers.[82] Similarly, in his self-serving *A Treatise on the Regular, Irregular, Atonic and Flying Gout* (1792), written for patients, the jobbing physician William Rowley (1743–1806) did not consider gout to be a form of arthritis – it was arthritis: 'Arthritis, vel *Morbus Articularis*, or what we call The Gout, is derived from αρθρός, articulus or joint'.[83]

We now know, however, that all that glistened in the past was not gouty gold. Today, most forms of arthritis can be distinguished through distinct clinical features and laboratory tests, although, occasionally, acute arthritis can cause diagnostic uncertainty. The blood urate level is not a faithful guide, as most people with a high level do not have gout (see above) and because the blood urate level can fall to the normal range during an acute gout attack.[84] Max Freudweiler had particularly stressed the value of polarising microscopy for detecting urate crystals, and Dan McCarty and Joseph Hollander sealed this as a diagnostic test:

> Since it is important to make the diagnosis of this most treatable disease in the field of arthritis with some degree of certainty, aspiration of gouty joints with microscopic examination of the synovial fluid for crystals, by a polarizing microscope if possible, should become the standard diagnostic procedure.[85]

Joint fluid crystal analysis is now a key component of the American College of Rheumatology/European League Against Rheumatism consensus diagnostic criteria for gout.[86]

Given all this, the actual frequency of true gout in Georgian times can be nothing but a guess. That said, all the bandaged feet in the cartoons, the ubiquitous gout stools in homes and private member clubs and the endless plausible descriptions of gout attacks in letters, newspapers and books, both by the victims and the physicians (and often they were the same), do leave one with the impression that true gout really was more common than it is today. I discuss possible lifestyle and environmental predisposing causes and triggers that may explain this in Chapter 12.

Reflections on Crystals and Inflammation

So, with all the knowledge that we have now, was Thomas Sydenham completely mistaken to accept the old humoral theory (see Chapter 2)? It is easy to be dismissive, and certainly Sydenham's notion that gout attacks prevent other diseases is quite wrong (although the same may not necessarily be the case for uric acid *per se*; see Chapter 13). However, as both Sydenham and Hunter realised, the point of inflammation is to protect and correct rather than to make things worse. Moreover, if we take uric acid to be the humour in excess, urate crystal formation and subsequent inflammation do give scientific substance to old beliefs.

The likes of Robert Kinglake were, however, partly correct in suggesting that gouty inflammation is not unique. Soon after conducting the experiments substantiating the inflammatory nature of urate crystals, McCarty and his group described a similar acute arthritis caused by calcium pyrophosphate crystals, which they named 'pseudogout'.[87] Furthermore, it has become clear that similar inflammatory responses can be induced experimentally by a number of other types of particle.[88] Importantly, the list has extended to cholesterol crystals and, probably, other forms of debris that make up the necrotic cores of arterial atherosclerotic plaques, which lead to heart attacks and strokes.[89] In some ways, an atherosclerotic plaque is comparable to a gouty tophus in that it is a sterile deposit of debris surrounded by connective tissue and has a variable degree of chronic inflammation. A very recent report suggests that atherosclerotic plaques can also contain plastic nanoparticles derived, presumably, from a polluted environment.[90]

Although inflammatory responses to different particles vary in intensity and duration, a common denominator is the activation in phagocytic cells of an intracellular protein complex, known as the NLRP3 inflammasome, and the subsequent release of IL-1β.[91] This is centrally involved during the elaboration of inflammation, with its direct and indirect actions including the induction of adhesion molecules for leukocytes on vascular endothelial cells and the attraction of leukocytes into and within the tissues. Testifying to the shared mechanisms between gout and athero-sclerosis, a recent cardiovascular clinical trial showed that a therapeutic antibody against IL-1β not only decreased cardiovascular events (i.e. heart attacks and strokes) due to atherosclerosis but also halved the number of attacks of acute gout.[92]

Chapter 10

From *Colchicum* to Colchicine

Now that the inflammatory nature of urate crystals is established, we can return to where we left off with *Colchicum* and the concerns over its safety (see Chapter 5). One of the driving ambitions of nineteenth-century organic chemistry was to isolate the active ingredients of medicinal plants to remove impurities and allow more consistent dosing. The first in line for this was the *principium somniferum*[a] of opium poppies, which Richard Mead (see Chapter 3) had described in 1708 as 'a volatile alcaline salt intimately mixd and combin'd with an oily sulphureous substance'.[1] Over the following 100 years, many chemists attempted to purify the principal further, and it was Friedrich Sertürner (1783–1841), a junior pharmacist in Paderborn in North Rhine-Westphalia, who succeeded where others had failed. In around 1804, he crystallised an alkaline factor, which he found to be highly effective in relieving his toothache, and named it morphium after Morpheus, the Greek God of dreams.[2] The name was adjusted to morphine by the Parisian chemist Joseph Louis Gay-Lussac (1778–1850), and it subsequently became customary to give other plant-derived 'alkaloids'[b] the suffix '-ine'. The list of purified alkaloids is now considerable, consisting of over 3,000 natural compounds, and many have been adopted into medicine as is or have provided leads for the synthesis of other useful compounds.[3] Many plants contain several alkaloids, the opium poppy being

---

[a] Soporific principle.
[b] An 'alkaloid' is a nitrogen-rich plant compound which has a physiological or pharmacological effect on animals.

a good example, since it harbours narcotine, codeine, thebaine, papaverine and narceine, in addition to morphine.

Early Attempts to Isolate the Active Principle of *Colchicum Autumnale*

The Parisian chemists Pierre-Joseph Pelletier (1788–1842) (see Figure 10.1(a)) and Joseph Bienaimé Caventou (1795–1877) were the international frontrunners in the early days of plant alkaloid chemistry. Among their many achievements were the first isolation of chlorophyll, the green leaf pigment of photosynthesis[4]; the isolation of quinine from *Cinchona officinalis* bark – the 'cortex' of Thomas Sydenham[5]; and the naming of caffeine.[c] Another plant they analysed for alkaloids was *Veratrum album*, the white hellebore that James Moore suggested was the active ingredient for *L'Eau Médicinale* (Chapter 5). In 1817, they announced the isolation of 'veratrine', which they concluded could also be found in *Colchicum autumnale*.[6]

One of the instigators of the move of pharmacy teaching and research from apothecary shops to university departments was Philipp Lorenz Geiger (1785–1836) (Figure 10.1(b)).[7] After his apprenticeship, Geiger settled in Heidelberg, where, in 1814, he purchased the university pharmacy. By 1821, he had established his own private lecture series, and he sold the pharmacy and manoeuvred himself with difficulty into a university lecturing position. Fending off the claims of the medics to own pharmacy, he moved it into a separate university discipline not subsidiary to medicine. His major scholarly contributions both date back to 1824: the first was his widely used *Handbook of Pharmacy to Accompany Lectures and for Self-Study by Doctors, Pharmacists and Chemists*,[d] and the second was his taking over the editorship of *Magazin für Pharmacie*. Geiger enhanced

---

[c] i.e. café-ine.

[d] Originally in German, *Handbuch der Pharmacie zum Gebrauche bei Vorlesungen zum Selstunterrichte für Ärzte, Apotheker und Droguisten.*

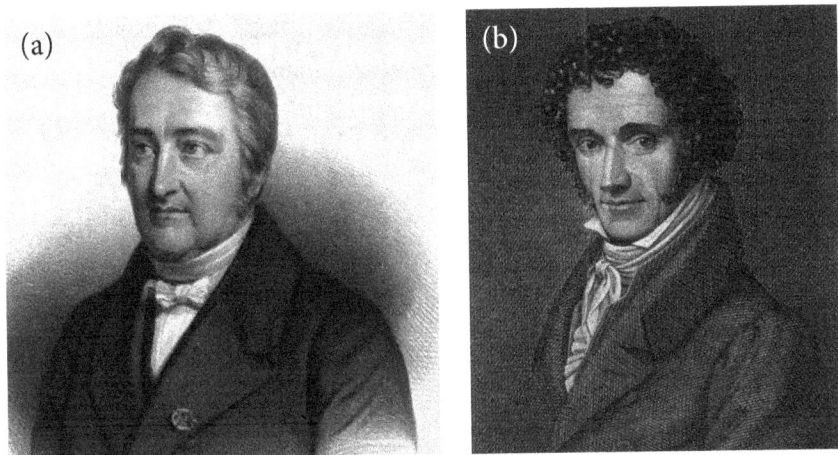

Figure 10.1.

(a) Pierre-Joseph Pelletier. Lithograph by Nicolas-Eustache Maurin.

(b) Line engraving of Philipp Lorenz Geiger by F. Rosmaesler after J. W. C. Roux, 1829.

Source: (a) Courtesy of the Wellcome Collection, public domain; (b) courtesy of the US National Library of Medicine, public domain.

the scientific image of the journal by adding '*and the underlying sciences*'[e] to the title and by inviting Justus Liebig to be his coeditor. They made a brave attempt to improve peer-review of submissions to the journal. This initially involved testing the repeatability of experiments, but that turned out to be unrealistic. Nevertheless, they set a path towards higher standards of scientific publishing. The *Magazin* merged in 1832 with *Archiv des Apothekervereins im nördllichen Teuschland* to become the *Annalen der Pharmacie*.

Geiger's presence in this chapter is through crystallising a compound from *C. autumnale*, which he called 'colchicine'. He realised that this was different from the veratrine described by Pelletier and Caventou, as it did not make him sneeze, while the substance he obtained from *Veratrum* species irritated the nose so badly that it was almost impossible to work with.[8] Geiger did not live to defend his discovery, as he died

---

[e] Originally in German, *und die dahin einschlagenden Wissenschaften*.

soon afterwards.[9] His contribution to the story also ended there, as it is doubtful that he isolated the main medicinal substance from *C. autumnale*. Nevertheless, the name stuck. After Geiger's death, Liebig built the journal they had edited together into one of the top chemistry journals, changing the title to *Annalen der Chemie und Pharmacie* and then, in 1874, to *Justus Liebig's Annalen der Chemie*. In 1998, it became the *European Journal of Organic Chemistry*. The sequence of journal titles tells a tale of pharmacy's gradual inclusion into mainstream chemistry.

Over the next 50 years, several other German and French chemists attempted to crystallise Geiger's substance from *Colchicum* but failed. They came up with various other factors they designated as colchicine, colchicëine and apocolchicëine; however, it was not clear whether these variants really existed within the plant or were just artefacts formed during the harsh laboratory procedures required for their isolation.[10] Crude *Colchicum* tincture remained the standard treatment for gout, with the *British Pharmacopoeia* published in 1864 by the new General Medical Council instructing *Vinum Colchici* to be made from four ounces of macerated *Colchicum* corm and one pint of sherry.[11]

Isolation and Chemical Identity of Colchicine

It was the French pharmacist Alfred Houdé (1854–1919) who worked out how to reliably isolate the alkaloid we now call colchicine in a crystallised marketable form. In the 1880s, he founded the pharmaceutical company Laboratoire Houdé to produce and market 'colchicine Houdé'.[12] The formulation can still be purchased today. Even after pure colchicine was available, unstandardised and potentially dangerous *Colchicum* wines and tinctures continued to be recommended by physicians well into the twentieth century.[13]

The three-ring molecular structure of colchicine was originally proposed by Adolf Windaus (1876–1959) at the University of Göttingen in 1924. Windaus later won the Nobel Prize for Chemistry for his work on cholesterol, vitamin D and related sterols (see Figure 10.2(a)).[14] He held that there were three benzene rings in the colchicine molecule, each composed of six carbons. In 1940, Aaron Cohen and colleagues at the Chester Beatty Research Institute in London (now the Institute of Cancer Research) proposed that Windaus's ring 2 might have seven carbons, and then in 1945, Michael Dewar (1918–1997) at the University of Oxford suggested that the

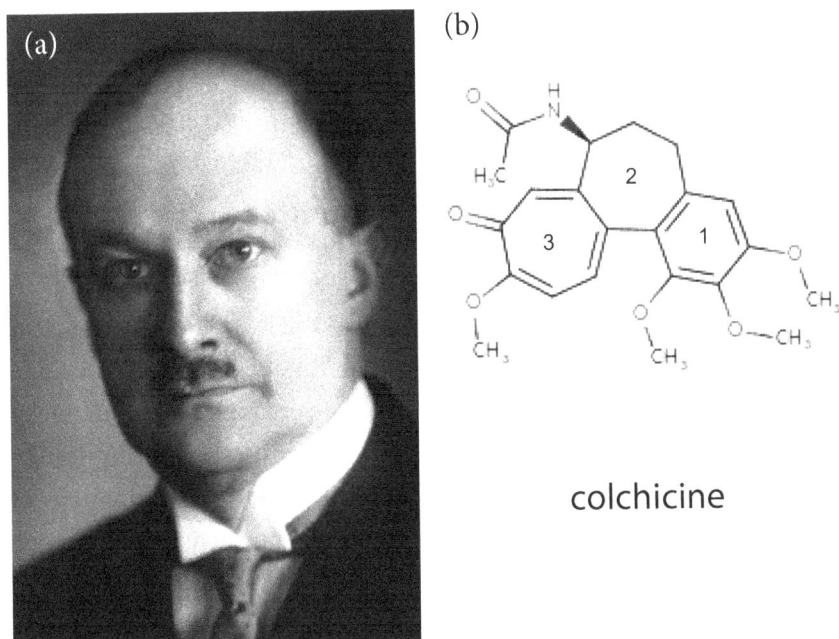

colchicine

Figure 10.2.

(a) Adolf Windaus was the first chemist to deduce the three-ring structure of colchicine. He went on to win the Nobel Prize for his work on cholesterol and vitamin D.

(b) Windaus proposed in 1924 that the colchicine molecule was composed of three six carbon rings. Later, Pepinsky and colleagues established using X-ray crystallography that Windaus's rings 2 and 3 (as numbered) each have seven carbon atoms (King *et al.*, 1952).

Source: (a) Courtesy of the Nobel Foundation via Wikimedia Commons, public domain.

same was the case for ring 3.[15] This made colchicine a 'tropolone'-derivative, after a name Dewar had previously coined for a similar ring structure in stipitatic acid, a metabolite of the *Penicillium stipitatum* mould.[16] Dewar's proposal was confirmed in 1952, when the exact structure of colchicine was solved through X-ray crystal analysis in the laboratory of Ray Pepinsky (1912–1993) at Pennsylvania State University (see Figure 10.2(b)).[17] Knowing this paved the way to the chemical synthesis of colchicine, a task that had previously proved elusive.[18] With modern analytical techniques, it has become clear that plants within the *Colchicum* genus also produce several colchicine variants in lesser amounts, perhaps explaining the inconsistent results of the many chemists who first attempted the isolation.[19]

Early Pharmacological Experiments

In March 1816, Everard Home (see Chapter 5) had communicated the results of his experiments with *Colchicum* to the Royal Society in London on behalf of 'The Society for Improving Animal Chemistry'. This was a dining club offshoot of the Royal Society and consisted of a small number of fellows interested in the links between chemistry and physiology.[20] Home reported some simple experiments designed along the lines of a similar study on the effects of opium, previously performed by his mentor John Hunter (see Chapter 9).[21] Injection of a *C. autumnale* extract directly into the jugular vein of a dog led to similar physiological effects to those seen after giving the drug by mouth, but with a faster action. From this, Home concluded that the drug acted after passing into the circulation rather than acting as a direct purgative on the stomach and intestine. Such was the public interest in *Colchicum* as the new treatment for gout that the work was reported as far and wide as the *Taunton Courier and Western Advertiser*.[22]

After that, various attempts were made to assess the effects of *Colchicum* derivatives on animals, and various erroneous conclusions were drawn. A prevalent view was that the drug was a poison, acting both on the central and peripheral nervous systems, and that its therapeutic action was as a pain killer.[23] However, as with most other pharmacological experiments at the time, interpretation was hampered by the lack of a pure compound.

Once Houdé's preparation became available, its effects could be established more precisely. Initial efforts were focused on understanding the toxic effects. In 1890, Carl Jacobj (1857–1944) reported that high doses of colchicine excited peristalsis in the gut and then paralysed breathing via an effect on the respiratory centre in the brain (Figures 10.3(a) and (b)).[24] This was at that early stage in Jacobj's career when he was working in Strasburg under Oswald Schmiedeberg (1838–1921), who was a driving force behind the success of the German pharmaceutical industry before World War II. Jacobj went on to become professor of pharmacology in Tübingen and is best remembered for pioneering pharmacology work using isolated perfused organs (see Figure 10.3(c)).

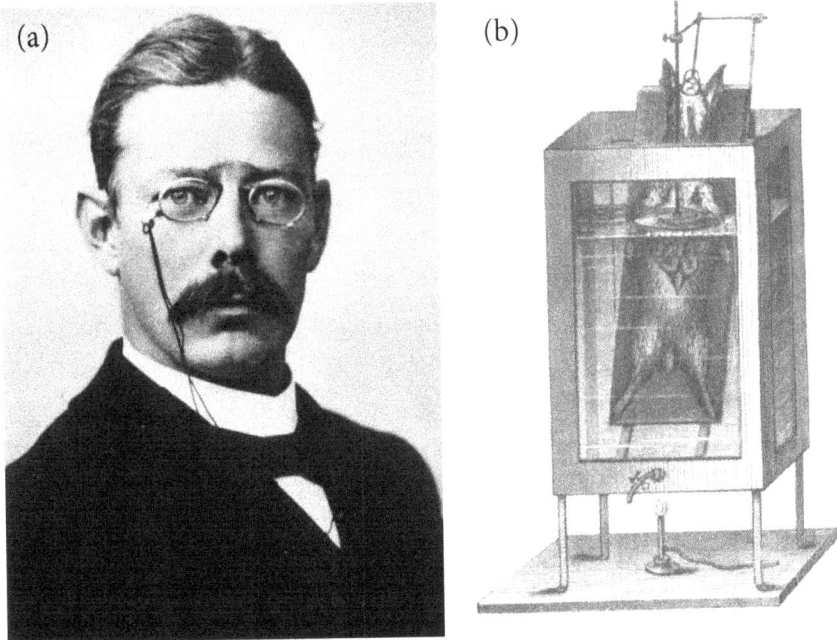

Figure 10.3.

(a) The early pharmacologist Carl Jacobj was the first to publish the effects of pure colchicine on animals but did so at a high dose to explore its effects as a poison.

(b) Jacobj's apparatus for studying the effect of colchicine on intestinal peristalsis.

(Continued)

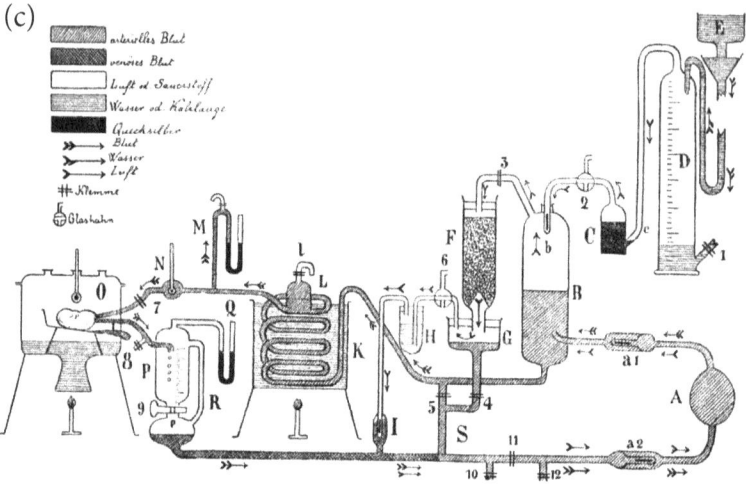

Figure 10.3. (*Continued*)

(c) Jacobj's elaborate apparatus for physiological studies on isolated organs. Jacobj's work was important to the development of heart–lung bypass systems for use in cardiac surgery.

Source: (a) and (c) Via Wikimedia Commons; (b) from Jacobj (1890); all are public domain.

Jacobj's view that colchicine primarily acted on the nervous system held sway for some years and fitted the neurological narrative to gout (see Chapter 9). An alternative mechanism emerged in 1908 when Walter Dixon (1871–1931) and Walter Malden (1858-1918) in Cambridge published similar experiments, in which they had set out to look for selective effects of colchicine on autonomic nerves that regulate the bowels.[25] They made the unexpected finding that injecting colchicine into rats, rabbits or dogs caused numerous immature cells in the process of dividing to appear in the blood[f].[26]

The significance of Dixon and Malden's observation was not clear at the time, and it took over 20 years for it to be followed up. These were the very early days of cancer chemotherapy, and Albert Pierre Dustin had been

---

[f] It later transpired that an Italian scientist named Pernice had published similar findings in a Sicilian journal earlier in 1889.

working for some years in Brussels to develop anti-tumour drugs. In the early 1930s, one of his medical students, F. J. Lits, injected colchicine into mice and observed a 'une véritable explosion de mitoses'[g] throughout the body.[27] These cells subsequently died in a manner similar to cells exposed to irradiation. Dustin followed up Lits' experiment with a study of his own and confirmed the observation.[28] Not long afterwards, the Hungarian plant biologist László Havas came to work with Dustin and demonstrated similar effects of colchicine on wheat seedlings, indicating that this was an effect of colchicine on a fundamental aspect of cell biology common to animals and plants.[29] Although Dustin had initially held the view that this was all because colchicine was a powerful cell stimulant, it became clear that colchicine freezes cells in the process of dividing. It does this by inhibiting the formation of the mitotic spindles that pull chromosomes apart during cell division (see the following).

Lits graduated from Brussels and took up a fellowship at Yale in the United States to study the effects of colchicine on tumours in mice.[30] Once there, he discussed his work with Edgar Allen (1892–1943), who saw the potential of colchicine for research on the effects of sex hormones. Allen had already made pioneering steps towards the discovery of oestrogens and had come to Yale as chairman of the Department of Anatomy in 1933.[31] The problem was that it was difficult to identify which cells were affected by hormones, as cell division is normally so rapid that few dividing cells can be seen in the snapshot of a tissue section mounted on a microscope slide. By pre-treating mice with colchicine prior to injection of theelin,[h] Allen was able to count the number of cells trapped in cell division over a fixed period. He established that the effects of the hormone on cells in the uterus, cervix and vagina were very much more extensive than previously appreciated and was also able to pinpoint the exact cell types that were involved.[32] Allen laid down some of the essential foundations

---

[g] 'A veritable explosion of mitoses'. Mitosis is the form of cell division that leads to two offspring cells that are identical to the parent cell.

[h] A natural ovarian hormone now called oestrone.

for our understanding of the endocrine functions of the ovaries and was nominated four times for the Nobel Prize over the course of a career that was terminated by a fatal heart attack at the age of 50. Following a talk by Allen at a meeting of the American Association for the Advancement of Science in 1936, several other US investigators became interested in colchicine as a cellular research tool.[33]

A Detour with Colchicine into Early Genetic Modification

What caused a much bigger stir at the time was the finding that colchicine could be used to double the chromosome count in cells.[34] To explain this, most animals and plants are 'diploid', with cells having one set of chromosomes from each parent. Prior to mitotic cell division, each of the chromosomes duplicates itself. The duplicates then separate under the guidance of fine spindles, resulting in a complete set of chromosomes entering each of the offspring cells. As mentioned, colchicine prevents spindle formation and hence prevents duplicated chromosomes from separating. If colchicine is washed away, the cells may resume division but with double the original chromosome count (i.e. tetraploid) (see Figure 10.4(a)).[35] If the brief colchicine treatment is repeated, there can be further doubling of the chromosome count. Cells with more than the regular diploid count are termed 'polyploid'.

All this happened before genes were found to be housed in DNA and at a time when genetic research was focused on understanding chromosomes. Colchicine now provided a valuable laboratory tool for working out how chromosomes segregate during cell division. At the forefront of the American effort was Albert Blakeslee (1874–1954), the director of the Carnegie Institution Department of Genetics at Long Island, New York, and a leading authority on plant genetics. He had made his career developing Jimsonweed (*Datura stramonium*) into a leading plant for genetic research.[36] Blakeslee saw changes in plant morphology associated with polyploidy as a way to substantiate the still-controversial contribution of chromosomes as the location of genes and heritability. Beyond that lay the hope of gaining

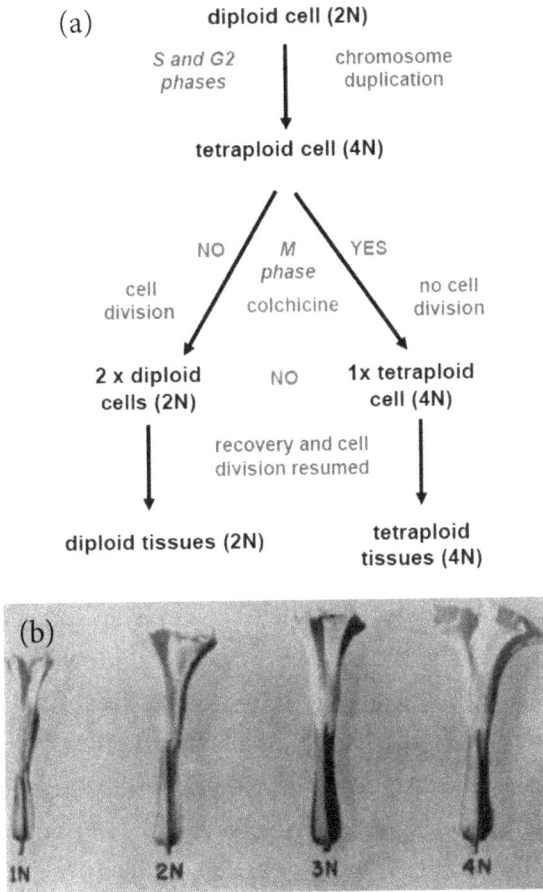

Figure 10.4.

(a) Mitotic cell division involves DNA synthesis and chromosome duplication (S phase) and nuclear breakdown (G2 phase), followed by the separation of duplicated chromosomes and the formation of two cells, each with its own nucleus (Meta- or M phase). In the presence of colchicine, the cell stalls in M phase with the failure of chromosome separation. If colchicine is washed away and the cells allowed to recover, cell division recommences starting with four sets of chromosomes, resulting in tetraploid (4N) rather than diploid (2N) tissues.

(b) Increased size of flowers of *Datura stramonium* according to complement of chromosomes. From left, 1*n* (haploid), 2*n* (diploid), 3*n* (triploid) and 4*n* (tetraploid). From Blakeslee (1939).

insights into how to cross-breed plants more effectively to create useful variants for horticulture and agriculture. Blakeslee had been trying, with very limited success, to induce polyploidy for years, and colchicine offered a brilliant opportunity.[37] He was able to induce polyploidy in his *Datura* and other seeds after soaking them briefly in a tap-water solution of colchicine. Seeds so treated with colchicine are easy to identify since they are larger, as likely are the genetically modified plants that grow from them.[38] There was now a reliable genetic way to 'improve' plants – all due to a drug for gout.

Colchicine was a cutting-edge talking point at the 7th International Congress of Genetics, held in Edinburgh at the end of August 1939 on the eve of World War II.[39] Blakeslee reported that he had succeeded in doubling the chromosome number of around 50 different plant species from 29 genera and 16 families.[40] Aside from being a shop window for colchicine, the conference is of particular interest in showing how genetics was entrapped at the time by febrile political ideologies.[41] The USSR delegates backed out, even though they were at the forefront of the field in the 1930s. The conference had originally been planned for Moscow two years earlier, under the presidency of Nikolai Vavilov (1887–1943), one of the world's leading plant geneticists. However, this was not accounting for the rise of the agronomist Trofim Lysenko (1898–1976), who had filled Joseph Stalin's ear with promises of ever better agricultural harvests by the application of his politically correct theories of environmental rather than genetic influences on inheritance.[42] The conference was postponed by the Soviet Politburo, after which the venue was shifted to the University of Edinburgh. Just 10 days before the opening of the meeting, Vavilov wrote that neither he nor any of the many other Soviet delegates would be attending. Ostensibly, this was due to the meeting having been taken away from the USSR, but the truth was that the geneticists were well out of kilter with Lysenko and had been forbidden by Stalin to attend. In the following years, Stalin denounced geneticists for their 'bourgeois' science. Vavilov was arrested in August 1940 and sentenced to death on a charge of rightist conspiracy. Although his sentence was commuted to 20 years in prison, he died in 1943 in the Saratov Gulag, officially of pneumonia but probably helped by starvation.[43] Many European and American geneticists were themselves communists and found themselves having to square their politics with the news of the purge on geneticists that filtered through from Moscow.[44] With regard to Lysenko, misguided and power-hungry as he unquestionably was, there is some irony in colchicine providing the first means by which humans can adapt the germline, albeit of plants. An article in the *Pittsburgh Post-Gazette* hailed Blakeslee as having 'thrown overboard the literal interpretation of the notion that acquired characteristics are not inherited' and explicitly linked him with Lysenko in pursuing a common noble goal of improving the farm.[45]

Many plants are naturally polyploid.[46] At an evolutionary level, the genetic redundancy offered by chromosome duplication can reduce the impact of dangerous mutations and facilitate genetic variation and the emergence of new species.[47] Obvious survival advantages provided by polyploidy include enhancing defence against herbivorous predators and attracting new pollinators through changes in flower size, pattern or colour.[48] Blakeslee found that tetraploid plants created using colchicine were usually more robust compared with diploids, with larger leaves, flowers, fruit and seeds (see Figure 10.4(b)).[49] He fully realised the agricultural and horticultural potential of colchicine treatment 'to improve life processes'.[50] There followed a gold rush of professional and amateur plant breeders keen to try their hand and create profitable variants without the slow slog of conventional crossbreeding.[51] As early as October 1939, the *Pittsburgh Post-Gazette* carried an enthusiastic feature with the title 'Drug aids in producing bigger and better plants – Colchicine becomes wonder drug in plant breeding'.[52] Again, in 1941, the same paper posted an article on 'Science speeding up evolution to grow finer food for us', informing the public of 'Astonishing short cuts that bridge years of growth, remove wrinkles from tomatoes, straighten out cucumbers and give beauty treatment and more vitamins to most garden products – all because a drug stops plant cells from dividing'.[53] In the United States, this was government sanctioned, demonstrated in 1961 by a self-help manual from the Department of Agriculture on how to use colchicine for genetic modification, all without any apparent consideration of potential ecological consequences.[54]

The ears of poultry breeders pricked up with the colchicine promise. Edna Higbee reported in *Science* her creation at the University of Pittsburgh of some giant chickens, with twice-normal-sized combs and wattles and elongated tail feathers.[55] Two years later, the *Pittsburgh Press* was able to report the generation of 'giants that tip the scales at nine or ten pounds and have silken plumage that would make an ordinary barnyard fowl green with envy'.[56] However, Higbee does not appear to have successfully bred from her freaky fowl. Early work in mammals likewise showed that while cell polyploidy was relatively easy to induce in the laboratory, subsequent animal development was hard to achieve.[57] In fact, spontaneous polyploidy in mammals is rare, probably because it usually results in the failure of embryonic development. Indeed, we now know that polyploidy in human embryos is seen in around one in five miscarriages.[58] Gösta Häggqvist, professor of anatomy and histology at the Karolinska Institute in Stockholm, succeeded in generating two giant rabbits using colchicine, one male and the other female.[59] Neither showed any interest in the opposite sex. The male was feeble, with libido that:

> ... was not very strong. If the female was averse, he soon got tired of mounting her and seated himself quietly in a corner without paying her any more attention. As for the super-female, she behaved very aversely. When mounted she cried, ran away and even attacked the males.

Both eventually had offspring, but these all died before or shortly after birth. Häggqvist also generated a giant pig, which grew to an enormous size of half a metric ton and 2.29 meters long but does not appear to have had offspring (see Figure 10.5).[60] Ultimately, the use of colchicine for bird and mammal genetic modification went nowhere, and farmers began to rely on hormones to make livestock larger.

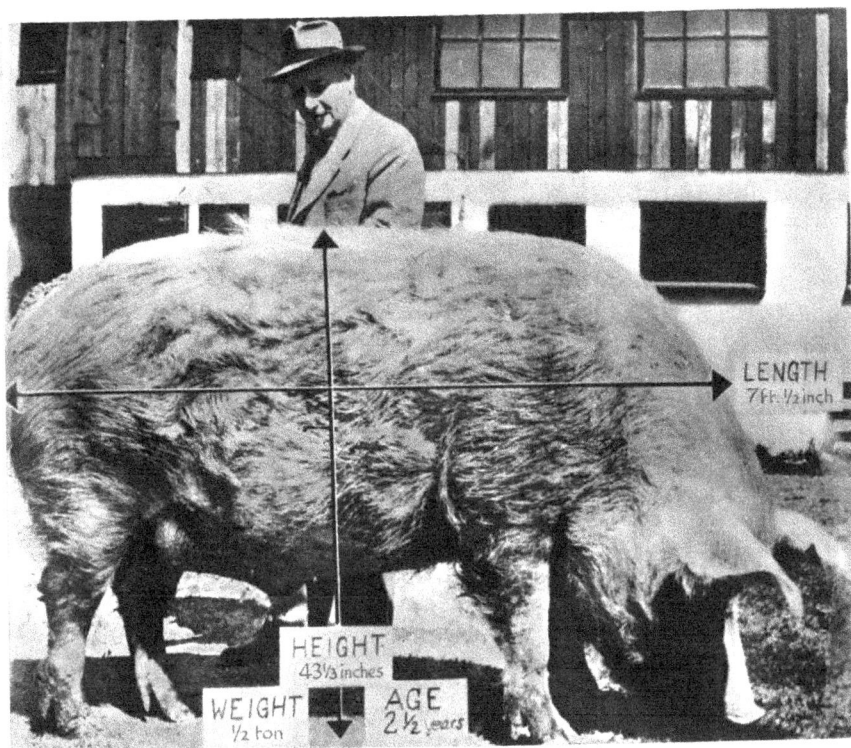

Figure 10.5.

Professor Gösta Häggqvist of the Karolinska Institute in Stockholm standing behind his giant pig created using colchicine. *Illustrated Sporting and Dramatic News.* 7 July 1954.

Source: Under licence @ Illustrated London News/Mary Evans.

Not everyone was so ecologically unconscious. The *Pittsburgh Sun-Telegraph* associated colchicine with *The Food of the Gods* by H. G. Wells (1866–1946), a dystopic novel in which scientists invent the growth-accelerant Heraklephorbia IV and test it on chicks, which become giant hens. The substance accidentally leaks into the environment, leading to, among many other plant and animal anomalies, rats as big as ponies and wasps that had to be hunted with shotguns.[61] Pandora's box had been opened, and environmental havoc ensued. In the words of the American Indian folklorist Arthur C. Parker (1881–1955): 'Unless mankind soon learns how to know itself, its knowledge of the universe and its mastery of energies may in the end contribute to the destruction of all humanity instead of its elevation'.[62]

In 1955, Orie Eigsti co-authored *Colchicine in Agriculture, Medicine, Biology and Chemistry* with Pierre Dustin, Albert Dustin's son and by then a distinguished pathologist in Brussels.[63] The book reviewed the hundreds of scientific papers published during the colchicine fad of the late 1930s and 1940s. Eigsti had conducted research on the chromosomal effects of colchicine as a postdoctoral researcher at the Carnegie Institution and had been instrumental in introducing Blakeslee to the drug.[64] A triploid plant can be created by back-crossing a colchicine-induced tetraploid with the original diploid plant, and Eigsti exploited the fact that such triploids tend to be seedless and sterile by founding the American Seedless Watermelon Corporation to promote more agreeable watermelons for the table. The idea took many years to catch on but was eventually successful, and the company was bought by Novartis when Eigsti was in his 90s.[65] For Pierre Dustin, the book was a tribute to his father, who, as president of the University of Brussels, had refused to open up the institution to the German occupation during World War II and had subsequently died in prison. Because of the university closure, the undoubted achievements of the Belgium group on colchicine were overshadowed by the American researchers who were able to continue working throughout the war.[66]

The Discovery of Tubulin

At the time that Orie Eigsti and Pierre Dustin's book came out, it was clear that colchicine affected the formation of the spindles that pull chromosomes apart during cell division, but what were the spindles made of? It was researching this fundamental cell biology question rather than a particular interest in a gout drug that led to the discovery of colchicine's action at a molecular level and indeed illuminated how mitotic spindles operate.[67]

Careful examination of various cell types under an electron micro-scope had shown that the spindles that pull chromosomes apart possess cylindrical structures, now called microtubules.[68] Furthermore, similar microtubules could be seen in cilia, flagella and spermatozoa tails, suggest-ing that they have evolved to play various roles in cell biology. Knowing that colchicine interfered with spindle formation, the biochemical question was to what exact molecular structure does it bind. Edwin Taylor and his team at the University of Chicago developed a technique for tracking mole-cules to which colchicine binds in cell cultures by labelling colchicine with tritium (^{3}H, a beta radiation emitter).[69] Having separated the cell extracts into fractions, they found that the colchicine-linked radioactivity was associated with a protein subunit of microtubules and that colchicine pre-vented subunit polymerisation.[70] Soon afterwards, Hideo Mohri, working at the University of Tokyo, published the amino acid composition of this colchicine-binding protein subunit and named it 'tubulin'.[71]

Colchicine, tubulin and cancer chemotherapy

Albert Dustin's interest in colchicine had, of course, been in its potential to kill cancer cells selectively by arresting their cell division – just as we have seen was attempted later by Hitchings and Elion using purine analogues (see Chapter 8).[72] Encouraged by an anecdotal report that cancer patients improved after treatment with *Colchicum* extract[73] and armed with the new insight that colchicine affects cell division, preclinical studies were performed to look for effects on experimental tumours, and it was found that tumour cells are particularly susceptible to the drug.[74] As early as 1935, Emmanuel Amoroso (1901–1982), working at the Royal Veterinary College in London, found that colchicine slowed down tumour growth in mice.[75] However, subsequent attempts to treat cancer patients with colchi-cine found that the gap between the dose that led to desired effects and the dose that was toxic (i.e. the 'therapeutic index') was too narrow to be practicable.[76] Efforts were made to identify *Colchicum*-derived chemical variants with similar effects on cell division but with less toxicity, and there was a ray of hope following the discovery of desacetylmethylcolchicine, which was developed for clinical use by Ciba Pharmaceutical Company with the trade name Colcemid. It was tested in a small number of patients with leukaemia; however, despite initial promise, unacceptable side-effects again prevented its widespread adoption.[77]

Although colchicine itself failed as an anti-cancer drug, inhibiting microtubule function remained a possibility as a cancer chemotherapy strategy. It then became clear that colchicine is not unique among plant alkaloids in interfering with microtubules and causing cell mitotic arrest. Some others have a more acceptable therapeutic index than colchicine and are now in routine clinical use as anti-cancer drugs (see Figure 10.6).[78] Vinblastine and vincristine both come from Rose periwinkle (*Catharanthus roseus*) and act like colchicine by disrupting microtubules. In contrast, paclitaxel (from Pacific Yew, or *Taxus brevifilia*) and laulimalide (from bacteria that live symbiotically on the Tongan marine sponge, or *Cacospongia mycofijiensis*) act by stabilising tubulin in the microtubules and preventing their dynamic disassembly.[79] Either way, these agents prevent cell division.

Coevolution of colchicine and the tubulin gene

Albert Blakeslee had found that algae are susceptible to colchicine.[80] It is curious that so many plant alkaloids affect tubulin, and this is probably an example of parallel evolution of a common defence strategy against herbivorous predators. Thus, it later transpired that the outer lining of aphid intestines is rich in microtubules.[81] Ingesting a tubulin inhibitor must be a powerful disincentive for them to continue with their meal. Since all plant cells have microtubules, why colchicine and other tubulin inhibitors do not poison the plants which make them has been a conundrum. As early as 1939, Albert Blakeslee had observed: 'The *Colchicum* plant is not affected by the colchicine in its own cells nor is there any swelling of roots or doubling of chromosomes evident when the roots are immersed in strong concentrations of the alkaloid colchicine. It is like a snake that is immune to its own venom.' Blakeslee thought that the *Colchicum* species might contain a chemical anti-colchicine, antibody-like agent for self-protection and tried hard to isolate one but without success.[82] Now that we have access to the gene sequences of plant tubulins, it has instead become clear that a plant that makes a tubulin inhibitor probably has a tubulin gene that has mutated such that the tubulin protein it encodes is not bound by the plant's

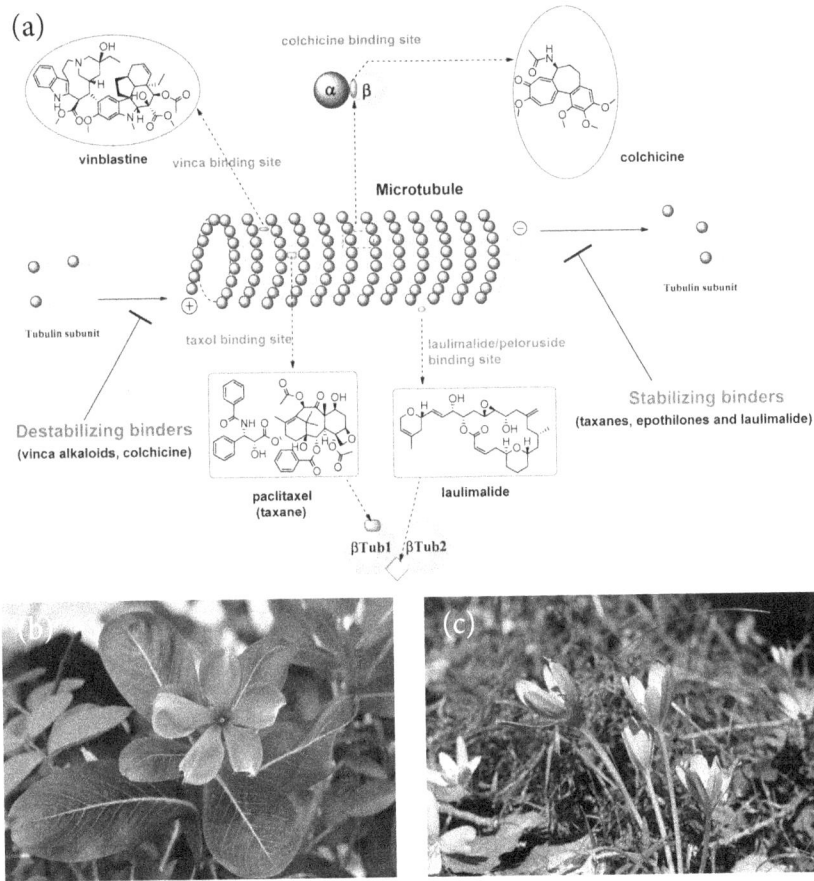

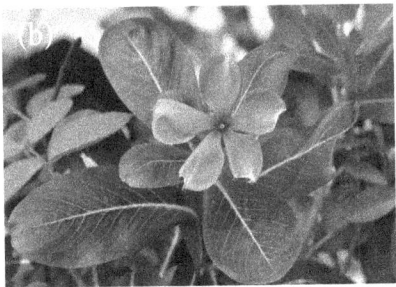

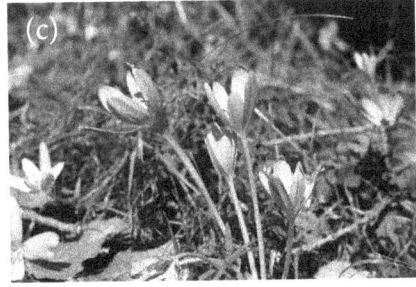

Figure 10.6.

(a) Numerous natural alkaloids interfere with tubulin function, either by destabilising or stabilising polymer assembly. From Banerjee *et al.* (2016) *Molecules* 21(11), 1468; doi: 10.3390/molecules21111468.

(b) Vinblastine derives from Rose periwinkle, *Catharanthus roseus*. Photograph by Joydeep.

(c) Colchicine derives from Meadow saffron, *Colchicum autumnale*, and other *Colchicum* species. Photograph by T. Kebert.

(*Continued*)

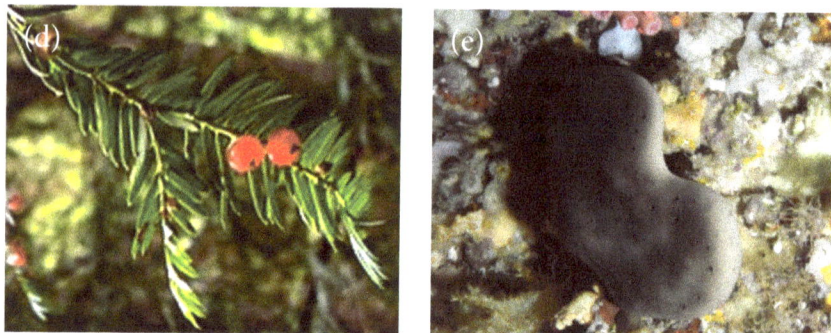

Figure 10.6. (*Continued*)

(d) Paclitaxel (taxane) derives from the Pacific Yew, *Taxus brevifilia*. Photograph by Jason Hollinger.

(e) Laulimalide derives from bacteria on the Tongan marine sponge, *Cacospongia mycofijiensis*. Photograph by Karen Stone and Dive Vava'u. From Miller *et al. Marine Drugs*, 2010;8:1059–1079.

Source: (a) and (e) Open Access Creative Common CC BY license; (b) and (c) via Wikimedia Commons, CC BY-SA 4.0; (d) via Wikimedia Commons, CC BY 2.0.

own tubulin-binding alkaloid.[83] This is a good example of how successful evolutionary adaptations often involve complementary parallel changes in more than a single gene.

Mechanisms of Action of Colchicine in Gout

Back to gout! Ten years after the introduction of probenecid as a urate-lowering agent (see Chapter 8), it was still not known why colchicine was so effective in treating acute attacks. There was still speculation that the primary site of action was on the nervous system or that it acted on an enzyme involved in purine metabolism.[84] While testing the effects of injecting urate crystals into the joints of gouty volunteers (see Chapter 9), Jay Seegmiller and colleagues took the opportunity of testing colchicine. They found that it was effective in attenuating inflammation if administered after the injection of crystals and that treating with colchicine before crystal injection largely prevented inflammation from occurring.[85] They also observed that colchicine prevented the phagocytosis of urate crystals by leukocytes, as well as the subsequent burst of leukocyte metabolic activity attributable to crystal uptake. Furthermore, colchicine was soon found to inhibit leukocyte migration, a necessary step for their entry into inflamed tissue (see Chapter 9).[86] Taken together, these observations helped establish the mechanistic basis of how colchicine is such an effective anti-inflammatory agent for preventing acute attacks of gout or treating them when they occur.[87] Once it was discovered that many of the inflammatory effects of urate crystals are due to activating the NLRP3 inflammasome (see Chapter 9), it was a small step to show that this is also inhibited by colchicine, presumably reflecting the need for microtubules.[88] These various anti-inflammatory effects of microtubule inhibition occur at just a tenfold lower concentration than that required to prevent mitotic cell division, explaining the narrow therapeutic window.[89] A further point is that neutrophils, the inflammatory foot soldiers among leukocytes, are particularly sensitive to colchicine, as they lack a transport mechanism for extruding it from the cell once absorbed.[90]

Unintended Consequences of Safety Regulation

Although pure colchicine seldom causes anything worse than loose bowels if used correctly, it is still potentially fatal in overdose and justifiably subject to regulation. How in the United States the Food and Drugs Administration (FDA) recently handled the licensing of colchicine illustrates the ongoing cat-and-mouse game in the profitable business of selling medicines. The 1984 US Waxman-Hatch Act had mandated that US market exclusivity should be awarded to newly approved drugs – a measure designed to encourage and reward the pharmaceutical industry for research and development. But newly approved drugs did not have to be new drugs, and the FDA let it be known that a short-term exclusive licence could be given to any company supplying data in support of the efficacy and safety of an existing, previously unevaluated generic agent. Suitably encouraged, a generic medicines company, URL Pharma, sponsored a small clinical trial to formally test the performance of its formulation of crystalline colchicine, Colcrys. Acute Gout Flare Receiving Colchicine Evaluation (AGREE) was a small study conducted on just 185 patients; nonetheless, such is the clear-cut effect of colchicine, the number of patients was sufficient to establish statistically what doctors and patients had known for years, namely that colchicine is effective at attenuating acute attacks of gout and that a brief treatment is as effective as a more prolonged one but has fewer side-effects.[91] AGREE was not even the first modern clinical trial that had shown the efficacy of colchicine in gout, as this had already been established by an Australian double-blind controlled study published in 1987.[92] It was, however, the first clinical trial of colchicine performed in the United States, and this enabled the company to gain FDA approval. Consequently, in July 2009, the FDA duly granted URL Pharma three-year exclusivity for the supply of colchicine for acute gout attacks. It also granted a three-year exclusive licence for the use of colchicine as an acute gout preventative, which had not been addressed by the AGREE trial. In addition, and remarkably, it granted a seven-year exclusive licence to the company under 'orphan drug' regulations for use in familial Mediterranean fever, a quite separate illness not tested in AGREE and again already an established indication for the drug.

Once exclusivity had been obtained from the FDA, URL Pharma promptly increased the cost of colchicine in the United States by fiftyfold, from around 10 cents to ~US$5.00 for each 0.6 mg tablet, arguing it had spent US$100 million on Colcrys development (of which ~US$50 million had apparently been paid to the FDA). It then initiated successful lawsuits to prevent five competitor companies from selling generic colchicine. In 2010, the FDA wrote to other US providers instructing them to stop marketing generic colchicine.[93] Although still substantially cheaper in real terms than *L'Eau Médicinale* had been in the early 1800s, the hugely ramped-up cost of colchicine was a blow to gout sufferers, although, considering their older age range, the substantial extra tab was largely picked up by the public purse. Reminiscent of Monsieur Delcroix's generous proposal to provide *L'Eau Médicinale* to the poor in 1812 (see Chapter 5), URL Pharma offered a three-month supply to low-income patients for US$15. Colcrys achieved a net sales of US$430 million in 2011, and the following year, URL Pharma was purchased for US$800 million by Takeda. Now that the exclusivity time has expired, colchicine is generic again, but it still costs about US$5 per pill in the US as generic drug companies set the drug at the new price. Colchicine can still be purchased for around 18p (~21 cents) per 0.5 mg tablet from generic suppliers in the UK and at similar low prices in most other countries.

The Colcrys pricing saga is by no means unique, as there are many other examples of companies price-hiking non-patent-protected generic drugs on the open market beyond reasonable affordability. An extreme example is that of Daraprim (pyrimethamine), a generic drug used to treat parasitic infections such as toxoplasmosis and malaria and which is on the World Health Organization's List of Essential Medicines. When Turing Pharmaceuticals took over marketing the drug, it raised the price from US$13.50 to US$750 per tablet and removed its competition by striking deals with the manufacturers to restrict access of other marketing companies to the drug.[94] Currently, there are class-action US lawsuits hanging over the heads of some 20 companies in relation to similar behaviour and conspiratorial price fixing.[95] The shenanigans are not just in the US, as several companies have been investigated and fined in the UK by the Competition and Markets Authority (CMA) for similar activities with other generic drugs, including enabling price hiking after paying off the competition.[96] It all goes to show that, without clear governmental control, *plus ça change* since *L'Eau Médicinale* commanded such high prices when it first came to London.

Colchicine in Modern Medicine

Colchicine has remained a mainstay for treating acute gouty arthritis and, since the early 1950s, has been widely used also for preventing flares of arthritis at the beginning of urate-lowering therapy (see Chapter 8). Its primacy for treating and preventing acute gout has not gone unchallenged, as salicylates and cinchophen became rivals in the late nineteenth century (see Chapter 9), followed by corticosteroids and Adrenocorticotrophic Hormone (ACTH) in the mid-twentieth century. The realisation that long-term use of corticosteroids or ACTH leads to serious untoward consequences led to a massive expansion in the so-called non-steroidal anti-inflammatory drugs (NSAIDs) in the latter half of the twentieth century. Up to 50 NSAIDs have been available at one time or another, testifying to the size of the market not only for gout but for many other inflammatory indications. Space does not allow for more details on their relative strengths and weaknesses, and many are still in general use. However, it is fair to say that NSAIDs, as a class of drugs, have followed the well-trodden track, from enthusiasm to disillusion. Consequently, for all the fearsome safety reputation of *Colchicum* extracts (Chapter 5), pure colchicine is a survivor.

For many years, colchicine was considered a 'specific' for gout, even to the point of the 'colchicine trial' being considered a diagnostic test when evaluating the cause of a difficult-to-diagnose arthritis.[97] While colchicine is unlike steroids or NSAIDs in modifying inflammation in general, its benefits are not confined to gout. Other conditions for which colchicine is now routinely prescribed include other forms of crystal-induced arthritis (e.g. 'pseudogout') (see Chapter 9), familial Mediterranean fever and pericarditis. A new and potentially very important application for colchicine may be in the affordable prevention of heart attacks and strokes due to atherosclerosis.[98] This is based on the relatively recent appreciation that atherosclerosis is a chronic inflammatory reaction driven by the innate immune system's response to particulate matter, such as cholesterol crystals and oxidised lipoproteins trapped in the walls of large- and medium-sized arteries, with both similarities and differences to the response to monosodium urate crystals in gout (see Chapter 9).

Chapter 11

In the Family

William Cadogan probably realised that he was overstating things when he wrote in 1771 that gout was all only about 'indolence, intemperance, and vexation' (see Chapter 3). Many saw this as not just insulting personally but offensive to the whole family. Gout was in the bloodline, similar to holding an aristocratic title. In Charles Dickens' *Bleak House*, written later in the 1850s, Sir Leicester Dedlock:

> … receives the gout as a trouble-some demon, but still a demon of the patrician order. All the Dedlocks, in the direct male line, through a course of time during and beyond which the memory of man goeth not to the contrary, have had the gout. It can be proved, Sir. Other men's fathers may have died of the rheumatism or may have taken base contagion from the tainted blood of the sick vulgar, but the Dedlock family have communicated something exclusive, even to the levelling process of dying, by dying of their own family gout. It has come down, through the illustrious line, like the plate, or the pictures, or the place in Lincolnshire. It is among their dignities. Sir Leicester is, perhaps, not wholly without an impression, though he has never resolved it into words, that the angel of death in the discharge of his necessary duties may observe to the shades of the aristocracy, 'My lords and gentlemen, I have the honour to present to you another Dedlock certified to have arrived per the family gout'.[1]

Quite apart from Sir Leicester's quaint obsolescence, Dickens had a point about the fatalism with which some people accept illness even today, particularly if it is deemed to be inherited. Whether that is so for gout is the subject of this chapter.

Mendelian Genetics

The science of genetics might be said to have begun with the work of Gregor Johann Mendel (1822–1884) (see Figure 11.1(a)), an Augustinian friar in what is now the South Moravian region of the Czech Republic. From around 1856, he cross-bred garden peas, analysing the heritability of simple characteristics, such as flower position, seed shape, plant height and colour. Several contemporaries, including Charles Darwin, were also using peas for hybridisation research, but what distinguished Mendel was his mathematical education and statistical approach to his results.[2]

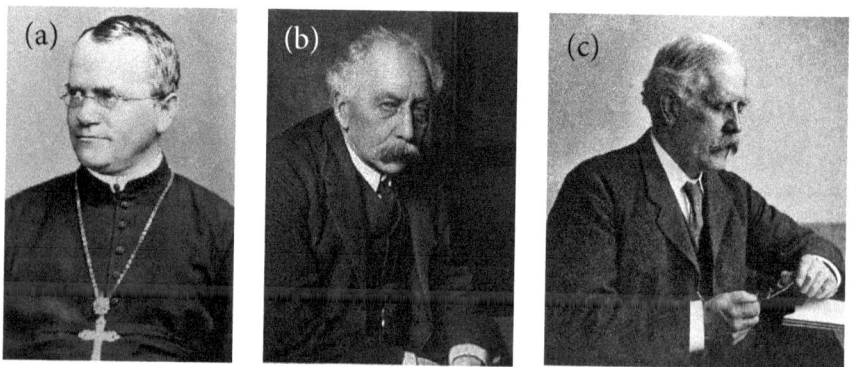

Figure 11.1.

(a) Gregor Mendel by an unknown photographer. Mendel initiated the field of modern genetics through his experiments cross-breeding peas but received little recognition for his work during his lifetime.

(b) William Bateson, who introduced Mendel's work to Britain.

(c) Bateson's influence came into medicine via Archibald Garrod, who discovered genetically inherited inborn errors of metabolism and thereby originated the field of medical genetics. Photographer unknown.

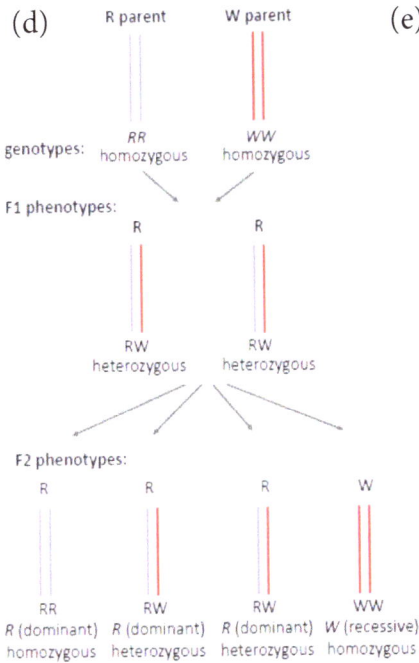

(d) R parent — W parent

genotypes: RR homozygous / WW homozygous

F1 phenotypes: R / R

RW heterozygous / RW heterozygous

F2 phenotypes: R R R W

RR R (dominant) homozygous / RW R (dominant) heterozygous / RW R (dominant) heterozygous / WW W (recessive) homozygous

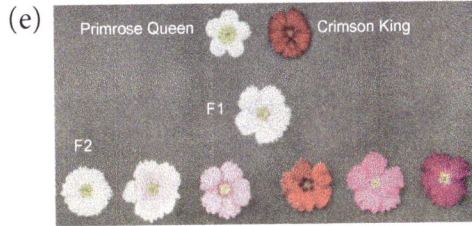
Primrose Queen / Crimson King / F1 / F2

Figure 11.1. (*Continued*)

(d) Mendel found that crossing plants with round (R) *versus* wrinkled (W) peas led to all first-generation (F1) plants having round peas, showing that the round trait was dominant. Inter-crossing these led to the re-emergence in the second generation (F2) of plants with wrinkled peas at a frequency of one in four. From this and other experiments, he deduced that W was a recessive trait.

(e) Both Mendel and Bateson based their fundamental genetic work on plant breeding. The image illustrates the crossing of two Primula varieties: Primrose Queen and Crimson King. All the F1 plants are the same and indicate that white is the dominant colour. However, the F2 generation formed from self-fertilising the F1 plants shows a greater complexity that can only be explained by the flower colour and pattern being attributable to dominant and recessive alleles of several genes being redistributed. The image is entitled 'Heredity in *Primula Sinensis*' and is the upper part of plate VI in *Mendel's Principles of Heredity*, William Bateson, Cambridge, 1909.

Source: (a)–(c) Via Wikimedia Commons: (a) and (b) public domain, (c) CC BY 4.0; (e) public domain.

Incidentally, there is no evidence that Darwin knew of Mendel's work, but Mendel was a keen follower of Darwin's.[3]

The conclusion that Mendel came to was not only the obvious one that some traits are inherited but also that some traits dominate over others. Thus, when a plant exhibiting a dominant trait was crossed with one bearing a non-dominant 'recessive' trait, all the offspring had the dominant characteristic. However, if a first-generation (F1) progeny was bred by self-fertilisation to form F2s, the recessive trait reappeared in one in four offspring. From this and similar experiments, Mendel laid down two laws of inheritance. The first, the law of segregation, is that each individual inherits two shares for a particular characteristic, one from each parent. A recessive trait cannot be expressed unless it is inherited from both parents (see Figure 11.1(d)). The second law, that of independent assortment, states that the two shares do not influence each other when passed on to the next generation. Mendel discontinued his plant studies in around 1868 when he was promoted to Abbot, and he died in 1884, largely unknown.

Mendel's observations challenged the prevailing view that crossing animals or plants leads to a simple blending of the differences between parents, like a cocktail. His legacy was championed in England by William Bateson (1861–1926) in Cambridge (see Figure 11.1(b)), and it was Bateson who coined the term 'genetics' in 1905 to cover the science of heritability that is independent of environmental influences.[4] Bateson received little support from his university colleagues, who were traditionally slow to adopt a new idea. He relied on female students to conduct his ambitious breeding programme: women at the time being on the fringe of academic acceptability themselves.[5] His main collaborator was Edith 'Becky' Saunders (1865–1945), who, as an undergraduate, became friends with Bateson's sisters at Newnham College. Bateson and Saunders together introduced the term 'allelomorph' (i.e. 'other form'; now simply 'allele') for an inheritable variant of a given characteristic.[6] The team's work on plant crossings substantiated Mendel's and showed that numerous dominant and recessive alleles are involved in the phenotypes of outbred strains (Figure 11.1(e)).

Inborn Errors of Metabolism

The Batesons were family friends with the Garrods, and William Bateson suggested to Alfred's fourth son Archibald (henceforth A. E. Garrod) (1857–1936) (see Figure 11.1(c)) that human diseases might be inherited in a similar fashion to the inherited characteristics of Mendel's peas.[7] A. E. Garrod had been born in 1857, just as Mendel was starting his experiments.[8] He obtained a first-class undergraduate degree at Oxford and then studied medicine at St. Bartholomew's Hospital in London. After that, he worked for some years in his father's Harley Street private practice while waiting for a hospital appointment, and under the wings of his father, he published *A Treatise on Rheumatism and Rheumatoid Arthritis* in 1890.[9]

Like so many who had come before him, A. E. Garrod focused his early research on the chemistry of urine as a window to diseases and published a series of papers using spectroscopy[a] to detect porphyrins in urine.[10] His paper, 'A contribution to the study of the yellow colouring of the urine' was read by his father to the Royal Society in 1894.[11] The relevance of porphyrins lay in their possible contribution to the formation and colouring of uric acid stones, and A. E. Garrod wrote papers on uroerythrin and urochrome as the causes of their rose and yellow tints.[12] All these were achieved alongside his chemist friend, Frederick Gowland Hopkins, who developed a widely adopted urine test for uric acid.[13] Hopkins went on to become the first professor of biochemistry at Cambridge and to receive the 1929 Nobel Prize for Medicine or Physiology for his work on vitamins. We meet him again briefly in Chapter 13, where he finds uric acid in butterfly wings.

Alkaptonuria is a rare condition in which the urine turns dark brown to black upon exposure to oxygen in the air. It was first described by Alexander Marcet (see Chapter 8) in 1823 and was so named in 1859 by the German pharmaceutical chemist Carl Bödeker (1815–1895), who detected an unusual reducing substance in affected urine that he called alkapton.[b,14] This was isolated in 1891 and renamed homogentisic acid. The oxidation of homogentisic acid in the skin, ears, eyes, joints and heart valves accounts for the dark colouration of tissues that is the signature of the condition and which Rudolf Virchow (see Chapter 9) referred to as ochronosis.[15]

---

[a] The scientific method of studying materials based on detailed patterns of wavelengths or colours.

[b] i.e. alkali-captured.

Initially, this was thought to be an inconsequential curiosity, but we now know that it causes early arthritis, kidney stones and heart valve failure.

In 1892, A. E. Garrod was appointed assistant physician at Great Ormond Street Children's Hospital. One of his young patients was an infant whose nappies had stained black the day after birth. Realising the child had alkaptonuria, he simplified the test for detecting homogentisic acid and started looking for other cases.[16] He discovered that most affected children had unaffected parents but that the parents were usually first cousins.[17] This was hard to square with the contemporary view that alkaptonuria was due to abnormal fermentation of the amino acid tyrosine by microorganisms in the intestine. Garrod instead proposed that 'alkaptonuria is what may be described as a "freak" of metabolism, a chemical abnormality more or less analogous to structural malformations'.[18] Through Bateson, Garrod realised alkaptonuria followed the rules of a Mendelian recessive inheritance.[19] He went on to discover three other familial recessive disorders: albinism, cystinuria[c] and pentosuria. Garrod summarised his findings to the Royal College of Physicians in his Croonian Lectures of June 1908, which were then published as his seminal *Inborn Errors of Metabolism*.[20] This was the launch pad for medical genetics.

The Search for a Single Gout Gene

The obvious next question was whether Mendelian genetics apply to gout. Being his father's son, A. E. Garrod must always have had this question on his mind and lectured on it at the British Medical Association Annual Meeting in 1904:

> as with the inborn errors hereditary plays a very important part in
> the aetiology of gout, and in families in which the tendency to gout
> is strongly transmitted the disease is apt to develop in members
> who have conformed to the strictest rules of living, and to develop

[c] Cystinuria causes cystine urinary stones, which had been discovered a century earlier by William Hyde Wallaston (see Chapter 6).

at earlier ages in succeeding generations ... there are comparatively few diseases in which the hereditary tendency is altogether absent, so that it is even possible to classify families according as their members afford good or bad soil for the exanthemata.[21]

However, A. E. Garrod did not actually conduct research into the genetics of gout, and there was little progress until the 1940s. Given the research challenges caused by the still vague clinical definition of gout, the simpler task was to study the inheritance of monosodium urate levels. John Talbott published evidence in 1940 that relatives of individuals with gout also frequently have relatively high urate levels in the blood while not necessarily having gout themselves.[22] Then, in June 1948, the results of three systematic family studies were presented at the American Rheumatism Association annual conference in Chicago. As they drew similar conclusions, the three groups then published a consensus in *Science* later that year, with further details of two being published separately later.[23] Overall, the results did not support a single culprit gene affecting urate levels, but this remained the working hypothesis. Deviations from a Mendelian distribution of urate levels within families were rationalised by assuming that a putative single genetic variant showed 'incomplete penetrance'.[24] Views did not change much over the next 10 years, with Charley Smyth, working at the University of Colorado in Denver (see Chapter 8), writing in 1957 that 'the dyscrasia known as "Classical Gout" is generally considered to be an inborn error of metabolism characterized by an increased concentration of uric acid in the blood and body fluids'.[25] This remained the dominant belief, with the zoologist Joan Keilin writing in an influential review two years later that hyperuricaemia 'is a genetically controlled disturbance of purine metabolism, a single dominant autosomal gene[d] probably being responsible for its transmission'.[26]

Come the 1960s, hyperuricaemia was still considered a single-gene inborn error of metabolism. Encouragement for this then came with the

---

[d] An autosomal gene is one not on an X/Y sex chromosome.

discovery of two distinct conditions in which a variant of a single gene caused gout. First, there was von Gierke's disease,[e] which has a recessive heritability and is due to a deficiency in the enzyme glucose-6-phosphatase. The enzyme is needed to extract glucose from glycogen stores in liver and muscle. When defective, low glucose levels result in a buildup of ketones and lactic acid, which, as we will see in Chapter 12, enhance urate reabsorption through kidney transporter channels. The condition tends to start in childhood, breaking Hippocrates' rule that gout does not occur before puberty in males or the menopause in females.

The second condition was identified in 1964 by Michael Lesch (1939–2008) and William Nyhan (1926–present) while the former was a medical student under Nyhan at Johns Hopkins in Baltimore.[27] Lesch–Nyhan syndrome has an X chromosome-linked recessive heritability, like classic haemophilia, and thus only occurs in males. It is a particularly unfortunate condition in which affected boys show mental retardation as well as cognitive and behavioural disturbances that include compulsive self-mutilation. In 1967, the defective enzyme was identified by William Kelley and Jay Seegmiller (see Chapter 9) at the National Institutes of Health in Bethesda as hypoxanthine guanine phosphoribosyl transferase (HGPRT). This acts to recycle hypoxanthine and guanine and hence reduce purine degradation to uric acid.[28] The same year, Kelley and Seegmilller reported on five gout patients from two families with histories of early-onset gout and renal stones but without obvious neurological features of Lesch–Nyhan syndrome. These patients had reduced but not absent HGPRT activity, suggesting that this could be one of the hereditary causes of common gout.[29] Two years later, the number of patients they had identified with what is now known as Kelley–Seegmiller syndrome had risen to 18.[30] A subsequent larger study conducted by Alexander Gutman and colleagues at the Mount Sinai Hospital in New York failed to confirm a more widespread involvement of HGPRT in gout. Among 425 individuals with a high

---

[e] Also known as Glycogen Storage Disease type 1.

urate level and gout and/or urinary stones, there were only seven cases of partial HGPRT, and five were in the same family.[31] Ultimately, therefore, discovering the genetic deficiencies of glucose-6-phosphatase and HGPRT did not take understanding the inheritance of common gout further forwards.

Renal hypouricaemia and urinary tract stones

Genetics can also cause a low level of urate in the blood (hypouricaemia). In renal hypouricaemia, there is an increased urate loss via the kidneys and a predisposition to uric acid stones. Two separate genes have been implicated as causing the problem, the first being *SLC22A12*, which is the gene for the URAT1 solute transporter channel introduced in Chapter 8. In the complex physiology by which the kidney deals with urate (see Chapter 8), URAT1 is the means by which the large majority of urate filtered by glomeruli is reabsorbed from the developing urine.[32] Loss of function mutations in the *SLC22A12* gene are mostly found in the Japanese population, but families among Iraqi Jews have also been identified.[33] Affected individuals do not respond to probenecid and other uricosuric agents, consistent with URAT1 being the main solute channel affected by these drugs. As might be expected from the low blood urate level, mutations of the *SLC22A12* gene protect against gout.[34]

Dalmatian coach hounds

The other genetic cause of renal hypouricaemia is a loss of function mutation in the *SLC2A9* gene, which is found in Japanese and Arabs and which encodes the GLUT9 solute transporter channel.[35] Mutation of the *SLC2A9* gene also accounts for the long-known urinary abnormality of Dalmatian coach hounds (see Figures 11.2(a)–(c)).[36] This was first reported by the clinical biochemist Stanley Benedict (1884–1936) (see Figure 11.2(d)), who is more remembered as the originator of Benedict's test, which was the first home test for diabetics to check the glucose level in their urines.[37] Realising that humans stand out from other mammals with respect to uric

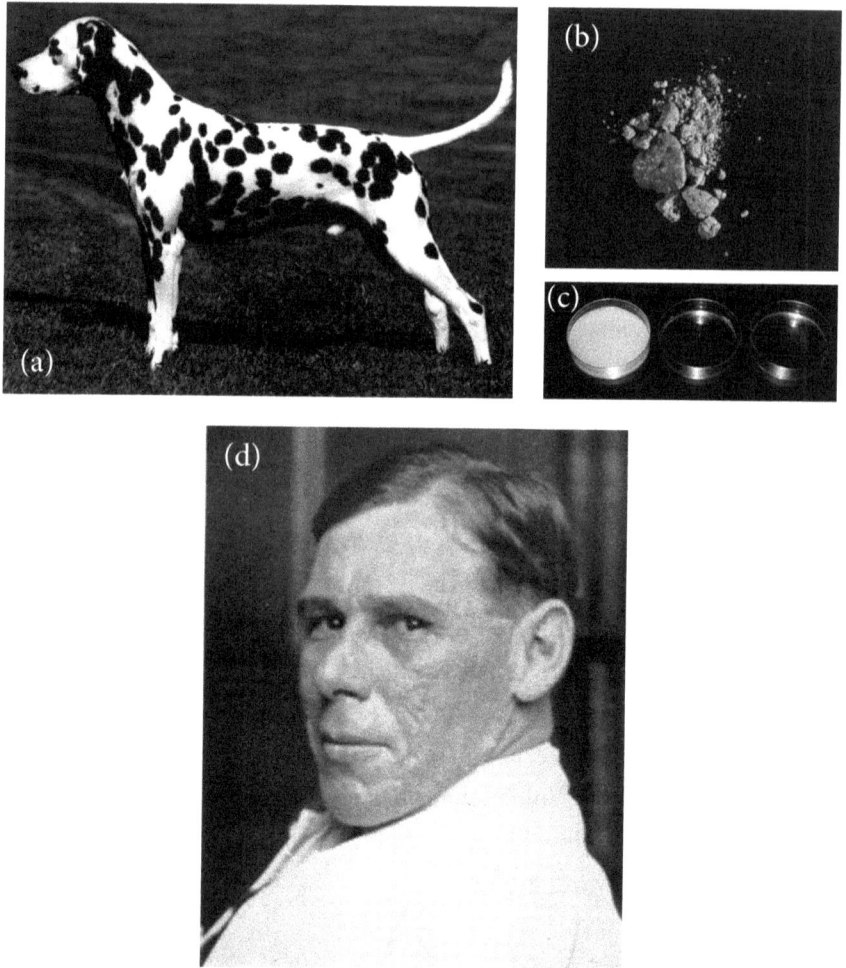

Figure 11.2.

(a) The Dalmatian coach hound with its characteristic black spots and patches.

(b) Uric acid urinary calculi from a Dalmatian.

(c) White uric acid crystallises out of Dalmatian urine (left dish), but not from urine from a Dalmatian–mongrel cross (middle) or from an unrelated breed (right).

(d) Stanley Benedict, who first drew attention to Dalmatian coach hounds having a genetic trait that leads to a very high urinary urate concentration. From a Biographical Memoir by Elmer Verner Mc Collum, National Academy of Sciences, Washington DC, 1952.

Source: (a)–(c) From Bannasch *et al.* (2008), public domain; (d) via Wikimedia Commons, public domain.

acid excretion (see Chapter 13), Benedict had been looking for a suitable animal with which to conduct clinically relevant research and stumbled on the Dalmatian coach hound, which passes much more urate in the urine than other dogs.[38] The high urate excretion makes them particularly liable to develop uric acid bladder stones, which commonly lead to obstruction to urine flow in the males.[39] The heritability of the abnormality was first addressed by Herbert Onslow at Oxford. He cross-bred a Dalmatian with a terrier for two generations and established that the abnormally high uric acid excretion likely followed a recessive Mendelian pattern of inheritance.[40] This was confirmed by a more extensive investigation by Clyde Keeler and Harry Trimble at Harvard, who, at the same time, showed through cross-breeding that the abnormality is not genetically related to the black on white coat spotting.[41] They did, however, find another interesting genetic feature, which is that whether Dalmatians run immediately behind the horse or further back behind the coach is related to genetically programmed 'bravery', albeit unconnected to uric acid excretion.[42] It has transpired that GLUT 9 is involved in the transport of urate into the liver as well as reabsorption from urine through kidney tubules, explaining the previous conundrum that the defect in Dalmatians can be cured by transplantation of a liver from an unaffected dog.[43] For owners, it is obvious if a dog is homozygous[f] for the variant gene, as its urine will result in white patches of crystallised uric acid on the lawn. However, a commercial DNA test is now available for anyone concerned that their mutt might be a carrier.

Physiological incompatibility with a single gout gene

Single-gene variants can thus certainly affect urate levels and gout, but discoveries emerged in the biochemical physiology of purines that posed serious problems for most gout being thus explained. As mentioned in Chapter 7, Ivan Horbachevsky (see Figure 11.3(a)) found that the glycine and urea can be combined to make uric acid – but all in a test tube.[44] The technical advances that enabled us to know just how uric acid is actually made in the body can be traced back to the discovery of deuterium

---

[f] i.e. affecting both the maternal and paternal copies of the gene.

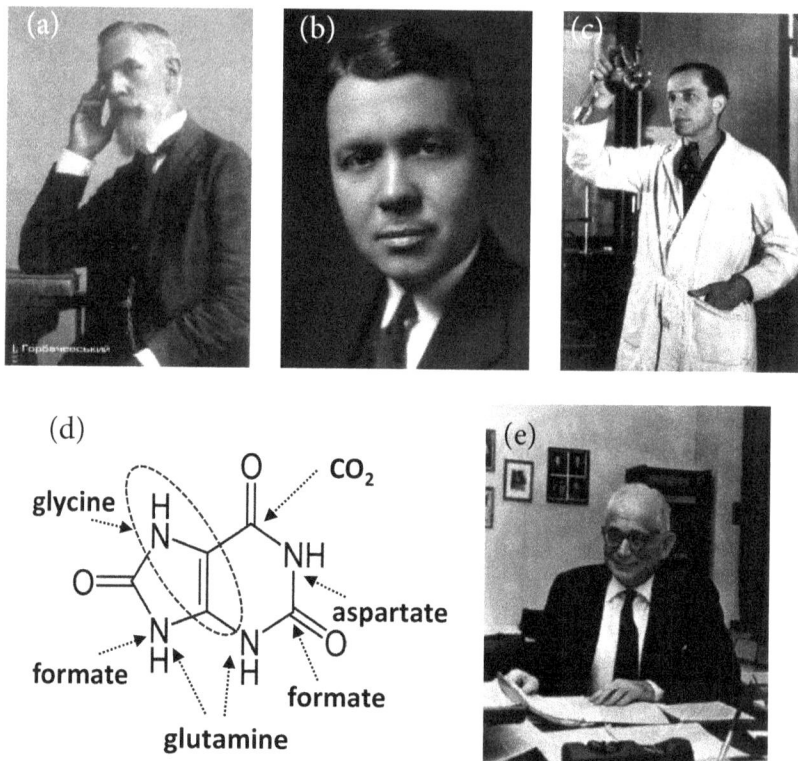

Figure 11.3.

(a) Ivan Horbachevsky, who first showed that uric acid could be synthesised in the laboratory from the amino acid glycine and urea.

(b) The radiochemist Harold Urey, who discovered deuterium (^{2}H, 'heavy hydrogen'), paving the way to the isolation of other stable isotopes.

(c) Rudolph Schoenheimer, who developed the technique of labelling organic precursors with stable isotopes for tracking the synthesis, distribution and degradation of purines in the body.

(d) Stable isotope labelling experiments enabled a map of the origins of the carbon and nitrogen atoms in uric acid. The amino acid serine is the chief source of the formate-derived carbon.

(e) DeWitt Stetten, who conducted his PhD studies under Rudolph Schoenheimer's supervision and applied the stable isotope tracer techniques to the study of uric acid physiology in humans.

Source: (a)–(c) Via Wikimedia Commons, public domain; (e) courtesy of the US National Library of Medicine, public domain.

by the Columbia University Professor Harold Urey (1893–1981)[g] (see Figure 11.3(b)). Deuterium (^2H, 'heavy hydrogen') is a stable, harmless isotope of hydrogen (^1H), and the two can be distinguished through mass spectrometry. It behaves chemically like hydrogen and can be introduced into organic compounds in the latter's place in the laboratory. The idea that compounds so tagged could be used as tracers to track the interconversion of organic compounds in the body was developed by the German biochemist Rudolf Schoenheimer (1898–1941) (see Figure 11.3(c)), working with Urey's PhD student David Rittenberg (1906–1970). Schoenheimer had carried out work in the late 1920s on cholesterol in atherosclerosis and provided some of the foundations for the discovery of statins.[45] In 1933, he fled Nazi Germany and became a colleague of Urey at Columbia.[46] Using deuterium-tagged compounds, Schoenheimer and Rittenberg performed seminal studies in rodents on the dynamics of body fat and cholesterol.[47] They established that fat and cholesterol are in a constant state of metabolic flux, marking a significant shift from the prevalent view at the time that tissues have a relatively fixed composition.

By 1937, Urey had succeeded in concentrating the stable isotope of nitrogen (^{15}N), which is approximately 0.4% of atmospheric nitrogen. This allowed Schoenheimer and Rittenberg to move on to studying the fate of nitrogen-containing compounds using the same approach.[48] The group published a series of papers establishing that amino acids can be synthesised from dietary ammonium and also that dietary amino acids provide nitrogen for incorporation into tissue proteins.[49] Sadly, Schoenheimer poisoned himself with potassium cyanide in 1941, much like Arthur Nicolaier would do a year later in Berlin (see Chapter 7) – both victims of Nazi oppression. His team members continued to add him as the last author on papers for another three years. One of these explored the incorporation of nitrogen into purines.[50] Refinement of the methods, as well as the use of the stable carbon isotope ^{13}C, soon led others to show that the atoms that

---

[g] For which Urey received the 1934 Nobel Prize for Chemistry. Not all radiochemistry is that innocent – Urey contributed significantly during World War II to the isolation of uranium-235 for use in the first atomic bomb.

make up uric acid mostly derive from the amino acids glycine, glutamine, aspartate and serine (Figure 11.3(d)).[51] Although much of this work was performed in pigeons due to the research convenience of high uric acid excretion in birds (see Chapter 13), the synthetic process was found to be similar in humans.[52]

It was DeWitt "Hans" Stetten (1909–1990) (see Figure 11.3(e)) who applied stable isotopes to the study of uric acid physiology. Stetten had previously worked in Schoenheimer's laboratory in Freiburg during a summer attachment, and now that Schoenheimer was at Columbia, he chose him as his PhD supervisor and learnt the stable isotope techniques.[53] After he moved to Peter Bent Brigham Hospital and Harvard in 1947, he and his colleagues established that the body pool of uric acid could be measured by determining the distribution and excretion rate of injected ^{15}N-labelled urate.[54] Not surprisingly, the pool was much higher in gouty subjects. Furthermore, they found that the urate in tophi was in a dynamic state, suggesting theoretically that it could be cleared by lowering urate levels and anticipating the effects of urate-lowering therapy once it became available (see Chapter 8).

With these new ways to study uric acid in the body, the key question was whether there is increased uric acid synthesis in gout. With this in mind, Stetton collaborated with Alexander Gutman and colleagues and found a more rapid transfer of ^{15}N from labelled-glycine into uric acid in some, but certainly not all, individuals with gout.[55] Other groups also had similarly variable results, such that no single physiological mechanism could be found, and hence a single hyperuricaemia gene was unlikely. The concluding durable statement on the matter came from Jay Seegmiller (see Chapter 8), who, in 1961, interpreted the observations of his own research group as follows:

> It seems unlikely that any single inherited disturbance of purine metabolism common to all gouty subjects would explain both an increased and a normal uric acid production. It may be more useful at this time to consider the hyperuricemia of gout to be the result of a variety of metabolic and physiological disturbances.[56]

Polygenic determinants of urate levels

Another problem for there being a single-gene variant causing hyperuricae-mia emerged from the large community studies conducted in the 1940s and 1950s, which showed that blood urate levels have a smooth, rather than a bimodal, distribution within populations after taking the effects of age and gender into account (for example, see Figure 11.4(a)).[57] There were hints in some studies of a small peak of higher readings, as would be expected from a single variant, but this was not generally the case.[58] Furthermore, the distribution curves of urate concentrations differed depending on the community. For instance, Filipinos and Polynesians were found to have increased urate levels compared to those of European origin, which for the Polynesians was irrespective of whether or not they were 'Westernised'.[59] Taken together, these new observations pointed towards any heritability of urate levels needing to be 'polygenic' with any number of genes potentially involved.

As mentioned at the start of the chapter, Mendel, Bateson and A. E. Garrod had no knowledge of the molecular basis of DNA or how genes are coded. The turn of the twenty-first century coincided with the first sequencing of the human genome,[h] an endeavour in terms of hard graft that was compared at the time to humans landing on the moon.[60] DNA technology has since advanced so rapidly that a human genome can now be sequenced in less than a day, and genomes of over a million humans have now been sequenced, not to mention those of many other animal and plant species, bacteria and viruses. Aided by computational data analysis, a genome-wide association study (GWAS) seeks to link genotypes[i] of individuals to phenotypes.[j] When this powerful approach was applied to blood urate levels in humans, the heritability was confirmed to be polygenic.[61] One way to illustrate this is with a 'Manhattan plot' (for example, see Figure 11.4(b)), in which the genome sequence is lined up chromosome by chromosome on the *x*-axis, and the probability of variation in a particular gene being

---

[h] i.e. all the genes.

[i] i.e. the precise genetic sequences.

[j] i.e. observable characteristics.

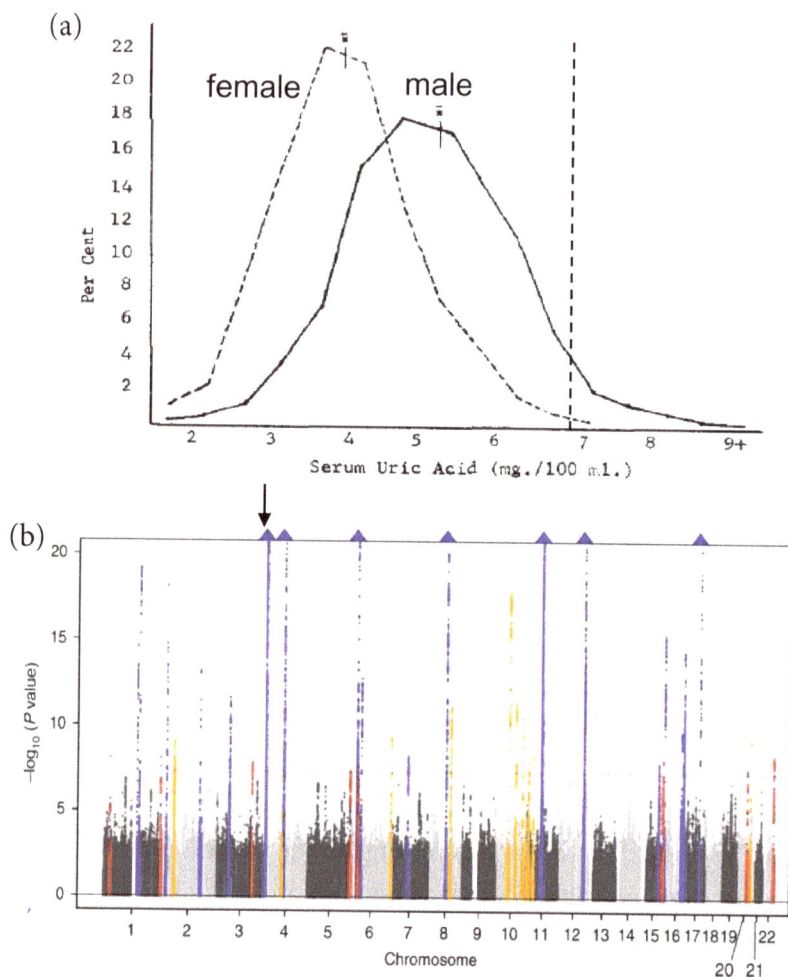

Figure 11.4.

(a) The distribution of monosodium urate levels in 32–64-year-olds in the Framlingham Heart Study population. Note the higher values in males. The vertical dashed line is the theoretical solubility threshold of monosodium urate in water (6.9 mg/100 ml, or 0.42 mmol/l). The normal distributions indicate that a single genetic variant as a cause of hyperuricaemia is unlikely. Adapted from Hall *et al.* (1967).

(b) Example of a Manhattan plot of the numerous genes influencing serum urate levels. From Nakatochi *et al.* (2019) *Commun. Biol.* 2: 115. The arrow points to *SLC2A9*.

Source: (a) Used with permission of Elsevier Science and Technology Journals, conveyed through Copyright Clearance Center, Inc.; (b) licensed under a Creative Commons Attribution 4.0 International License.

linked to a given phenotype, such as blood urate level, is shown on the *y*-axis. A predetermined horizontal line is set for statistical significance, and variants of genes above the line are deemed to be positively associated with the chosen phenotype.

If genetic inheritance was a card game, uric acid levels and the propensity to gout would be influenced by the whole hand dealt rather than holding, say, the two of clubs. To extend the analogy, modern statistical techniques and the analyses of very large numbers of genomes have led to a bad hand becoming increasingly large and complex, with variants of many genes being linked to urate levels.[62] Several of the proteins involved that have been linked to urate levels in humans are solute transporter channels (see Chapter 8). One of the strongest genetic associations is with variants of the *SLC2A9* gene (see above) that presumably influence the protein's quantity or function in kidney or liver.[63] However, the impact of *SLC2A9* genetic variation is still quite small, and indeed, the cumulative effect of *SLC2A9* and 34 other implicated genes associated with urate levels in Europeans only accounts for 6.9% of the variance between individuals.[64] Clearly, there may well be other genetic influences on urate levels that remain to be identified. Now that we have a good idea of the most important genetic sequence variants that make a difference, the next step will be to explore whether there are additional inherited 'epigenetic' factors that are not directly encoded in the genes but which affect the levels at which genes are expressed.

It is important to understand that finding an association between a genetic variant and disease does not directly establish that one leads to the other. However, there is a statistical technique known as 'Mendelian randomisation' that can address the issue of causation. This method involves randomising a group of subjects according to the presence or absence of a particular genetic variant and determining whether there is a phenotypic difference between the groups. As an example, using this approach, a *SLC2A9* variant has been found to causally increase the blood urate level, but only by a modest amount (0.022 mmol/l, or 0.37 mg/100 ml); however, it has been found to increase the tendency for gout by around 1.5-fold.[65]

Polygenetic predisposition applies potentially not only to the propensity for a high urate level but also to whether a high urate level leads to gout. This may well depend on any number of further heritable variables that govern the ease of urate crystallisation and the reactivity of the immune system to urate crystals once formed (see Chapter 9). Much remains to be determined, but the trend in gout, as well as in many other diseases, is towards resolving all the genetic variables into a single 'polygenic risk score'. Progress in this has been made, and a polygenic risk score has already identified variants linked to the age of onset of gout in men and the likelihood of developing tophi.[66] It is still early days, as an ultimate polygenic risk score will need to factor in influences of genetics on responses to lifestyle influences as well as ethnic variations (see Chapter 12).

Genetics and Responses to Drugs

Genetics can also influence responses to treatment. We do not know much about how genes affect the ability of drugs to do what is intended of them in treating gout, but it would be surprising if they turned out to have no influence. What we do know is that genetics can predispose to side effects, and this is well illustrated by allopurinol (see Chapter 8). The risk of developing a severe and potentially fatal adverse reaction is up to 12 times higher in Blacks, Asians and Native Hawaiians/Pacific Islanders than in Caucasians.[67] The reason for this, in large part, is a link with the *HLA B*5801* gene, a variant of the Class I D major histocompatibility complex, which has also long been known to be involved in the rejection of organ transplants. There is a strong case for testing for the presence of *HLA B*5801* before treating individuals in susceptible groups with allopurinol and choosing the more expensive febuxostat in those that are positive.[68] This exemplifies the influence of a single gene on the response to a drug; however, in the future, polygenic risk scores may be able to provide not only the likelihood of a disease but also the chances of positive and negative responses to particular agents and thereby enable more effective personalised medicine.

Reflections on the Genetics of Gout

Summarising this chapter, the recent explosion of new information stemming from genetic research has certainly confirmed that gout has a strong hereditary component, but not in the simple 'father-to-son' manner that Sir Leicester Dedlock might have imagined in the nineteenth century. Nor did gout turn out to be attributable to a variant of a single gene as one of A. E. Garrod's 'inborn errors of metabolism'. It turns out that the genetics of gout are very complicated, in the first instance due to a polygenic inheritance affecting the urate level and then by virtue of still-to-be determined genetic influences that translate a high urate level into gout. Beyond the immediate task of creating an ever more detailed picture of the multiple genes that affect urate levels, there is the challenge of integrating the genetics with lifestyle factors. We go on to this in the next chapter.

Chapter 12

Triggers and Protectors

Almost everyone in the old days who ever put pen to paper on the causes of gout considered the contribution of lifestyle to be obvious, and many delivered a harsh judgement on the gouty. The typical gout patients under Thomas Sydenham (see Chapter 2) were 'old men as, after passing the best part of their life in ease and comfort, indulging freely in high living, wine, and other generous drinks, at length, from inactivity, the usual attendant of advanced life, have left off altogether the bodily exercises of their youth'.[1] Forty years or so later, in 1726, Richard Blackmore emphasised that 'it is the dissolute and voluptuous indulgence of sensual appetites, that administer to the blood the seeds of gout by oppressing nature with too great plenty of rich supplies'.[2] However severe these words, physicians needed to keep their patients and may not always have laboured such views or challenged the favoured view that gout is familial (see Chapter 11).

Not all doctors were prepared to go along with such a doctor–patient collusion. For example, the late eighteenth-century anti-colonialist system-bucking Thomas Beddoes (see Chapter 6) seems to have almost celebrated what he saw as payback for the expanding merchant class: 'To be visited by the GOUT, the DROPSY, the PALSY – by the BLUE and other COLOURED DEVILS lodged in the system, that compensates business by boisterous pleasures, and privation by gross indulgencies! … and here too does not gold bring with it plaques?'[3]

Before we go on, I do need to make it very clear that all of this is part of history, and we now know that gout is not usually due, in Beddoes's words, to gross indulgencies, nor usually a just dessert for misbehaviour.

Many people are probably so genetically predisposed to a high urate level that it does not take much 'indulgence' to trigger acute gout (see Chapter 11).[4] The measured nineteenth-century physician Charles Scudamore realised the interplay between heredity and behaviour:

> We may rest satisfied with the fact, that some individuals possess in their constitution an hereditary disposition to gout, which comes into action in proportion as it is called forth by the influence of the predisposing and the exciting causes.... Very frequently, however, the gout is wholly acquired, there being no trace of its existence in any preceding generation, by those persons who use animal food to excess, drink freely of wine, or indulge in the use of strong malt liquor together with sprits, and commit other irregularities.[5]

A good way to gauge the relative contributions of inherited and environmental influences is to study twins.[6] Differences between identical (monozygotic) twins should be largely due to the environment. In contrast, both genetic and environmental factors contribute to differences between non-identical (dizygotic) twins. A study conducted at Stanford University assessed the levels of uric acid and the incidence of gout in over 500 middle-aged male twin pairs. Identical twins had more similar urate levels to one another than did non-identical twins, which comes as no surprise given what we now know about the genetic determinants of blood urate levels (see Chapter 11). In contrast, there was no difference in concordance for gout between identical and non-identical twin pairs.[7] This result is entirely consistent with hyperuricaemia alone being a poor predictor of actual gout (see Chapter 9) and supports an extra non-genetic contribution.

The Importance of Urate Level Fluctuations

While the probability of an acute gout attack increases with the amount of urate in the blood, a sudden change in urate level probably often

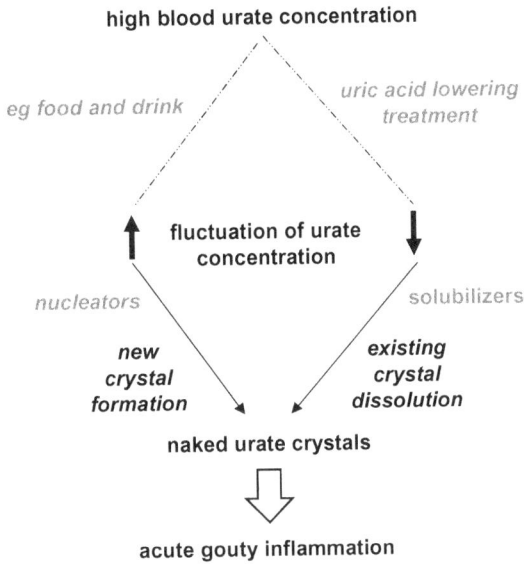

high blood urate concentration

eg food and drink   *uric acid lowering*
                                   treatment

↑   **fluctuation of urate**   ↓
    concentration

nucleators   *solubilizers*

new   ***existing***
crystal   ***crystal***
formation   ***dissolution***

naked urate crystals

⇩

acute gouty inflammation

Figure 12.1.

Acute gout attacks are triggered by naked monosodium urate crystals rather than by simply having a high blood urate level. This can happen either when the urate crystalises as the urate concentration rises or when established crystals that are masked by a protein coating and connective tissue start to dissolve, as during the initiation of urate lowering therapy.

provides the critical spark, and this may be the most important link to the dietary factors discussed in the following (see Figure 12.1). As mentioned in Chapter 9, urate crystals forming in the body are much less inflammatory once they become coated in the body by proteins and encased by connective tissue. Inflammation is particularly incited by 'naked' crystals, which are most likely to occur when the blood urate level suddenly changes, either increasing or decreasing. On the one hand, a rise in urate level may lead to the precipitation of fresh naked crystals. On the other hand, a sudden drop in blood urate level, as occurs upon the commencement of urate-lowering therapy (see Chapter 8), leads to solubilisation of the surface of crystals with release of protective proteins and a return to nakedness. A drop in the urate level through the dilutional effect of bleeding may well explain Sydenham recommending doctors not to use the treatment for gout: 'If blood be taken during an intermission, however, long after a fit, there is danger lest the agitation of the blood and humours bring on a fresh one, worse than the one that went before it'.[8] The principle of not allowing urate levels to suddenly change evokes what eighteenth-century physicians called 'regimen', a regular plan of eating, drinking and other measures to be adhered to at all costs. In Sydenham's words, 'between fits, every point of regimen is to be looked to with no common attention'.[9]

As should by now be clear, purine metabolism and the synthesis and elimination of uric acid are complicated, and it is hard to predict how different foods and drinks will fluctuate plasma urate levels in an individual. Although it is common to think of dietary purines as being quintessentially to blame, dietary proteins can potentially enhance urate level by providing the nitrogen for purine synthesis (see Chapter 11), and fructose also increases uric acid production (discussed in detail later in this chapter).[10] Aside from things that fluctuate urate levels, there may be additional unknown factors in what we eat and drink that promote the nucleation of urate crystals and/or the inflammatory response to them. Conversely, many foods and drinks contain substances that are directly protective, such as polyphenols in red wine, or which stimulate the body's own anti-inflammatory defences, such as sulforaphane in broccoli and other cruciate vegetables. In addition, attacks of acute gout may be influenced by the balance between anti-inflammatory and pro-inflammatory substances released by the 'microbiome' in the gut. Lastly, there is the paradox that uric acid itself has anti-inflammatory properties by virtue of being an antioxidant (see Chapter 13).

The Difficulty of Establishing Causation

A further difficulty is scientifically establishing dietary, behavioural or environmental links to uric acid and gout over and above personal experience. William Cadogan (see Chapter 3) realised the methodological difficulties as far back as 1771: 'Thus one error brings on another, and when men have eaten too much, they drink too much also by a kind of necessity'.[11] To give another example of Georgian excess, we can consider the eccentric gouty George Fordyce (1736–1802), who lectured on medicine and chemistry at London's St. Thomas's Hospital. He had the same dinner every day at Dolly's Chophouse for more than 20 years:

> His research in comparative anatomy had led him to conclude that man, through custom, eats oftener than nature requires, one meal a day being sufficient for that noble animal the lion. He made the experiment on himself at this, his favourite house, and finding it succeeded, he continued the following regimen.... At four o'clock, his accustomed hour of dining, he entered, and took his seat at a table always reserved for him, on which were instantly placed a silver tankard full of strong ale; a bottle of port wine, and a measure containing a quarter pint of brandy. The moment the waiter announced him, the cook put a pound and a half of rump steak on the gridiron, and on the table a delicate trifle as a *bon bouche*, to serve until the steak was ready. This morsel was sometimes half a broiled chicken, sometimes a plate of fish: when he had eaten this, he took one glass of his brandy, and then proceeded to devour his steak. We say devour, because he always ate so rapidly that one might imagine that he was hurrying away to a patient, to deprive death of a dinner. When he had finished his meat, he took the remainder of his brandy, having, during his dinner, drunk the tankard of ale, and afterwards the bottle of port. He thus daily spent an hour and a half of his time, and then returned to his house in Essex Street, to give his six-o'clock lecture on chemistry. He made no other meal until his return next day....[12]

Was it overeating or overdrinking that gave Fordyce gout? Or did overeating and overdrinking simply signify having the personal resources to live a life with other gout-giving luxuries?

Meat eating

Let's start with meat eating, a deeply ingrained culprit in our minds. Sydenham instructed his gouty patients to have only one type of meat at a meal and only once a day. This would have involved some significant personal sacrifice for the better-off, particularly at feasts. In *The English House-Wife*, a mainstay seventeenth-century domestic manual, Gervais Markham (see Figures 12.2(a) and (b)) instructed hosts how to prepare 'a humble feast, or an ordinary proportion which any good man may keep in his family, for the entertainment of his true and worthy friends'. A 'full service' should have 32 dishes, 'which is as much as can conveniently stand on one table', including roasted beef, pig, goose, turkey, swan, venison and a kid with a pudding in it.[13] Well-mannered guests could not have been expected to sample more than a few of these, but the plan gives you the general idea that if you could afford meat, you might eat a lot of it. In contrast, meat was a luxury for the poor, who may only have eaten a small portion once a week, if at all. This meat fest of the better-off calmed down over the years, but traditional mixed farming, together with country shooting and fishing, ensured a plentiful availability of meat, poultry and fish if you could afford it.

George Cheyne (see Chapter 3) went further than Sydenham and argued that complete abstinence from meat was necessary to lessen the intake of gout-provoking salts.[14] He warned that this drastic course of action was not without risks, and:

> never to be undertaken but with great caution, and in the last extremity; first, because an entire vegetable diet weakens all the digestive powers, and all the functions of life, impoverishes the whole mass of the fluids; impairs the strength, and dispirits the man: and thereby necessarily begets the worst kind of hysterical and hypochondriacal disorders, and all their black and dismal consequences (at least until the body has become long accustomed to it) which is a disease far worse than the Gout itself.[15]

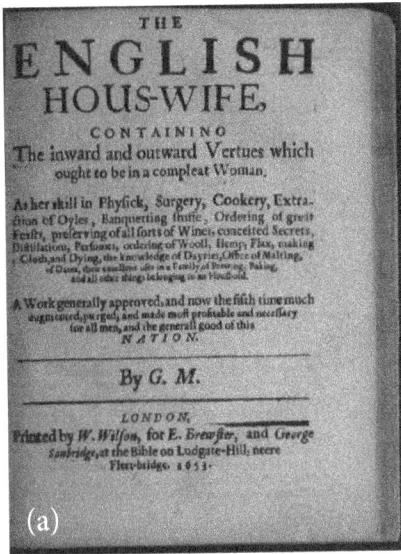

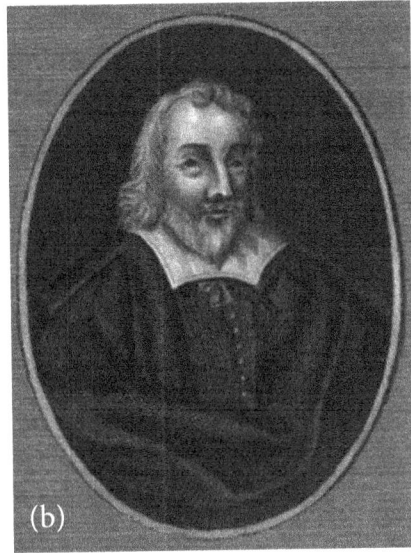

Figure 12.2.

(a) It would be hard to come up with many title pages more out of line with today's views on gender roles, but it sold very well in its day. Gervase Markham's *The English House-Wife Containing the Inward and Outward Vertues Which Ought to Be in a Compleat Woman* was first published in London in 1615 and went through nine editions, the last being in 1683. It provides an excellent insight into recipes and menus in the seventeenth century, many of which would have endured well into the nineteenth century. Meat featured prominently.

(b) Line engraving of Gervase Markham by Burnet Reading, after Thomas Cross.

Source: (a) Courtesy of the Wellcome Collection; (b) via Wikimedia Commons. Both public domain.

Such was the entrenched view that meat was needed for health. Cheyne was an expert on the link between lifestyle and mental health, and his bestselling *The English Malady* of 1733 was one of the first books to address it.[16]

Modern analysis of data from the US Third National Health and Nutrition Examination Survey has shown that eating meat and seafood is statistically associated with a high blood urate level.[17] Furthermore, the Health Professionals Follow-up Study based at Harvard has addressed whether meat eating actually leads to gout. This is a prospective study designed to test connections between various aspects of nutrition and disease and involves 51,529 male dentists, optometrists, osteopaths, pharmacists, podiatrists and veterinarians. Of these, 47,150 were assessed at the start of the study on the basis that they did not have gout. Gout developed in 730 of the men over 12 years, enabling statistical confirmation that attacks of gout are indeed linked to eating meat, with beef, pork and lamb standing out as particularly blameworthy.[18] However, this risk of meat eating is not simply a matter of ingesting more purines and proteins, as eating purine-rich vegetables such as cauliflower, mushrooms, oatmeal, peas, beans, lentils and spinach is not linked to gout. Why not is unclear, but possibly vegetables do not stimulate gout because they also provide protective anti-inflammatory compounds. Also, in the case of meat, animal fat can lead to the generation of ketones that enhance urate retention from the urine and thereby raise blood urate levels further (see the following). Lastly, the high iron content in meat might play a role, as iron is known to associate with urate and that may enhance crystal formation or the subsequent inflammatory response (see Chapter 9).[19] Consistent with this, iron depletion was found to reduce the frequency and severity of acute gout attacks, although this needs confirming in a modern controlled trial.[20] Recent support for the role of iron in gout comes from a Mendelian randomisation study (see Chapter 11) that has indicated a causal link between genetically-determined high iron levels and gout.[21]

Sugar

Less well appreciated than meat is the contribution of sugar. Importation of sugar was an integral component of the eighteenth-century slave-trade triangle and catered to a sweet-toothed market. Whether sugar is good or bad for you was controversial from the start. Thomas Willis (see Chapter 3), who first detected sweetness in urine and coined the term diabetes mellitus, considered sugar to be caustic and held it responsible for scurvy and consumption.[22] The sugar advocate Frederick Slare (ca. 1647–ca. 1727) then published his successful *Vindication of Sugars Against the Charge of*

Dr. Willis: Other Physicians, and Common Prejudices. Dedicated to the Ladies, commending the sugar trade and arguing the benefits of sugar for children on the basis that breast milk is sweet and healthy.[23] Another sugar enthusiast was the physician Thomas Short (1690–1772),[a] who started his chapter on sugar in *Discourses on Tea, Sugar, Milk, Made-Wines, Spirits, Punch, Tobacco with Plain and Useful Rules for Gouty People* of 1750 with 'tea without sugar makes a very ordinary tipple to most people' and listed sugar's many health benefits, including acting as an internal soap to disperse fatty, oily and viscous juices.[24] Fast forwarding to the late nineteenth century, Alfred Garrod (see Chapter 6) conceded that sugar is fattening but dismissed its role in gout.[25]

'Sugar' is an umbrella term to cover sweet-tasting monosaccharides, which include glucose, fructose and galactose. Traditional table sugar is mainly sucrose, which is a combination of glucose and fructose, both of which contribute to becoming overweight and, therefore, indirectly raise urate levels and promote gout (see Chapter 14). However, it has also been shown that fructose, but not glucose, raises urate levels directly.[26] This has been attributed to an increase in turnover of purines during fructose metabolism.[27] To give a real-life example, drinking a single can of 'Sprite' containing 15.8 grams of fructose is enough to significantly raise the blood urate level within 30 minutes.[28] Prospective studies in the United States have established that consumption of sugar-sweetened soft drinks is associated with increased urate levels and increased gout in both men and women.[29] It is worth noting that the same considerations apply to the consumption of fructose in fruits and fruit juices, showing that these do not escape blame just because they are 'natural'.

Paradoxical effects of fasting

You might think that not eating would help blood urate levels – certainly; the German clinical scientist Heinrich von Ranke (1830–1909) documented in 1858 that fasting lowers the urate content of urine, the most obvious

---

[a] Not the same Thomas Short to whom Thomas Sydenham dedicated his *Treatise on the Gout and Dropsy*.

explanation of course being reduced food intake.[30] However, the actual reason for this became clear with the work of the neurologist William Lennox (1884–1960) during his epilepsy research. Lennox originally trained to be a medical missionary and, early on in his career, worked as one in China. He returned to the United States after his daughter developed epilepsy and set up a neurology unit at Harvard specialising in its treatment. Over the years, he made a major contribution to patient care, not least by introducing the electroencephalograph (EEG) to clinical practice. He was the corecipient of the Lasker Award in 1951. One imagines the mental struggles that he must have had squaring his Christian foundations with the long suffering of some of his institutionalised patients with severe untreatable epilepsy and mental incapacity, as well as with the costs to society. These led him to become an outspoken exponent in the euthanasia and eugenics movements. He was not alone, as this had widespread support among physicians and scientists in the United States and Western Europe before World War II.[31]

Lennox was working in an age before anti-convulsant drugs.[b] Fasting as a treatment for epilepsy dates back to Hippocrates or before and was recorded by St. Mark as recommended by Christ.[32] Lennox found that while food withdrawal did indeed lower urate in the urine, this was unexpectedly accompanied by a rise rather than a fall in blood urate level.[33] This was quickly corrected by eating carbohydrate or protein but not by eating fat.[34] It turned out that it was ketones that were responsible.[35] These are what make the breath smell fruity during a fast and derive from the breakdown of fat to provide energy in the absence of carbohydrates. Later, it was discovered that direct intravenous infusion of ketones increases renal retention of urate.[36] We now know this is due to the passage of ketones into the urine via solute carrier transporters in the renal tubules being in exchange for urate influx and thereby enhancing urate retention (see Chapter 8).[37] Not unexpectedly, the same rise in blood urate follows a high fat 'keto' diet to help lose weight.[38] Actually, in most people, the increase in urate levels due to fasting or a keto diet does not lead to acute

---

[b] Phenytoin was the first and was introduced in 1936.

gout, which is likely to be due to ketones or other metabolic consequences of fasting suppressing urate crystallisation or the inflammatory response to urate crystals.[39]

Alcohol

There can be no greater longstanding popular and medical belief than that gout is a consequence of heavy drinking. While Sydenham blamed meat, he considered alcoholic drinks to be even worse:

> simple gluttony, and the free use of food, although common incentives, by no means so frequently pave the way for gout as reckless and inordinate drinking. This annihilates the ferments due to the different digestions, it throws down the digestions themselves, and through the over-abundance of adventitious vapours subdues and disperses the natural spirits. Then at one and the same time the energy of the spirits which are the instruments of digestion is diminished. Then also a vast mass of humours oppresses the blood ... Little progress will be made unless there is a total and complete abstinence from all (even the weakest) fermented liquors.[40]

Although concluding that Sydenham's own destruction by gout disqualified him from preaching, John Ring, writing in 1811, was broadly in agreement: 'For it is an unquestionable truth, that a man who indulges himself in the liberal use of alcohol, under any form, has not only the vulture perpetually gnawing his liver, but is also, in general, tortured with the gout'.[41] Forwarding 50 years, Alfred Garrod agreed that:

> there is no truth in medicine better established than that the use of fermented or alcoholic liquors is the most powerful of all the predisposing causes of gout; nay, so potent, that it may be a question whether the malady would ever have been known to mankind had such beverages not been indulged in.[42]

Abstinence from alcohol was widely held to be the reason Moslems rarely suffered from gout. William Cadogan pointed out: 'There are whole nations of active people knowing no luxury, who for ages have been free from it, but have it now since the Europeans have brought them wine and spirits' and that the people of India 'living in the most temperate simplicity, chiefly upon rice, have no such thing as the gout, or indeed any other chronic disease among them'.[43] Similarly, Hester Stanhope wrote to Joseph Banks from Lebanon (see Chapter 5) that:

> I have been assured by a physician who practiced above thirty years in Turkey, that from the Danube to the Euphrates he had never seen a gouty Turk. I have also been informed by some of our ministers who had resided many years at Constantinople, that the Gout, and other diseases of the same class, were not uncommon at court, but the courtiers, it seems, were not as good Mahometans as those who lived in the country; for they drank wine, drams, liqueurs of all sorts, without restraint.[44]

Indeed, it became so widely accepted that Moslems were exempt that, in 1910, the physician Dyce Duckworth reported a case to the Royal Society of Medicine.[45] The patient was the exception that proved the rule, being a Mandalay cook and a 'free drinker' of rum, whisky and beer – as well as a big meat-eater.

There was some mitigation for high alcohol consumption before town and city councils took charge of sewage, as public water was both obnoxious and unsafe. While Alfred Garrod was working on his thread test, the immediate threat to life in London was water-borne infections. Between 1830 and 1860, there was a series of cholera outbreaks, the third of which hit Britain in 1853–1854. This accounted for 23,000 lives, of which around 10,000 were in London. The risk of cholera contagion was believed to originate from the putrid 'miasma' in the air until John Snow and others incriminated the water supplied by public pumps.[46] These were the days before bacteriology, but the resemblance of River Thames water to sewage was well illustrated by Arthur Hill Hassall (see Chapter 4) (see Figure 12.3(a)). Clean water was desirable but was not readily available, and only the well-off could afford to purchase fresh bottled water. Consequently, beer was widely drunk and often throughout the day. The day-to-day drink was 'small beer' of low alcohol content, but much more alcoholic special brews were made for celebrations. Wine was more a drink of the middle and upper classes and, like beer, was consumed in large amounts.[47]

Several aspects of alcohol bear discussion. The first is the triggering effect of intoxication. Drunkenness had historically been a reforming

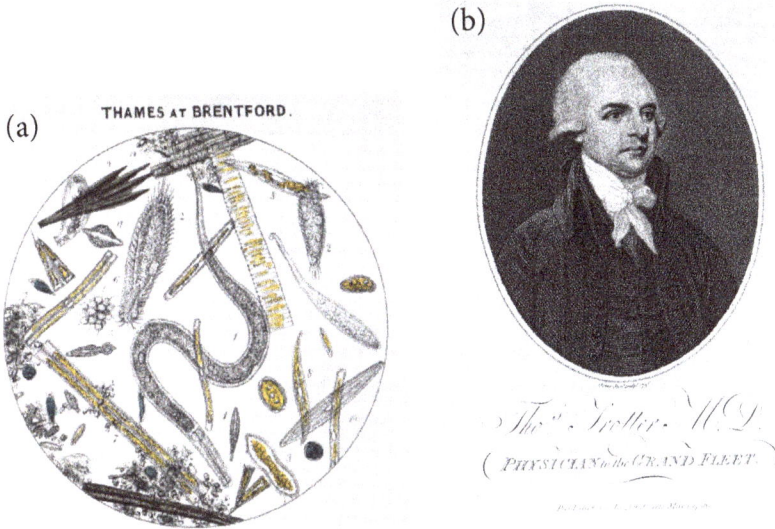

Figure 12.3.

(a) Wine and beer were widely held to be healthier options than public water. This view of what Arthur Hill Hassall saw under the microscope of River Thames water in 1851 was similar to sewer water. Hassall recognised 'vibriones' in the faecal discharges of patients with cholera but did not make the link to their being responsible for the disease.

(b) Thomas Trotter, the naval physician who first recognised alcoholism as a disease. Trotter sided with his contemporary, Thomas Beddoes, in viewing gout and other chronic diseases politically as largely consequences of national and personal wealth. Portrait by Daniel Orme.

(Continued)

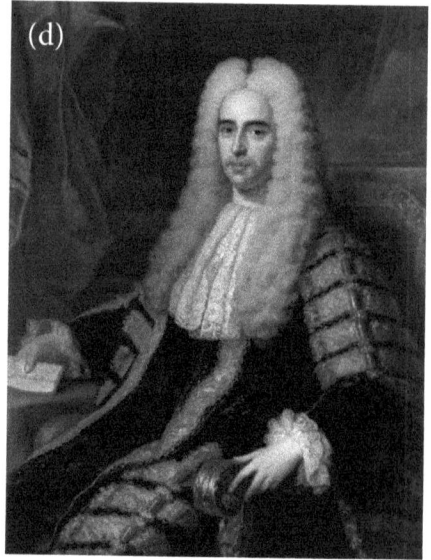

(c)	purines (mmol)
Beer -pint (4%; 568 ml)	127.8-650.8
Wine - glass (12%, 175 ml)	5.0-18.9
Whisky - shot (40%, 25 ml)	0.2-0.5

Figure 12.3. (*Continued*)

(c) Beer has the highest purine content of alcoholic drinks, followed by wines. Data from Kaneko *et al.* (2009).

(d) John Methuen's 'Port Wine Treaty' of 1703 between England and Portugal was instrumental in bringing affordable wine to England. This was fortified with brandy to prevent fermentation at sea, hence the origin of port. Lead and other contaminants were common. Portrait of Methuen as Lord Chancellor of Ireland by Adrien Carpentiers.

Source: (a) and (b) Courtesy of the Wellcome Collection: (a) public domain; (b) CC BY 4.0; (d) via Wikimedia Commons, public domain.

province of the clergy, but it became medicalised towards the end of the eighteenth century, following the work of Benjamin Rush in the United States and Thomas Trotter in Britain (Figure 12.3(b)).[48] The devastating effects that chronic alcohol abuse has on the liver were once considered to be due to concurrently eating poorly, and it was Charles Lieber (1760–1832), professor of medicine at New York's Mount Sinai School of Medicine, who first persuaded people that the effects were the direct result of alcohol itself.[49] He found in the early 1960s that drunk patients tended to have an increase in blood urate levels. He went on to administer alcohol to volunteers (I pity their hangovers) and showed that the rise in blood urate was linked to a fall in urinary urate excretion. He also found that alcohol intoxication raised blood lactate levels and reproduced an earlier observation that a reduction in urate excretion followed the administration of sodium lactate.[50] It became clear that lactate enhances urate retention through the renal tubular solute carriers in much the same way as ketones (see above).[51] Indeed, as people often neglect to eat while intoxicated, lactic acidosis and ketosis will complement each other in acutely raising blood urate levels and potentially triggering a gout attack.[52]

Whether or not more 'social' drinking affects uric acid and gout is a more complicated matter.[53] Alcohol can stimulate uric acid synthesis in the liver by enhancing purine metabolism, but some drinks are worse than others as gout triggers, irrespective of alcohol content.[54] Writing in 1859, Alfred Garrod considered that, 'A considerable difference, however, exists between these various fermented liquors in their power of inducing gout … distilled spirits, when exclusively taken, appear to exert little or no power in inducing gout, whereas wines, strong ales, and porter, are potent agents'.[55] His views on distilled spirits were based on knowing that gout was not a particular feature of the English gin craze, which held down the poor in the early 1700s.[56] He also knew that gout was rare in Scotland, where nerves were calmed by whisky rather than wine. The early toxicologist Robert Christison wrote to him, saying that Edinburgh Royal Infirmary had seen just two cases of gout in nearly 30 years, both in overfed butlers. However, spirits may not be as neutral as Garrod thought, as the Health Professionals Follow-up study based at Harvard has shown that those who drink spirits regularly are indeed at slightly increased risk of gout.[57] In the same study, a moderate intake of wine did not link to gout, whereas drinking beer certainly did.

Alcoholic drinks are made by fermentation with yeasts, which convert sugars into alcohol and release purines. Yeasts do not contain xanthine oxidase and so do not generate uric acid.[58] However, yeast purines can readily be converted to uric acid in the body once ingested. Beer is much richer in purines than wine or distilled spirits, and the major purine is guanine (Figure 12.3(c)).[59] This probably explains why, of all drinks, beer is the most successful in raising urate levels.[60] Indeed, just over one pint of regular beer has been found to raise the blood plasma urate level by as much as 6.5% – probably enough to activate urate crystallisation and trigger acute gout in someone with a critically high urate level already.[61] It therefore comes as no surprise that the strong link between beer and gout holds up under modern epidemiological scrutiny.[62]

The intriguing question is why wine, which was universally blamed in the past, should nowadays escape much censure. Certainly, the purine content of wine is far less than that of beer, and also, wine, particularly red wine, contains polyphenols with anti-inflammatory properties, which might suppress the inflammatory reaction to urate crystals.[63] However, a major factor accounting for the historical perception that wine led to gout might be that its sugar content used to be much higher. In Sydenham's time, wine merchants exploited the prevailing sweet-tooth and liking for a sparkle by adding in some sugar or molasses to stimulate a secondary fermentation and release carbon dioxide. Christopher Merrett, the career-doomed Harveian Librarian at the College of Physicians (see Chapter 2), reported to the Royal Society in 1662 that 'Our Wine-coopers of latter times use vast quantities of Sugar or Molasses, to all sorts of wines, to make them drink brisk and sparkling.'[64] It certainly looks as if the English were enjoying sweet, sparkling wine some 50 years before Champagne became fashionable in France. This was because the English were ahead of the French in making glass bottles that were strong enough not to burst from the pressure of the bubbles.

Of all the wines historically linked to gout, port wine always comes out top. At the beginning of the eighteenth century, wine drunk in England was mostly imported, and the closest source was France. However, the ongoing standoffs and wars with France meant that its wine was often difficult to obtain, and the fallbacks were the distant vineyards in Portugal and Spain. The 'Port Wine Treaty' of 1703 was a gouty landmark, being the second of three treaties between England and Portugal that were negotiated by the

British Ambassador John Methuen (Figure 12.3(d)). The treaty allowed the Portuguese to export wines to England at a third less duty than imposed on wine imported in peacetime from France. It was a win-win for England, as, in return, the wool traders were able to export cloth to Portugal duty-free.[65] The main distributors to England were located in Oporto and traded wines from the rocky Alto Duoro valley. The challenge the vintners faced in transporting wine all the way by sailboat was that the wine continued to ferment along the way, and it often arrived in England as vinegar. To counter this, from about 1715, they fortified the wine with more alcohol to stop further fermentation *en route*.[66] Ostensibly, they used brandy but, in practice, often just added alcohol distillations from corn, potatoes or other sources. To cater for sweet tastes, the spirit was often added to halt fermentation before the grape sugars had fully fermented, and molasses were sometimes also added in to enhance the sweetness further. In addition, the manufacturers might have added elderberry, bilberry or black-cherry juice for colouring, all contributing more fructose. The fortification process of the sugary, strongly alcoholic beverage did not necessarily end in Portugal, as more sugar and spirit might have been added by the British vintners, again to appeal to the market.

Port became the standard drinking wine in Britain. In 1810 alone, 6,450 thousand gallons were imported, and that was just what went through customs.[67] There were fabrications and imposters, as a bottle of 'genuine Old Port' might well not have come from Portugal. Thus, 'wine brewers' created imitations from home-made wine or spoilt cider and passed them off as the real thing.[68] Port was drunk by the better-off before, during, after and between meals, and there were one, two, three or four bottle-men. The British Prime Minister William Pitt, for whom Hester Stanhope had kept house (see Chapter 5), routinely drank three bottles a day.[69] As a bottle in those days contained five-sixths of a pint (474 ml), this amounted to around 1.4 litres of port a day, and given the sugar load, it is hardly surprising that Pitt suffered from gout from an early age. Even today, at 120–220 grams sugar/litre, port wine has substantially more sugar than dry unfortified wine at a mere <10 grams/litre.

Alcohol consumption by the 'more polite classes of society' in Britain fell substantially in the latter part of the nineteenth century, partly because improvements in sewage disposal led to greater confidence in drinking water and partly because of the increasing influence of the Victorian temperance movement.[70] Another reason was the growing appreciation of the contamination of wines by the artifices of the wine trade, with port developing a particularly poor reputation.[71] This may be one reason why gout stools started disappearing from London private member clubs during the late nineteenth century.[72] The modern equivalent to mass consumption of beer and wine is non-alcoholic sugary beverages (see above).

Lead pollution

Sugar is not the only reason why wine caused gout, as it often also contained lead. Lead poisoning has been a public health issue since the Ancient Egyptians and was described by Hippocrates.[73] It may have contributed to the fall of the Roman Empire.[74] Lead was also a serious problem in Georgian and Victorian times. The issue of contamination of food and drink generally with lead and other toxic ingredients was first drawn to the British public's attention by Fredrick Accum (see Chapter 4) in his *Treatise on adulterations of food and culinary poisons* (1820), prefaced by the Old Testament quote 'There is Death in the Pot'.[c,75] Such was public interest and concern that the book went to four editions over two years. The issue was taken up more systematically in the 1850s by *The Lancet's* Analytical and Sanitary Commission (see Chapter 4).[76] Arthur Hill Hassall and Henry Letheby documented a scandalous level of lead contamination, often wilful to raise sales, cut costs and increase profits. They catalogued toxic quantities of red lead[d] being used as colouring in 13/28 samples of Cayenne pepper, 8/26 samples of curry powder and 9/43 samples of snuff (in one at 4.6%). Lead chromate was found to provide the yellow colouring of custard powders and other desserts.

---

[c] 'There is Death in the Pot': II Kings chap. 4, verse 40.
[d] Lead [II,IV] oxide.

Wine had long been known to be liable to adulteration with lead, and Hassall and Letheby found that this was still the case in the 1850s.[77] It was not unusual for manufacturers to add the 'sugar of lead'[e] to wine, partly to sweeten it and appeal to the sweet-toothed clientele, partly to precipitate solids and partly to arrest fermentation towards vinegar.[78] Bearing in mind that <10 micrograms/l is the current acceptable level of lead in public drinking water in England, readings as high as 1.9 milligrams/l obtained when Georgian-era wine was assessed by modern analysis are on the high side.[79] The use of lead presses and lead-glazed storage vessels led to the adulteration of traditional cider.[80] Rum was also famously contaminated.[81] Judging from the analysis of bones in a fleet cemetery in Antigua, lead poisoning from the daily grog and other sources must have been common in the Royal Navy.[82] Sometimes, lead in wine was just an accidental contaminant, left behind by a lead shot used for cleaning scale off bottles, or a consequence of 'breathing' claret or port in leaded crystal glass decanters. Enjoying the wine with desserts would have boosted the lead intake yet further, as, besides being coloured and sweetened with lead salts, these were often prepared in lead moulds.[83]

Apart from being common in food and wine, lead was everywhere else in the 1700s and 1800s. It was in the paint on the walls; water was conducted in lead pipes and kept in lead tanks; printers relied on lead type; early Georgian men and women 'of class' whitened their faces with lead salts to distinguish themselves from sun-tanned labourers; children played with lead soldiers; and lead was prescribed as a medication for consumption and diarrhoea and as a sedative for 'hysteria'. Hassall and Letheby even found lead contaminating the colouring on the famous Penny Red postage stamps: 'The colour is easily removed and the hands and lips, if the stamps be moistened with the lips, quickly become much stained'.[84] The stamps had to be withdrawn, adding to their collector value. Lead also assimilates in plants for recycling in the food chain.[85]

---

[e] Lead acetate.

Lead is toxic to many parts of the body, not least the nervous system. Children exposed to lead may suffer lasting brain injury, with learning difficulties and emotional problems. It also affects the peripheral nerves and was responsible for the limp wrists of painter-decorators. It causes gastrointestinal symptoms, such as indigestion, vomiting, abdominal pain ('lead colic') and constipation. As with mercury poisoning, there may occasionally be an increase in saliva, and this is distinguished by a bluish tinge. More commonly, the gums develop 'Burton's lines', the linear blue-grey discolouration near the teeth due to lead sulphide deposition that are eponymously named after the physician Henry Burton, who first noticed them in 1840.[86]

Gout associated with lead poisoning is known as 'Saturnine Gout', from the alchemical link between lead and the planet Saturn.[87] It was described by several eighteenth-century doctors, of whom the West Country physician William Musgrave (1655–1721) is thought to have been the first.[88] However, it was Alfred Garrod who brought the connection between lead and gout to more widespread attention. He observed that about a quarter of the gouty patients under his hospital care had been exposed to lead, and most were painter-decorators or plumbers, working with lead paints and lead pipes.[89] In pointing out to Garrod that gout was rare in Edinburgh, Robert Christison also mentioned that he seldom saw obvious lead poisoning. He offered an explanation:

A journeyman, who had been a house-painter for seventeen years, a part of which he had spent in London, was well acquainted with lead-colic and lead-palsy, as occurring in his fellow-workmen in the capital. He assured me that neither he nor any painter of his acquaintance in Scotland had ever known either disease among painters who had worked only in Edinburgh. He ascribed the difference between London and Edinburgh to the circumstances, that in Edinburgh they are never so far from their homes as to be prevented from going thither to their meals; that they therefore take off their working-dress, or overalls. And wash their hands and faces before going to meals; but that in London, workmen are so far from home or their master's establishment, that they cannot go home for breakfast or dinner; that they therefore take their meals where they work, and do not take the trouble of changing their dress before they feed.[90]

There are at least two mechanisms underlying lead poisoning and gout. The first was mentioned in Chapter 9 and is the potential of lead to combine with urate, crystallise as insoluble lead urate and nucleate secondary monosodium urate crystallisation. The second mechanism is through lead injuring the kidneys and reducing urate excretion.[91] Garrod had observed this in two hospital patients being treated with lead acetate,[f] in whom the urinary urate dropped and the blood urate rose.[92] The effect of lead on the kidneys was studied much later as a consequence of illicit alcohol. Moonshine derives its name from whisky smuggling into Britain by the light of the moon but came to mean the product of illegal distillation in the Southeastern United States during the prohibition years.[93] Automobile radiators were commonly used to condense or store the whisky, and lead solder would leech into the brew. Lead plates were sometimes added in to sweeten the taste. The practice continued after the end of prohibition, and a 1969 report on three patients in Birmingham, Alabama, set the sad scene:

Case 1. A 36-year-old social derelict who began drinking moonshine heavily in his early teens … Case 2. A 40-year-old man had intractable alcoholism that was already well established by the age of 34 … Case 3. A 46 year old man admitted drinking a pint jar of moonshine almost daily for many years.[94]

---

[f] Lead acetate was used in the old days as an astringent, but it is not clear why Garrod's patients were given it.

We do not know the exact reason for the reduced urate excretion in chronic lead poisoning, but the most likely mechanism is dysfunction or destruction of the renal tubular solute transport channels (see Chapter 8).[95]

The Lancet's publications were instrumental in the passing of the Adulteration of Food and Drink Act of 1860, and public health measures since then have gone a long way in reducing lead pollution, not least with the introduction of lead-free petrol. In high-income countries, lead is unlikely to be a major factor in everyday gout; however, in many parts of the world, lead toxicity has not gone away.[96] According to the World Health Organization, it accounts for three in a thousand deaths in low- and middle-income countries.[97] It is also entirely possible that other pollutants may have similar adverse effects, perhaps explaining surveys in the People's Republic of China and in Taiwan that have linked environmental air pollution to gout.[98] A recent study in China has suggested that the other heavy metals that pollute the environment, such as cadmium and arsenic, may have additive effects with lead on urate levels.[99]

Gout Protectants

Many gout patients choose not to use urate-lowering drugs if they can avoid them (see Chapter 8), very reasonably preferring to try a dietary adjustment.[100] Obviously, care can be taken to lower meat, sugar and alcohol intake, as above. Moreover, many dietary options probably have protective properties against gout, although it is fair to say that the field has not been exhaustively studied.

Sydenham was a great believer in cow's milk, which 'represses that turgescence or virosity of blood to which gout is due; so that those few with whom it agrees are free from gout as long as they take it exclusively'. However he recognised the difficulty: 'whoever, then, would put himself under a milk diet must seriously consider within himself whether he is likely to persist in it all his life long. Resolute as he must be, he may fail in this'.[101] I suppose this applies to most serious dietary regimens. A milky diet was a standard treatment recommended by George Cheyne, and

Joseph Banks wrote in 1804 that he hoped it would enable him to regain the use of his legs.[102] In modern studies, diary product consumption has been inversely correlated with serum urate level and likelihood of gout.[103] The mechanism underlying this is not clear but may be related to enhanced urate excretion.[104] Furthermore, compounds in both the protein and fat components of milk may have anti-inflammatory properties.[105]

A promotional text of 1845 published by the Patent Concentrated Tea Company recommended coffee as 'a great restorative to constitutions emaciated and worn down by gout, rheumatism, and paralytic affections'.[106] Similarly, Alfred Garrod noted that coffee 'may possess the power of preventing gout, seeing that in countries where it is extensively drunk, as in Turkey, gout is scarcely known' but qualified this with 'but it must be remembered that, in such countries, little wine or malt liquors are taken'.[107] In fact, recent studies in which alcohol and other confounding factors are taken into account have substantiated coffee as being associated with lower serum urate levels and less frequent gout.[108] As for tea, the Patent Concentrated Tea Company promotional text proposed that 'persons of a phlegmatic and melancholy temperament, *gouty* and *rheumatic* patients, and above all those prone to *calculous diseases* (of the lithic acid diathesis) will find tea the least objectionable article of common drink'.[109] However, in contrast to coffee, drinking tea does not appear to either alter urate levels or influence gout, despite containing caffeine.[110] Probably, one or more of the many phenolic compounds contained in coffee is responsible for its protective quality, but as with dairy products, the precise mechanism is unknown.

There are, of course, abundant chemical compounds within plants that could fend off gout, bearing in mind that their actions need to be balanced against the urate-raising effects of plant purines, proteins and sugars. I have touched on this earlier in relation to the possible anti-inflammatory effects of polyphenols in wine.[111] The plant extract supplement trade for gout is going strong, and in the United States, an internet-based survey showing that around 50% of self-selected respondents with gout take one or more. Of these, cherry extract and cherry juice are by far the most common.[112] In fact, this practice has the support of studies which have related consumption of whole cherries or concentrated tart cherry juice to significant reductions in acute gout attacks.[113] The mechanism of protection could involve one or more inflammatory mediators, including an inhibitory effect of cherry anthrocyanins on the release of IL-1β by monocytes in response to urate crystals (see Chapter 9).[114] Cherry extract has been found to modestly lower urate levels in the short term.[115] However, a recent randomised controlled study against a placebo found that drinking tart cherry juice twice a day over 28 days did not affect blood urate levels.[116] Cherry extract may be an alternative to the use of colchicine or an NSAID for preventing gout flares during the introduction of urate-lowering therapy (see Chapter 9).

Another supplement that has received attention is vitamin C, which can modestly increase urate in the urine and lower the serum urate level in some people.[117] However, vitamin C does not appear to lower serum urate in those with gout.[118] Furthermore, a Mendelian randomisation study (see Chapter 11) was unable to show a link between a genetically determined high-plasma vitamin C and a low-plasma urate.[119] It remains possible that the antioxidant function of vitamin C may help prevent gout flares.

Reflections on the Place of Food and Drink

To conclude this and the previous chapter, we now have a fairly good idea of the predisposing and immediate causes of gout attacks, including genetic, environmental and behavioural factors. Modern studies addressing the latter were well summarised in a systematic review in 2011, and there have been several other reviews since.[120] Certainly, the scientific evidence supports flipping the everyday habits of a George Fordyce (see above) towards a more varied and light diet.[121] The general recommendation of reducing meat, sugar and alcohol consumption has been suitably sanctioned in the British Society for Rheumatology guidelines for treating gout and by guidelines from similar organisations in other countries.[122] I will return in the final chapter to one of the most important associations of hyperuricaemia and gout, which is a high body weight. In the meantime, we move on next to address the significance for gout of simply being human!

Chapter 13

The Humanness of Gout

To understand why gout is particular to humans among other mammals, we need to begin with some long-recognised differences between species in the use and handling of nitrogen and uric acid. George Pearson had asserted in his Royal Society presentation of 1798 (see Chapter 6) that uric acid, or uric oxide as he called it, was present in the urine and urinary stones of humans but not those of dogs, rabbits or horses.[1] Pearson was correct, as most mammals pass very little urate out in their urine and instead excrete allantoin.[a] Regardless, uric acid or allantoin accounts for only around 5% of the nitrogen in mammalian urine, the major part being in urea. In striking contrast, Pearson's Parisian contemporaries, Antoine de Fourcroy and Louis Vauquelin (1763–1829), found that the semi-solid excrement of an ostrich is mainly composed of uric acid rather than urea.[2] Soon after, the London physician and chemist William Prout (1785–1850) discovered that the excrement of a 16-foot boa constrictor being exhibited on the Strand and fed a live rabbit once a month was also mostly uric acid.[3] The same turned out to be the case for all birds and terrestrial reptiles: urate is the white in pigeon droppings that force you to clean your car and which coat the statues of forgotten statesmen in public places.

---

[a] The word allantoin derived from '*l'acide allantoique*', which was found first in the allantoic fluid of cow embryos.

Justus Liebig's Sub-Oxidation Theory

As introduced in Chapter 8, Friedrich Wöhler (see Figure 13.1(a)) and Justus Liebig (see Figure 13.1(b)) were pioneers in replacing vitalism with organic chemistry. Not content with simply identifying and measuring organic compounds, they explored whether one could be converted to another. Wöhler had already shown that urea could be assembled in a test tube from simple ammonia. But could urea also be formed by the disassembly of uric acid? He showed, along with Liebig, that it could indeed, as uric acid could be oxidised to allantoin, which in turn could be broken down to urea and then urea degraded to ammonia.[4] However, this was test-tube stuff, and their claim that chemical compounds could interconvert in the body met with some stern opposition, as for example from the London physician William Gairdner (1793–1867): 'I receive

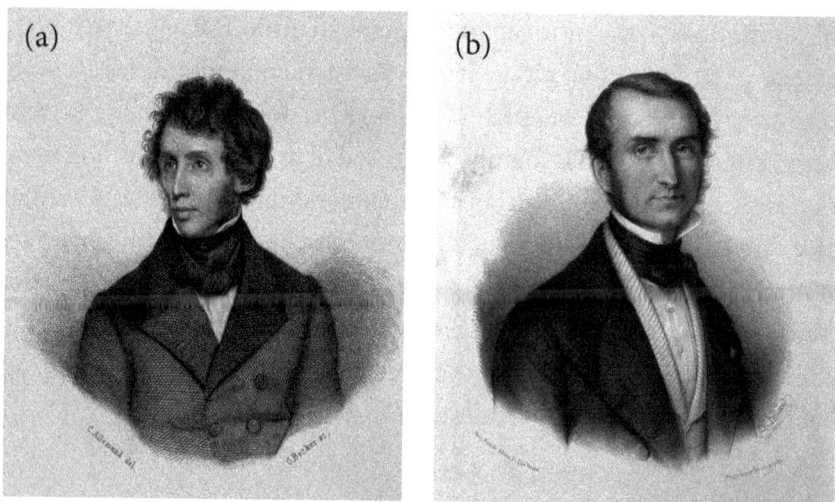

Figure 13.1.

(a) Friedrich Wöhler, who originated organic chemistry by synthesising urea from inorganic potassium cyanate and ammonium sulphate. This is an engraving after an original by Conrad L'Allemand.

(b) Justus Liebig. Lithograph by Zéphirin Belliard.

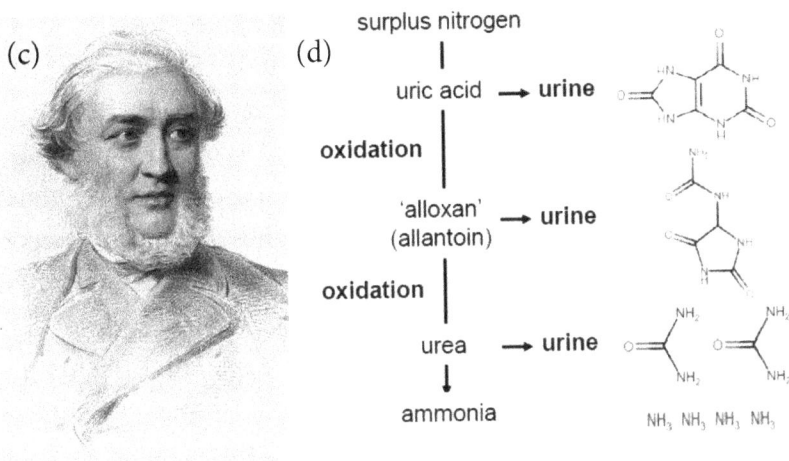

Figure 13.1. (*Continued*)

(c) Henry Bence Jones by George Richmond. Bence Jones studied under Liebig in Guessen in 1841.

(d) When Bence Jones returned to London, he published the application of Justus Liebig's flawed 'sub-oxygenation theory' to gout. The figure illustrates the simple scheme envisioned by Liebig of how one uric acid molecule containing four nitrogen atoms brakes down in the human body form four molecules of ammonia. The buildup of uric acid and gout could be explained by insufficient oxygen to allow the oxidation steps. The structures on the right were not known at the time and serve to help illustrate the process.

Source: (a) and (b) Courtesy of the Wellcome Collection, public domain; (c) via Wikimedia Commons, public domain.

this opinion with great difficulty, because it implies the admission of the convertibility of organised principles, of which I have already pointed out the great objection.'[5]

Liebig was prone to stray from his academic patch and to massage attractive chemical theories into physiological facts without doing the necessary experiments; we encounter this weakness again in his agricultural venture in Chapter 14. He had advanced his career by establishing a prestigious training laboratory in Giessen, which became the 'go-to' place for aspiring chemists internationally. In 1841, he hosted for six months a young English physician, Henry Bence Jones (see Chapter 9 and Figure 13.1(c)). Bence Jones is remembered today for his classic paper describing an abnormal urinary protein in a patient with bone cancer, written well before the discovery of antibodies.[6] What are now known as Bence Jones proteins turned out to be free immunoglobulin (antibody) light chains, and their presence in the urine is a diagnostic feature of myeloma. Bence Jones had been recommended to Liebig by Thomas Graham, who was professor of chemistry at University College London and would have been teaching Alfred Garrod at the time (see Chapter 6). Upon returning to London, Bence Jones got a job at St. George's Hospital, where he was asked to analyse the chemical composition of urines and urinary stones (an interest at the hospital since George Pearson). Making good use of his time in Giessen, Bence Jones soon published *On Gravel, Calculus, and Gout: Chiefly an Application of Professor Liebig's Physiology to the Prevention and Cure of These Diseases* (1842).[7] As Liebig believed that 'nothing enthuses young people more than to see their names in print', typically he did not put his name on work published by his students.[8] Nevertheless, the ideas in the book were clearly Liebig's, as admitted by Bence Jones in the preface: 'I have assumed that the theories of Professor Liebig were probably true, because most of them seemed to me to be founded on facts which are well known and possess the evidence of simplicity in a high degree'.

The presence of urate in urine was taken by Liebig, via Bence Jones, to indicate an inadequate supply of oxygen to allow urate oxidation to allantoin and thence to urea and ammonia, as in the test tube (see Figure 13.1(d)): 'The disappearance of uric acid and the production of urea plainly stand in a very close relation to the amount of oxygen absorbed in respiration'.[9] The lack of urate in the urine of meat-eating mammals could be explained by the copious oxygen inhaled while chasing prey, whereas the urate-rich excrement of Prout's boa constrictor, eating similar food, was due to the snake spending most of its time coiled up and breathing slowly.[10] Translating to humans, the gouty were deemed oxygen deficient, with tissues around joints being particularly vulnerable to urate deposition owing to reduced local oxygen supply. Conversely, a low urate concentration in the urine was a sign of adequate overall oxygenation and good health. Gouty patients could enhance their oxygen intake by taking more exercise, reading aloud, sleeping 'only so far as is necessary' and by avoiding hot rooms since 'air is expanded by heat and contracted by cold, and, therefore, equal volumes of hot and cold air contain unequal weights of oxygen'. Iron treatment was suggested to enhance the oxygen-carrying capacity of the blood, and fruit and non-nitrogenous foodstuffs full of starch or fat were discouraged to reduce consumption of the precious oxygen needed for their digestion. If these simple measures were inadequate, Bence Jones recommended oxygen in nitrous oxide water.[11] Distancing himself from the jollity of laughing gas (see Chapter 6), he cited Thomas Graham as stating 'when in solution, it possesses none of those stimulating properties which it exercises when absorbed as a gas'.[12]

Reading a contemporary review of Bence Jones's book in the *American Journal of Medical Science*, one is immediately struck by the awe that mid-nineteenth-century physicians must have felt with the arrival of professional chemists, such as Liebig, onto the medical scene. There was also a sense of professional foreboding:

> the very nature of the new doctrine calls medical men to make themselves acquainted with that which bids fair to explain so many important points in physiology and pathology, and to add the daring hope of a large accession to our means of successful practice in curing and preventing disease. Either the physician must travel out of the record of his former proceedings, and assume the responsibility of pronouncing opinions in chemistry, the science so long existing exclusively by the labours of his predecessors, and which may be said to have been discovered by them, or he must now expect to find the chemist adopting a parallel course, and becoming his competitor in the practice of medicine and hygiene. It is impossible, indeed, to do justice to the various important diseases which complicate or produce real health, without the full employment of this philosophy, so characteristic of the age.[13]

302 *The Gout: A Medical Microcosm in a Changing World*

The Liebig sub-oxidation theory influenced the interpretation of gout by many doctors for some years. However, confidence was not universal. Why did birds, which obtained enough oxygen to maintain a relatively high body temperature (~105°F/~40°C *versus* 98°F/37°C in humans), excrete uric acid and very little urea? Why did housing a sparrowhawk in an oxygen chamber not lead to urea excretion?[14] The most obvious flaw was, of course, the simplicity of a single biochemical process careering nitrogen in organic waste towards ammonia as fast and as far as the availability of oxygen allowed. Being able to measure urate in the blood, Alfred Garrod found that there was no obvious relationship between blood levels of urate and urea (see Chapter 6).[15] Expanding on this, the physician Edmund Parkes (1819–1876) wrote in his massive *The Composition of the Urine* (1860):

> Considering the apparent independence of each other of urea and uric acid, it would seem more probable, that each is produced by the metamorphosis of a definite structure or substance: and that, under ordinary circumstances, there is no conversion of uric acid to urea. Physiology will doubtless be able to indicate whence the uric acid is derived, at present it is mere guess work to hazard an opinion.[16]

Garrod came to regard the kidney as the site of uric acid synthesis and proposed that different cells in the kidney are responsible for urea and uric acid production and that species differences might be explained by the relative numbers of these putatively specialised cells.[17] However, this idea did not catch on, not least because it became clear that the liver is the main site of uric acid synthesis. A. E. Garrod (see Chapter 12) modified and modernised his father's views in his 1908 Croonian Lectures to London's Royal College of Physicians:

> Nowadays, very different ideas are in the ascendant. The conception of metabolism in block is giving place to that of metabolism in compartments. The view is daily gaining ground that each successive step in the building up and breaking down, not merely of

proteins, carbohydrates, and fats in general, but even of individual fractions of proteins and of individual sugars, is the work of special enzymes set apart for each particular purpose. Thus the notion of general sub-oxidation is reduced to very narrow limits....[18]

John Davy and Charles Darwin

We have Humphry Davy's younger brother John Davy (1790–1868) (see Figure 13.2(a)) to thank for extending observations on the composition of urine within the animal kingdom. John was taught chemistry in 1811

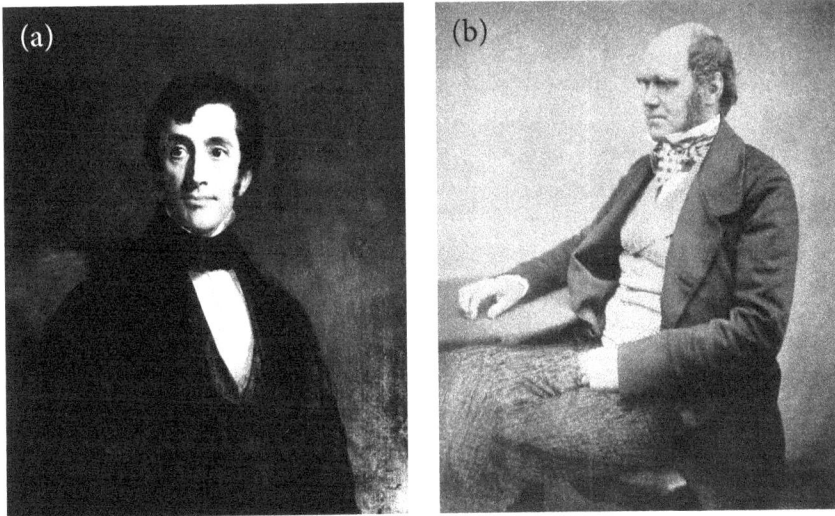

Figure 13.2.

(a) John Davy, Humphry Davy's medical brother. John posted from the West Indies the results of meticulous analyses of the composition of insect excrement, which he concluded was mainly uric acid. He fully appreciated the importance of uric acid excretion by insects, birds, reptiles and, to a lesser extent, mammals for maintaining plant fertility and was among the first to write about the nitrogen cycle. Artist unknown.

(b) Davy shared a love of angling with Charles Darwin. This photograph of Darwin was taken in 1860, just after their correspondence on the distribution of salmon eggs. Davy's work helped shape Darwin's views on the geographical distribution of species.

Source: Both courtesy of the Wellcome Collection, CC BY 4.0.

while staying with his brother at the Royal Institution and then went on to study medicine in Edinburgh. Having obtained an MD degree in 1814, he joined the army as a hospital assistant and was posted in 1815 to Brussels, where he helped treat the horrendous wounds of soldiers brought in from the nearby battleground at Waterloo. After that, he was made an assistant surgeon and posted to Ceylon,[b] from where he wrote to the Royal Society that he had added to the finding that Prout had made on the captive boa constrictor. All the snakes he examined in Ceylon expelled an excrement that was composed mainly of uric acid, and the same was the case for all species of lizards. On the other hand, frogs and toads excreted mainly urea:

> Perhaps additional facts are not required to prove, that the secretion of the kidneys of animals depends more on the intimate and invisible structure of these organs, than on the kind of food the animals consume; were such facts wanting, there would be no difficulty in furnishing them. How different is the urine of the brown-toad and that of any species of small lizards! yet flies are the favourite and common diet of both animals.[19]

Davy's subsequent career as an army doctor and prolific work as a naturalist can be the subject of another story. Fast forwarding, his final three-year posting was as inspector general of army hospitals in the West Indies, to where he travelled in 1845 by a paddle steamer. He was an obsessive data collector and kept detailed records during the 20-day voyage to Barbados, showing, among many other things, a drop in the uric acid content of his urine while at sea. He concluded that seafaring might be useful for gout and urinary stones: 'Gout is, I believe, almost unknown amongst sailors, and calculous complaints far from common. May not this be owing in part to an influence such as that alluded to, tending to check the lithic acid diathesis.[c,20] Once in the West Indies, Davy wrote a series of fine letters during his three-year posting, reporting his methodical chemical

---

[b] Now, Sri Lanka.
[c] Note the continued use of 'lithic acid' for uric acid during the mid-nineteenth century.

and microscopic analyses of the excrement of grasshoppers and numerous other invertebrates. While concluding that they mainly excreted uric acid (see the following), he found spiders to be different, as 'this acid is either assimilated, so as to form a part of the nutritive fluid, or is altered and converted into some other compound'.[21] He considered this to be xanthine (still known then as xanthic oxide), but it turned out to be the substance isolated the same year from guano (see Chapter 14) by the German chemist Julius Unger (1819–1885) and hence named guanine.[22]

After the West Indies, Davy retired to the Lake District in Northwest England. Humphry had died, leaving him a substantial legacy, including his fishing tackle and the royalties on *Salmonia*, his popular book on trout and salmon fishing that had been published in 1828.[23] John also loved fishing and, in 1857, published *The Angler in the Lake-District, or Piscatory Colloquies and Fishing Excursions in Westmoreland and Cumberland*, a very readable account of angling on the beautiful rivers and lakes thereabouts.[24] He corresponded with another fisherman, the vice-president of the Royal Society. This was none other than Charles Darwin (1809–1882) (see Figure 13.2(b)), 20 years returned from his voyage on the *Beagle*. Darwin was particularly interested in the geographical distribution of freshwater fish and suggested to Davy that fertilised fish eggs might be transported by birds inadvertently between lakes and rivers.[25] With his characteristic spirit of enquiry, Davy set to work, experimenting on the durability of salmon eggs procured from a local hatchery, and in March 1855, he wrote back to Darwin that his eggs had survived for a considerable time at a cool temperature and in moist air. He concluded that it was possible for salmon to spread to rivers in different valleys by the fertilised ova travelling on the feathers, beaks or legs of birds but that the eggs would be destroyed in birds' warm and acidic stomachs. Darwin responded, 'With many such experiments as yours, Geographical Distribution would become in my opinion, a very different subject to what it is now. Allow me again to thank you for the great interest I have received from your Memoir & for the honour you have done me'. He forwarded the letter for communication to the Royal Society.[26]

The issue of the geographical spread of species and their adaptation to new environments was, of course, central to Darwin's thought process. Three years later, papers from Darwin and Alfred Wallace were presented at the Linnean Society of London, announcing their independent thoughts on the natural selection of species as the basis for evolution.[27] Darwin followed this up with his seminal *On the Origin of Species.*[28] As is very well known, Darwin and Wallace transformed our understanding of creation by proposing a competitive world in which species that are most in tune with their environment survive and those that cannot adapt to change do not. In the process of adapting, species beget new varieties and, in due course, new species. The controversial implication was that all lifeforms are positioned in an evolutionary ancestral tree rather than lined up in a vertical hierarchy with humans at the top.

The Evolution of Nitrogen Disposal

Evolution provides the framework for understanding the differences between branches of the animal kingdom in the use of uric acid for the disposal of waste nitrogen (see Figures 13.3 and 13.4). Carbon can be safely accommodated in fat, but there is no animal equivalent for storing the nitrogen surplus that derives from the breakdown of proteins and purines. Enzyme systems emerged in ancestral single-cell organisms that degrade these to ammonia, similar to what Liebig and Wöhler had shown can be achieved for purines in the laboratory. Ammonia so formed simply diffuses into the aqueous surroundings. The long evolution of aquatic single-cell organisms into terrestrial multicellular animals which cannot so simply dispose of nitrogen required various biochemical and anatomical adaptations, as ammonia is toxic and cannot be allowed to accumulate.

Bacteria

The ancient biochemical pathways that result in ammonia formation from protein and purine digestion remain intact in most bacteria today. The breakdown of nitrogen-rich organic material to ammonia by soil bacteria

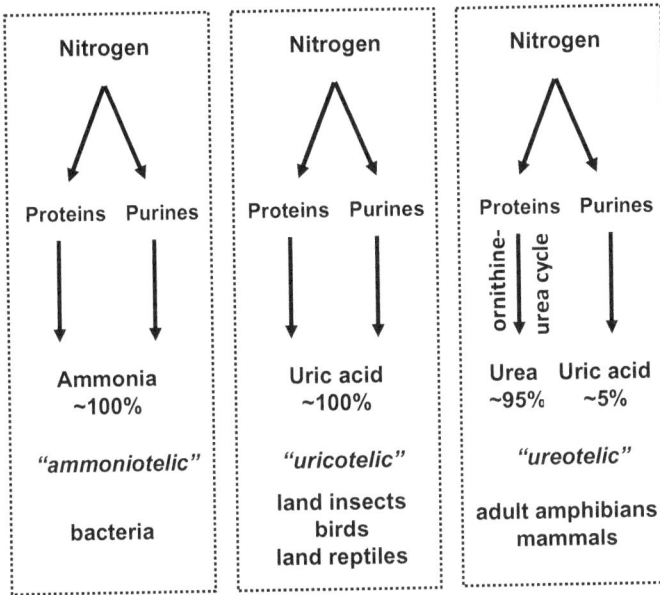

Figure 13.3.

Nitrogen is needed for the synthesis of proteins and purines in all living cells, but free nitrogen cannot be stored by animals for risk of toxic ammonia formation. Single-cell organisms, such as bacteria, degrade surplus proteins and purines to ammonia, which then diffuses out of the cell. In terrestrial animals, nitrogen elimination is more complex. 'Uricotelic' animals (e.g. birds, land reptiles and land insects) conserve water by excreting the large majority of surplus nitrogen contained in insoluble uric acid. In 'ureotelic' animals (e.g. mammals), ~95% of urinary nitrogen derives from proteins and other non-purine sources and is in the form of water-soluble urea. Purine degradation provides the ~5% urinary nitrogen excreted via uric acid. Uric acid is converted to allantoin before it appears in the urine in mammals other than hominid primates, including humans. Likewise it is converted further from allantoin to urea in adult amphibians (see Figure 13.4).

is of fundamental importance to the nitrogen cycle, about which I will write more in the following chapter. Bacteria use the enzyme urease to degrade urea to ammonia, which then forms ammonium salts that provide nitrogen for bacterial proliferation and for passing nitrogen on to plants. As if that were not important enough, bacteria are also integral to the internal

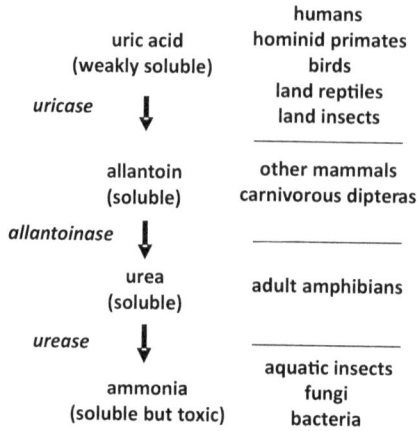

	humans
uric acid (weakly soluble)	hominid primates birds land reptiles land insects
uricase ↓	
allantoin (soluble)	other mammals carnivorous dipteras
allantoinase ↓	
urea (soluble)	adult amphibians
urease ↓	
ammonia (soluble but toxic)	aquatic insects fungi bacteria

Figure 13.4.

Simplified flow diagram of the enzymatic steps in degrading uric acid to ammonia. Gradual upstream attenuation of the enzyme pathway in different branches of the animal kingdom over the course of time has altered how uric acid-derived nitrogen is expelled in urine. Thus, humans and other species that have no uricase excrete uric acid, whereas other mammals and carnivorous dipteras have no allantoinase and excrete allantoin, etc. Some intermediate enzymes are not shown.

environment of animals, as the number of organisms in intestinal 'micro-biomes' is estimated to be around 10 times greater than the number of cells in animal bodies.[29] Stable isotope labelling studies performed in the 1950s on human volunteers (see Chapter 11) had shown that around one-third of uric acid leaves the body via the gastrointestinal tract rather than via the kidneys, and this proportion is higher in those with reduced kidney function.[30] Once within the gastrointestinal tract, uric acid is degraded by bacteria, both by the canonical route by which nitrogen ends up in ammonium salts and by a newly discovered biochemical pathway which contributes to the generation of short-chain fatty acids that are known to have anti-inflammatory properties.[31] A study in China has found that the microbiome profile of individuals with gout differs from normal, and it is possible that its exact composition is a factor determining whether or not hyperuricaemia leads to inflammation (see Chapter 9).[32] This new information on the importance of intestinal bacteria has obvious therapeutic implications, both for developing probiotics to promote a healthy microbiome and for being aware of the untoward consequences of changing the microbiome with antibiotics.[33]

Amphibians

Fish remove ammonia via their gills. A major adaptation that allowed multicellular species to live on land without gills was the development of an enzyme system in the liver known as the ornithine-urea cycle. This converts the ammonia derived from the degradation of proteins into less-toxic urea. The enzymes involved existed for different reasons in single-cell organisms and were repurposed for nitrogen waste disposal early during animal evolution.[34] The ornithine-urea cycle accounts for most of the urea in the urine of adult frogs and toads, with the remainder coming from purine breakdown via uric acid.[35] Tadpoles live, of course, in water and excrete ammonia like fish, and ornithine-urea cycle activity commences during metamorphosis into an adult amphibian – a good example of embryonic development sometimes recapitulating evolution.[36] Interestingly, the adult African clawed frog *Xenopus laevis*, which now has a watery existence, has largely reverted to ammonia excretion.[37]

Evolutionary adaptations are often due to the loss or silencing of genes rather than the gain of new ones.[38] Thus, ammonia generation from urea was prevented during the transition to terrestrial living by the loss of urease activity.

Reptiles and birds

As mentioned, birds and most reptiles release a semi-solid excrement rich in uric acid. Birds, of course, all descended from reptilian dinosaurs, a connection proposed by Thomas Huxley (1825–1895)[d] but not actually

---

[d] Huxley was a staunch defender of Charles Darwin's controversial theory and is often referred to as 'Darwin's Bulldog'.

proven until later.[39] During reptile evolution, the ornithine-urea cycle was silenced, and both protein and purine-derived nitrogen became shunted into uric acid. Furthermore, the expression of uricase, the enzyme that initiates the conversion of uric acid into allantoin, was also lost, resulting in uric acid being the major carrier of nitrogen into the urine. These changes are thought to have been water-conserving adaptations to arid climactic conditions and occurred in parallel with anatomical changes allowing urine to be concentrated within the cloaca and rectum. As uric acid has a very limited solubility in water, it compacts into an inert solid.[40] An obvious evolutionary benefit for birds retaining water by excreting uric acid is not needing to land for a drink while migrating. The Hudsonian godwit, for example, fuels up with protein from insects, molluscs and worms prior to a non-stop, nine-day flight of 10,000 km or so between southern South America and the Arctic.[41] Subsequent nitrogen excretion during flight via uric acid solidification then saves enough water for the journey. Along similar lines, terrestrial reptiles are able to live in sun-soaked deserts.

High urate levels in birds explain the observation made by the seventeenth-century Italian naturalist Ulisse Aldrovandi on hawks: 'a hard gypsum-like swelling around the fingers and palms, an evil of prime importance that hinders prey and for the most part incurable'.[e,42] Blood plasma urate levels can rise up to 1.8 mmol/l (31.6 mg/dl) after a meal in the peregrine falcon, which is impressive even accounting for the greater urate solubility at the higher body temperature of birds.[f,43] Given this, it is surprising that gout is not more common in carnivorous birds, and robust mechanisms must exist to prevent urate crystallisation (see Chapter 9). Nowadays, not many people keep birds of prey, but farmed poultry can also develop gouty tophi if inappropriately fed too much protein or if they

---

[e] Originally, '*Quae quidem nihil aliud est quam tumor durus, ac gypso similis, circa digitorum articulos, esque malum maximi in racabibus momenti. Impedit enim quo minus praedam captare possint, et incurabile plerumque est, quicquid decant alii*'.
[f] The theoretical limit of solubility of uric acid in avian blood plasma at 43°C is ~0.6 mmol/l (10.1 mg/dl).

have kidney problems. Curiously, gout in birds is somewhat different to humans, as it predominantly consists of tophi in the kidneys and other internal organs, hence the term 'avian visceral gout'.[44] That said, gout of the claws ('avian articular gout') can occur in genetically susceptible chicken strains (see Figure 13.5(a)), probably due to a reduced capacity of renal tubular solute carriers – as is the case for many humans with gout (see Chapter 11).[45] Reptiles can also develop gouty tophi, which are more often visceral than articular.[46] Actually, some of the dinosaurs probably also suffered from gout, as hinted by the eroded forefoot metacarpal of Sue, a *Tyrannosaurs Rex* which lived 65 million years ago (MYA) and whose fossilised bones are now in the Field Museum of Natural History in Chicago (see Figure 13.5(b)).[47] Alfred Garrod's drawing of a human metacarpal bone with a gouty erosion can be seen in Figure 13.5(c) for comparison.

Insects

John Davy found that a wide variety of insect larvae and adult insects in the West Indies also excrete most of their surplus nitrogen as uric acid. This does not apply to all insects, as, like snakes and amphibians that have reverted to living in water, aquatic insects release ammonia rather than uric acid or urea. Besides using uric acid as a means for nitrogenous waste disposal, terrestrial insects are interesting in the other uses to which they have evolved to put excreted uric acid. The concept of 'storage excretion' dates back to Frederick Gowland Hopkins (see Chapter 11), who early on in his career combined his love for butterflies with his chemical expertise to show that the wings of the Cabbage White (*Pieris brassiccae*) are rich in uric acid.[48] Many types of insects are now known to store uric acid in granules in 'urate cells' in the epidermis of their outer body. Uric acid, or one of its chemical derivatives, is responsible for white or opaque insect colouring, which contributes to camouflage from predators and mating identity and also serves an important protective role against sunburn. Insects that are genetically unable to make uric acid or prevented from doing so with allopurinol have reduced lifespans when subjected to oxidative stress or

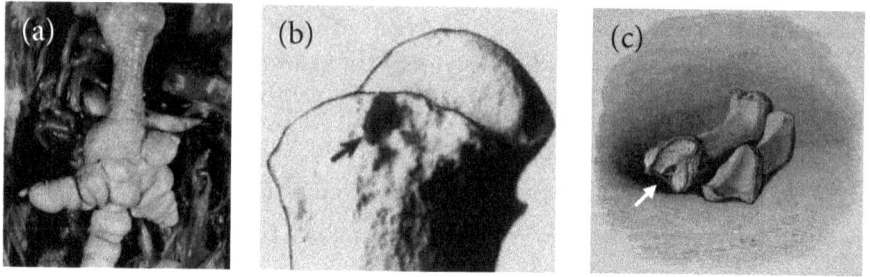

Figure 13.5.

(a) Gouty tophi on the left claw of a genetically predisposed chicken. From Cole and Austic (1980).

(b) A fossilised metacarpal bone of Sue, the Tyrannosaurs Rex that lives in the Field Museum of Natural History in Chicago. The arrow points to a bone erosion that could well have been due to a gouty tophus. From Rothschild *et al.* (1997).

(c) Drawing of two metacarpal bones by Alfred Garrod. The arrow points to an erosion surrounded by sodium urate incrustation. From *The Nature and Treatment of Gout and Rheumatic Gout* (1859).

Source: (a) Used with kind permission of Elsevier Science and Technology Journals; (b) used with kind permission of Springer Nature BV. Permission for (a) and (b) conveyed through Copyright Clearance Center, Inc.; (c) public domain.

ultraviolet radiation.[49] Other applications of uric acid by insects include providing the sheen of the wings of the scarab beetle and forming granules that reflect the flash out of the light organs of fireflies.[50]

Mammals

Although Liebig was correct that uric acid can be converted to urea in a test tube, the main reason that his sub-oxidation theory was wrong is that urea in mammalian urine does not derive from uric acid. Because of the ornithine-urea cycle, protein nitrogen goes directly into urea. In most mammals, purine-derived nitrogen, which accounts for only about 5% of total nitrogen excretion, is excreted as allantoin. This is because mammals have lost allantoinase that breaks down allantoin to allantoic acid. That humans are not alone amongst mammals in excreting uric acid rather than allantoin was discovered in the early 1900s by Wilhelm Wiechowski (1873–1928) at the German Institute of Pharmacology in Prague. He developed the first method for accurately measuring allantoin, which allowed him to establish that Max, Moritz and Lizy, three chimpanzees that he had befriended in a Viennese variety theatre, also excreted uric acid rather than allantoin.[51] In contrast, rhesus macaques and baboons excreted allantoin similar to other mammals.[52] In the United States, Gideon Wells (1875–1943) at the University of Chicago tested whether liver extracts could convert urate to allantoin in a dish. He found that livers from various mammals, including the rhesus macaque, rapidly did so, whereas human, chimpanzee and orangutan liver extracts failed.[53] Taken together, the implication from these studies was that uricase is not only missing in humans but also in great apes.

Reviving the Ancestral Uricase Gene

The arrival of DNA technology has led to the discovery of the genetic sequences for the uricase enzyme of mice, rats, pigs[g] and many other mammalian species.[54] These have been found to be very similar to that of soybean uricase, attesting to the common biochemical origins of animals and plants.[55] As uricase is not present in humans, one might have supposed that its gene would likewise be absent, but it turned out to still exist in the human genome as a vestigial inactive 'pseudogene' – part of 'junk DNA'.[56] Initial inspection of its sequence appeared to offer an explanation for its absence, as there is a mutation that disrupts the transcription of the gene into messenger RNA (mRNA), the chemical intermediary from which the protein enzyme is translated from the genetic code.[57] As this mutation was not found in gibbon uricase DNA, it must have occurred after the divergence of the gibbon and the human lineages, i.e. 18–12 MYA in the early-mid Miocene era.[58] At face value,

---

[g] From which the therapeutic Pegloticase is derived.

this finding favoured a critical one-off dramatic evolutionary event that led to the loss of uricase in all hominid descendants. However, the story is not that simple.

Palaeontology and geology have been recurrent interests among the cast of characters in this story, including Christopher Merrett, William Stukeley, John Hunter, Thomas Beddoes and James Parkinson. They all speculated on the origin and age of fossils in different rock strata and worried how their conclusions squared with the dates of Biblical creation. If they had possessed electron microscopes, they could also have seen fossilised bacteria and dated them back two billion years.[59] Similarly, fossilised pigmented subcellular organelles, known as melanosomes, have been used to infer the feather colours and plumage patterns of Jurassic dinosaurs that lived more than 175 MYA.[60] Despite these microscopic wonders, most fossils do not contain DNA, and so we know much more about the anatomies of ancient organisms than their genes. DNA is sufficiently stable to catch the perpetrators of legacy crimes, but it does not last forever, and the oldest archaic mammalian DNA fragments are from the teeth of mammoths preserved in Siberian permafrost around 1.65 MYA – just the other day on the evolutionary timeline.[61] The oldest DNA from an early human relative comes from Neanderthal remains found in a cave in Spain and dated at a mere 430,000 years ago.[62]

Enter the relatively new scientific discipline of paleogenomics. High-throughput technology has already given us the sequences of whole DNA genomes of numerous existing animals, plants and microorganisms.[63] These can now be aligned computationally to infer the common ancestral DNA at nodes of evolutionary divergence.[64] Once an ancestral sequence is deduced, it can then be used to synthesise in the laboratory the protein that the gene would have been translated into, and the function of this can then be tested.[65] For example, this approach has been used to determine that rhodopsin, a protein involved in night vision, was functional in detecting light in archosaurs, ancient reptiles that lived more than 240 MYA and which gave rise to birds and crocodiles. This suggests that archosaurs could see in the dark and may have been nocturnal.[66] In much the same way, the DNA sequences of ancient uricase genes have been inferred and ancestral uricase enzymes synthesised and tested for activity. It transpires that the gene was not suddenly lost by a single mutation, as had initially been supposed, but underwent a much slower sequential process of multiple minor changes. Based on the estimated dates of species divergence, this started more than 40 MYA in the Eocene epoch and resulted in a gradual reduction in enzyme activity and a functionally inert enzyme by the beginning of the Miocene epoch (20–15 MYA), well before the relatively recent mutation that prevents the gene being transcribed into mRNA.[67]

Has a High Uric Acid Level Benefited Humans?

As we have seen, reptiles, birds and insects have used uric acid for water conservation, and insects have put it to all sorts of other good uses. Has the climb in human blood urate levels due to diminishing uricase activity over the millennia done more for our race in its struggle for survival than simply and unjustly predispose us to gout? Apparently damaging genetic mutations can certainly have beneficial trade-offs, with the most commonly cited example being sickle cell anaemia. In that case, disease-causing mutations of the haemoglobin beta gene have survived because they confer a degree of resistance to malaria.[68] Many theories have arisen on the possible benefits to humans of a high uric acid level; however, before I go on, I must point out that none are proven.

Intelligence and drive

The first theory to mention concerns drive and intelligence, which some may say are the keys to our success as a species. The physicist and metallurgist Egon Orowan (1902–1989) wrote to the science journal *Nature* in 1955 suggesting that uric acid acts as a brain stimulant. His point was that many alkaloids that are variably found in coffee, tea and other plant products are purines with chemical similarity to uric acid. Caffeine, for example, is trimethyl-xanthine (see Figure 8.4(b)) and, after ingestion, is initially metabolised to monomethyl-xanthine and then further metabolised by xanthine oxidase to methyl-uric acid.[69] Orowan proposed that a high uric acid level might have a caffeine-like effect on the brain that might have been an advantage to our evolutionary ancestors.[70] The geneticist Jack Haldane (1894–1964) soon reminded *Nature* readers that the potency of any such effect of urate must be slight, as a relatively high concentration of urate in the body does not prevent us from feeling the impact of a much lower concentration of caffeine once we drink coffee.[71] There is probably nothing to Orowan's theory, as we now know that caffeine and other plant purines act on specific receptors in the brain, heart and other tissues, and these receptors do not appear to respond to uric acid.[72] An alternative take on caffeine as a purine is that inhibiting xanthine oxidase with allopurinol or other inhibitor drugs may well enhance the effects of a cup of coffee by preventing caffeine degradation to inert methyl-uric acid.[73]

The notion that gout is linked to high mental function was actually around long before Orowan, with Thomas Sydenham having famously consoled himself for his own severe gout as follows:

> For humble individuals like myself, there is one poor comfort, which is this, viz. that gout, unlike any other disease kills more rich men than poor, more wise men than simple. Great kings, emperors, generals, admirals, and philosophers have all died of gout. Hereby Nature shows her impartiality: since those whom she favours in one way she afflicts in another – a mixture of good and evil pre-eminently adapted to our frail mortality: *Nihil est ab omni beatum*.[h,74]

---

[h] '*Nihil est ab omni beatum*' is from Horace, Odes 2.16, and translates as 'Nothing is blessed in every way'.

The belief survived into the twentieth century, with the physician and sex-psychologist Havelock Ellis noting in his *A Study of British Genius* (1904):

> There is, however, a pathological condition which occurs so often, in such extreme forms, and in men of such pre-eminent intellectual ability, that it is impossible not to regard it as having a real association with such ability. I refer to gout.[75]

A number of mid- and late-twentieth-century studies attempted to address this matter scientifically. DeWitt Stetten (see Chapter 11) and the mathematician John Hearon (1920–2009) at the US National Institute of Health found that blood urate levels in a group of young male army recruits eating the standard camp diet showed a small but statistically significant correlation with results from the Army Classification Battery psychological aptitude tests.[76] Following this, a number of studies have been published in prominent journals showing, for instance: that urate levels were higher in company executives than in blue-collar workers; that serum urate concentrations correlated with measures of drive, achievement, and leadership amongst university professors; and, in male high school students, with persevering with education and with grade achievement.[77] Modern sensitivities over what constitutes intelligence and its heritability, and indeed the perceived social injustice of the questions, make organising a definitive project on this subject difficult, and in any case, it would require a large number of participants to enable a robust statistical analysis to exclude the very many possible confounding lifestyle variables causing spurious correlations.

Uric acid as an antioxidant

The next theory to bring up concerns uric acid being an 'electron donor' and acting as an antioxidant. This may be as much responsible for uric acid's life-prolonging function in insects as providing a physical barrier to solar irradiation (see above). Our most obvious antioxidant is ascorbic acid (vitamin C), which back in time could be synthesised within the body. More than 61 MYA, well before the loss of uricase, serial mutations of the gene encoding the enzyme L-gulen-gamma-lactone oxidase led to our primate ancestors losing the ability to synthesise ascorbic acid. This may not have mattered much when the ancestral diet contained plenty of ascorbic acid in fruit and vegetables; however, since then, it has been a necessary dietary supplement.[78] It has been suggested that, over time, uric acid has taken on some of the antioxidant load from ascorbic acid.[79] It is now twice as plentiful in the human body as ascorbic acid and contributes over 50% of the antioxidant capacity of blood plasma.[80] This raises the question of whether uric acid, if not gout (see Chapter 2), has a salutary benefit.

There may be a particular protective role for uric acid in the brain, which is particularly sensitive to oxidative stress.[81] The first hint that high urate levels might protect against brain disease came from a study showing that those with multiple sclerosis had significantly lower blood urate levels and lower incidences of gout than those without multiple sclerosis.[82] Since then, high urate levels have been correlated with protection from various other neurological and psychiatric problems, including Parkinson's disease, schizophrenia, Alzheimer's disease and depression.[83] In the case of Parkinson's disease, this association only seems to apply to men.[84] Post-mortem examination of brains from Parkinson's disease patients has revealed a relationship between low urate concentrations and reduced dopamine, the principal neurotransmitter deficient in the disease.[85] However Mendelian Randomization studies, using variants of genes affecting urate levels (see Chapter 11), have not offered much support for a direct causal relationship between a low plasma urate and Parkinson's or other neurological diseases.[86] Furthermore, a large clinical trial which tested the effect of increasing urate levels by administration of inosine, a precursor of uric acid in purine degradation, failed to show any benefit to Parkinson's disease patients.[87]

Fat deposition

Moving from the brain to metabolism, another theory for the advantages of a high urate level is that it contributes to the laying down of fat (see Chapter 14).[88] Nowadays, fat is mostly unwelcome, whereas, for our ancient primate ancestors, it might have been a lifesaver in providing an energy store to help through winters and other periods of food scarcity. The evolutionary changes in the uricase gene may therefore have contributed to what has been called the 'thrifty genotype', a controversial term used to encompass a group of genetic changes that accelerate fat deposition as an insurance against future famine.[89] Curbing enthusiasm for this story is the distinct disadvantage for our ancient ancestors of being overweight when it came to chasing prey or avoiding predators.[90]

Just genetic drift?

The risk of squeezing genetic changes in general into a natural selection framework was highlighted in *The Spandrels of San Marco* (1979), in which Stephen Gould (1941–2002) and Richard Lewontin (1929–2021) pilloried the evolutionary speculations over the previous 40 years in Britain and the United States, pointing out that basing species change solely on natural selection was overinterpreting Darwin's message.[91] In the final edition of *Origin of Species*, Darwin himself asserted:

> As my conclusions have lately been much misrepresented, and it has been stated that I attribute the modification of species exclusively to natural selection, I may be permitted to remark that in the first edition of this work, and subsequently, I placed in a most conspicuous position – namely at the close of the Introduction – the following words: 'I am convinced that natural selection has been the main, but not the exclusive means of modification.' This has been of no avail. Great is the power of steady misinterpretation.[92]

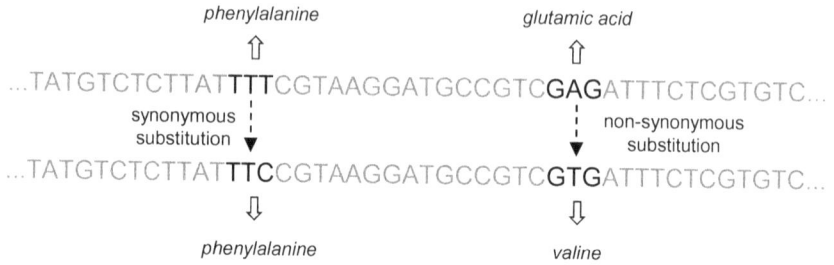

phenylalanine   glutamic acid

⇑   ⇑

...TATGTCTCTTAT**TTT**CGTAAGGATGCCGTC**GAG**ATTTCTCGTGTC...

synonymous   non-synonymous
substitution ▼   ▼ substitution

...TATGTCTCTTAT**TTC**CGTAAGGATGCCGTC**GTG**ATTTCTCGTGTC...

⇩   ⇩

phenylalanine   valine

Figure 13.6.

DNA is made up of a string of purine (adenine, A; guanine, G) and pyrimidine (thymine, T; cytosine, C) nucleotide subunits. Each three nucleotides form a 'codon' that is transcribed into messenger RNA and then translated into a particular amino acid, which is then incorporated sequentially into a protein. A 'non-synonymous substitution' describes a nucleotide mutation that changes the amino acid translated from a codon. On the right of this figure, an A-to-T mutation results in valine rather than glutamic acid, which will in turn alter the protein. As some amino acids are translated from more than one codon, a 'synonymous substitution' describes a mutation that does not alter the amino acid and leaves the subsequent protein unchanged. On the left of this figure, phenylalanine is encoded by either TTT or TTC, so the T-to-C mutation does not matter. A high ratio of non-synonymous to synonymous substitutions provides evidence for positive evolutionary selection of a gene. This evidence is lacking in the case of the uricase gene.

The banal possibility is that, over the course of time, the rise in urate levels has just been through neutral genetic drift, as the precise level of uric acid prior to reaching the saturation point did not matter much. Adaptive selection in a gene is more likely if the number of non-synonymous mutations[i] exceeds the number of synonymous mutations[j] (see Figure 13.6). In the case of the uricase gene, this is not the case, making neutral drift entirely possible.[93] Similar considerations apply to the finding that parallel genetic mutations in the URAT1 solute channel (see Chapter 11) have

---

[i] i.e. mutations that alter amino acids in the translated protein.
[j] i.e. mutations that do not alter amino acids in the translated protein.

led to an increased efficiency of urate reabsorption from the kidney back into blood.[94] However, if these were both due to genetic drift, a parallel conundrum is what has prevented similar genetic drift in the uricase genes of non-hominid mammals that have maintained uricase activity?

Reflections on Evolution and Gout

Whatever the reason, the definite conclusion of this chapter is that human evolution is one of the most important causes for the urate concentration in humans being so close to its saturation point and causing crystal formation and gout (see Figure 13.7). However, one only has to look at chimpanzees to realise that a loss of uricase does not in itself cause gout. Chimpanzees have a urate concentration of 0.18–0.24 mmol/l (3–4 mg/100 mol), well

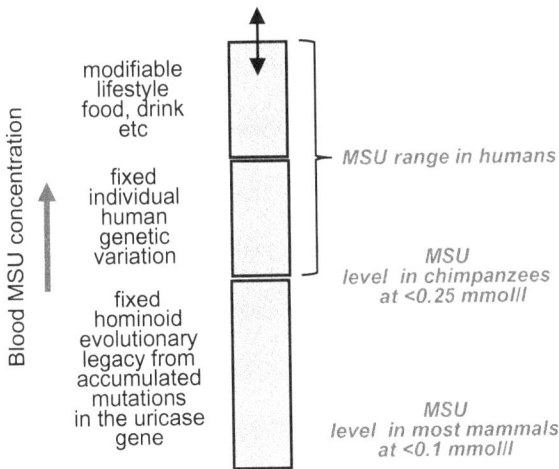

Figure 13.7.

Our evolutionary legacy is one of the most important reasons for blood monosodium urate (MSU) levels being close to the saturation level. We vary genetically one to another in uric acid handling, placing some more than others in the danger zone for gout. Levels can then fluctuate due to lifestyle, most obviously related to food and drink. It is the fluctuations that trigger acute gouty inflammation.

below the notional saturation level of 0.41 mmol/l, and appear to be gout-free.[95] As outlined in Chapter 11, humans have developed many further genetic variations that increase urate levels, but again these are mostly not enough to lead to gout without a further environmental influence, however small, taking us out of kilter with the lifestyle our genes equipped us for. For instance, humans only started eating meat about 1.5 MYA, millions of years after the loss of uricase, and drinking beer many many years after that! We now turn to the final chapter to look at much more recent environmental considerations.

Chapter 14

Food, Gout and Global Health

The link between body weight and gout has long been recognised, as in 1825 by Charles Scudamore:

> Most commonly, we find upon enquiry that the patient traces a gradual enlargement of the abdomen, joined with various indications of an increasing fulness of habit; ... the whole of the abdomen is unduly distended; and the muscles are usually covered with an accumulation of fat.... In a few words there is too much abdominal corpulence.[1]

Corpulence and gout in Scudamore's time were the province of the rich and well-fed, but no longer is that the case. This last chapter takes an ecological look at how changes in food supply and consumption have led to weight gain and have moved gout into being a sentinel of ill health in the general population.

Food Insecurity

A large population used to be considered desirable for national survival. In the mid-1700s, the same Thomas Short who recommended sugar (see Chapter 12) delved into English parish records for shortfalls in baptisms *versus* burials and determined that a higher birth rate was needed for the nation to be competitive in the battle for resources. He recommended taxing bachelors – similar to the *Lex Papia et Poppaea* that the Emperor

Augustus imposed in Ancient Rome in 7 AD and to the laws of national expansion introduced later in the twentieth century by Joseph Stalin in the USSR and Benito Mussolini in Italy.[2]

The notion that countries cannot expand indefinitely without resorting to war only started being taken seriously with the publication of the cleric Thomas Malthus's *Essay on the Principle of Population, as it affects the Future Improvement of Society*. This came out in 1798, around the time William Hyde Wallaston was discovering sodium urate in gouty tophi.[3] Malthus realised that the size of any population depends on the availability of the food required for its sustenance. Put starkly, a population can expand until there is not enough food, at which point there will be civil disorder. Malthus's essay immediately separated romantics from realists. Optimists such as Samuel Taylor Coleridge and Robert Southey, who came together in Thomas Beddoes' Bristol set (see Chapter 6), dismissed Malthus's gloomy predictions as self-evident in the absence of political reform: 'It remains to be seen whether human institutions, or the laws of nature be in fault'.[4] On the other hand, the Malthusian struggle for existence later became one of the premises for Charles Darwin's theory of natural selection.[5]

The backdrops to Malthus's essay were the harvest failures and the high cost of living in Western Europe that led up to the revolution and its bloody aftermath in France in 1789, as well as to food rioting in England in 1795.[6] Thomas Beddoes had delayed fundraising for his Medical Pneumatic Institution (see Chapter 6) 'partly from the necessity of contributions to keep the poor alive this hard winter'.[7] He wrote a public letter to the prime minister William Pitt castigating him for doing so little to prevent hunger and offering a raft of advice for diversifying food production and consumption to meet the challenges.[8] James Parkinson in London was also a campaigner, that is, when not writing about gout, describing the shaking palsy or collecting and cataloguing fossils (see Chapter 6). Wisely using the pseudonym 'Old Hubert', he had published *An Address to the Hon. Edmund Burke from the Swinish Multitude* (1793), reproaching Edmund Burke (1729–1797) for his negative *Reflections on the Revolution in France* and taking particular exception to his writing that 'learning will be cast into the mire, and trodden under the hoofs of the swinish multitude,'[9] Parkinson concluded that, as far as Burke was concerned, the swinish multitude could always eat acorns. He followed up two years later with *Whilst the Honest Poor Are Wanting Bread*, contrasting the sufferings of the poor with the excesses of the wealthy.[10] As a member of the secret anti-establishment London Corresponding Society, Parkinson sailed close to the political wind and ended up being investigated and cross-examined by the Privy Council in 1795 for his knowledge of the 'Popgun Plot', a trumped-up intrigue to assassinate King George III with a poison dart.[11]

Food availability and pricing remained a big problem in Britain throughout the late 1700s and early 1800s and threatened political stability. Following the Battle of Waterloo on 18 June 1815 and the end of the long Napoleonic wars, resumption of trade led to an influx of cheap foreign corn and a fall in wholesale prices. To appease the landowners (who largely constituted the very limited electorate), the government passed protectionist Corn Laws, which imposed an importation tariff that prevented a fall in bread prices. The problem was then conflated by the fallout from the massive volcanic explosion of Mount Tambora in the Dutch East Indies (now Indonesia) in April 1815, the largest eruption on historical record, releasing around 60 megatons of sulphur into the Earth's atmosphere. It is said that the heavy rains and mud attributable to the eruption exhausted Napoleon's troops marching towards Waterloo and helped the Duke of Wellington and the Prussian allies win the battle.[12] The sky was still overcast in 1816 and led to 'the year without a summer' with crop failures, further increased food prices and riots throughout the world.[13] In addition, there were epidemics of infectious diseases, such as typhus and cholera. All these underlined the rapid effects that even brief climate change can have.[14] On a brighter note, the brilliant sunsets due to the atmospheric ash over Europe are said to have inspired the colourful skyscapes of contemporary painters such as J. M. W. Turner and Caspar David Friedrich.[15]

The maintained high price of food, together with the lack of suffrage of the working class, led to the protest at St. Peter's Field in Manchester in August 1819, at which government cavalry killed 18 protesters and wounded hundreds more. George Cruikshank (1792–1878), the inheritor of James Gillray's legacy, castigated what has become known as the 'Peterloo Massacre' (Figure 14.1(a)) and then three days later published *The Royal Embarkation*, showing the Prince Regent looking particularly out of touch while being carried from a bathing hut to his barge (Figure 14.1(b)).[16] The future George IV was an old-fashioned high-living gouty stereotype (and a regular consumer of *Dr. Wilson's Tincture* – see Chapter 5) and the epitome of Hanovarian self-indulgence. He had suffered his first attack of arthritis in 1811 at the age of 49 years.[17] The episode was put down to a sprained ankle, and there was a court cover-up to prevent it being viewed as the first sign of his having inherited his father George III's madness. In the words of the historian Arthur Bryant,

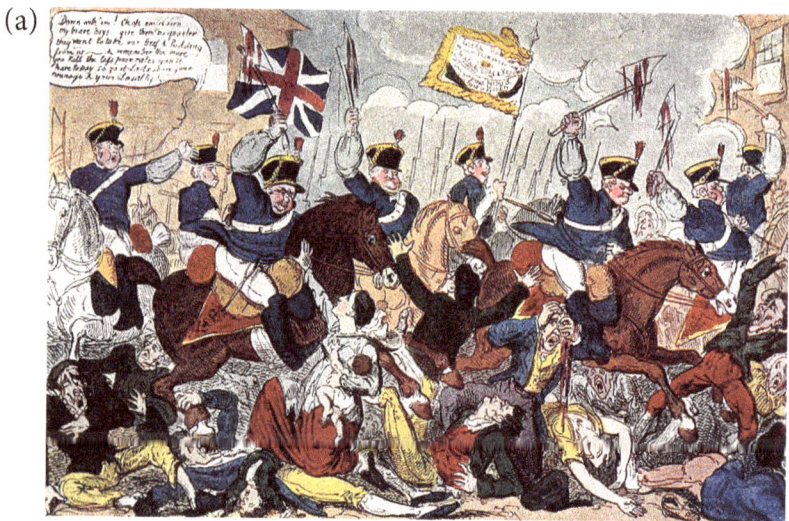

Figure 14.1.

George Cruikshank was James Gillray's successor as top British satirical cartoonist.

(a) His *Massacre at St. Peter's or BRITON'S STRIKE HOME!!*, as depicted soon after food riots in Manchester in 1819, during which government cavalry killed 18 protesters and wounded hundreds. The cavalry captain exclaims top left: '*Down with 'em! Chop em down my brave boys: give them no quarter. They want to take our Beef and Pudding from us___& remember the more you kill the less poor rates you'll have to pay so go it Lads and show your courage & your loyalty!*'

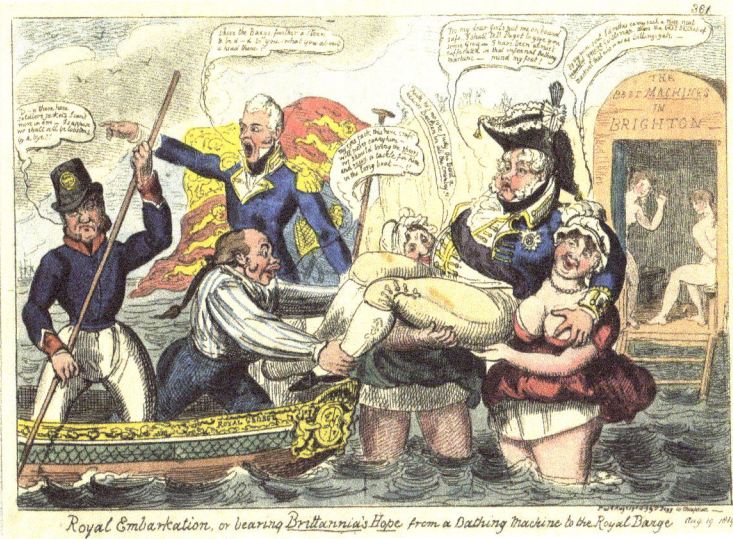

Figure 14.1. (*Continued*)

(b) Three days later, Cruikshank published *The Royal Embarkation, or Bearing Brittannia's Hope from a Bathing Machine to the Royal Barge*. Note the Prince Regent's bandaged right foot, indicative of gout and all its social and political connotations. The bathing machine is named '*Best Bathing Machine in Brighton*' and is shown with its attractions top right.

Source: Both via Wikimedia Commons, public domain.

the Regent was 'at once a national scandal, a national disaster, a national achievement, and a national entertainment'[18] – entertainment for his lifestyle; achievement for his building Brighton Pavilion and Regent's Street in London; disaster for his political mishandling of the nation; and scandal for the combination of the three.

The Board of Agriculture

The riots emphasised a pressing need in Britain for more food security. Novel farming techniques, land drainage and new crops were being introduced with the 'Agricultural Revolution' from the mid-1600s, but gains in food production were modest.[19] It was Humphry Davy, already famous for his laughing gas experiments with Beddoes (see Chapter 6), who introduced chemistry to British farmers. Davy's move from Bristol to London came three years after the publication of Malthus' essay. Joseph Banks arranged for him to conduct soil analyses and deliver lectures on chemistry for the Board of Agriculture and Internal Improvement.[20] This was what today we would call a 'quango', established by an act of parliament in 1793, with the early statistician John Sinclair (1754–1835) as founding president. The agricultural writer Arthur Young (1741–1820) was chosen as secretary in light of his *Example of France: a warning to Great Britain* (1793), in which he recounted eyewitness experiences of the anarchy, bloodshed and famine across the Channel.[21] The Board's aims were to provide previously unavailable quantitative information on the state of agriculture in England, improve the productivity of farming, increase the availability of affordable food and benefit the domestic manufacturing industry – all towards obtaining food security and preserving the political *status quo*.[22] In Sinclair's words:

> The people having thus the necessaries of life cheaper, must be better satisfied with the government under which they live than otherwise they would be, and must have more money to lay out on superfluities.... Hence, both the peace and quiet of the country, and the resources of the state depend upon the progress of our agricultural improvements.[23]

Davy delivered six agricultural lectures annually from May 1803, with the content maturing over 10 years.[24] He published his lectures in 1813 as *Elements of Agricultural Chemistry*, which was the first systematic book on the subject. It is a very readable account of the 47 chemical elements that had been identified to date and of the simple ways in which they combined with one another. The book went into some 23 editions by 1847, including translations into French, Italian, German and Russian.[25] That chemical elements cycle between animals and plants had already been made clear by Joseph Black, who showed the conversion by animals of oxygen to carbon dioxide, and Joseph Priestley, who showed the reciprocal conversion by plants of carbon dioxide to oxygen.[26] Reflecting on the carbon cycle, Davy wrote that plants and animals 'seem to be connected together in the exercise of their living functions, and to a certain extent made to depend upon each other for existence'.[27] He conducted experiments which showed the improved growth of plants fed with nitrogen via ammonia dissolved in water but had little idea how nitrogen achieved this or how plants obtained nitrogen naturally.

Liebig's Law of the Minimum

Davy's book remained the standard text on the subject in Britain and North America until the arrival onto the agricultural scene of Justus Liebig (see Chapters 8 and 13).[28] Liebig published his foray into food production in 1840 as *Organic Chemistry in Its Application to Agriculture and Physiology*.[29] His 'law of the minimum' advocated that the growth of plants is primarily limited by whichever essential chemical is least plentiful in the soil. As part of his demolition of vitalism, Liebig dictated that crop improvements could be achieved cheaply by dressing the fields with a cocktail of essential elements. He teamed up with commercial partners in Britain and, around 1845, started marketing a panel of six fertilisers, each designed to provide only what he considered necessary for particular crops.[30] While Liebig realised that plants needed nitrogen, he viewed its presence in his fertilisers as unnecessary since he mistakenly believed plants could perfectly well take it up directly from the air, as they do carbon dioxide, or have it delivered dissolved in rainwater. Just as Liebig was not a physiologist, he was not a practising farmer. He unwisely considered experimental field trials unnecessary, even though the methodology for these already existed.[31] Without nitrogen, his fertilisers were a disaster, and Liebig rapidly moved from saint to sinner among the many farmers who had wasted their money.[32] Ironically, the lack of nitrogen had inadvertently demonstrated his law of the minimum.

Liebig later made various other commercial nutritional ventures, perhaps the best known being his *Extractum Carnis,* which was derived from South American beef and marketed as a kind of superfood. In Liebig's words, *Extractum Carnis* 'derives its value as a nutrient for the nations of Europe, provided it can be produced in large quantities and at a cheap rate from countries where meat has no value'.[33] One pound of the extract was claimed to have as much soluble nitrogen as 32 pounds of lean, fresh beef meat. The assertion came to the attention of the food analyst Arthur Hill Hassall (see Chapters 4 and 12) and others, who found that some preparations had plenty of salt but none had much utilisable nitrogen.[34] The battle was thrashed out in the correspondence section of *The Lancet,* Hassall's home turf. In due course, the sales pitch for *Extractum Carnis* was changed to its benefits as a nerve tonic and then to just flavouring, becoming the precursor of kitchen stock cubes today.[35]

Nitrogen Processing in the Soil

We now know that a strong thunderstorm can cause some atmospheric nitrogen to enter rainwater as nitric acid, but the amount is not substantial. Whether or not nitrogen in the air can be taken up by plants had been addressed in the late 1830s by the French chemist Jean-Baptiste Boussingault (1801–1887). Crop rotation, including a season of growing legumes, is a very old farming practice, going back at least as far as the Romans. Boussingault obtained experimental evidence that legumes can assimilate nitrogen from the air, whereas cereal plants cannot.[36] Actually, legumes and other 'nitrogen-fixing' plants do not directly fix nitrogen but depend on 'diazotrophic' bacteria. Very early on in Earth's history, strains of bacteria developed the capacity to convert atmospheric nitrogen (N_2) to ammonia (NH_3) using an enzyme called nitrogenase that presumably evolved to operate under low oxygen conditions underground – indeed nitrogenase is inhibited by contact with oxygen.[37] In a symbiotic arrangement,[a] these bacteria isolate themselves

---

[a] i.e. mutually rewarding.

from oxygen in easily visible nodules on the roots of the plants, where they have access to plant sugars that provide the energy needed for nitrogenase to function.[38] Fixed nitrogen then transfers from the bacteria into the plant root, where it is incorporated into organic compounds for distribution to the plant above ground. In peas and beans, the primary starting point for distributing nitrogen is via purines, synthesised by the same ancient enzyme series introduced in Chapter 8. Uric acid is then generated via xanthine oxidase and digested via uricase to soluble allantoin and allantoic acid (see Chapter 13), which then pass up the plant to the leaves, flowers and fruit.[39] While this is the most efficient way in which plants can acquire nitrogen naturally, they also do so via the actions of soil microorganisms degrading dead plant and animal organic material (see Chapter 13).[40]

Guano and the nitrogen cycle

The other traditional way to fertilise the soil and improve crops is to add animal dung. Humphry Davy had given an excellent account of the various types of manures that farmers used in the early nineteenth century.[41] Although not yet available, he realised the potential of guano, made up from the excrement and carcases of mammals, birds, insects and spiders and deposited in vast amounts on the rainless Chincha islands and other coastal sites off Peru.[42] Guano was highly valued as a soil conditioner by the Incas, who protected its sustainability by law. The German explorer Alexander von Humboldt (1769–1859) had acquired a sample while visiting Peru in 1802 to observe a transit of the planet Mercury. Once back in Paris, he had passed it on to the chemists Antoine de Fourcroy (see Chapter 6) and Louis Vauquelin, who found that at least a quarter by weight was uric acid – hardly surprising in view of the origin of the material.[43] Later analyses showed guano to have a very high nitrogen content, originating not only from uric acid but also from urea, guanine, proteins and their various products degrading into ammonia, as well as being rich in phosphates, sulphates and 'potash'.[b] Imitating guano, Davy organised a trial of

---

[b] i.e. potassium salts.

local seabird dung in Merionethshire in North Wales and found that it had a powerful effect on the growth of grass.[44] His army surgeon brother John (see Chapter 13) later presented a paper to the Royal Society, indicating that the crucial environment for Peruvian guano was the absence of rain that would wash away the nitrogen and the strong sunlight that promoted uric acid degradation.[45] This was well before the digestion of nitrogenous compounds in animal excrement by soil bacteria was understood.

It was probably through his brother's interest in guano as a soil supplement that John Davy conducted his painstaking analyses of insect and spider excrement while posted in the West Indies (see Chapter 13). Just four years before he travelled there, Boussingault and Jean-Baptiste Dumas (1800–1884) had published their *Essai de statique chimique des litres organists*, which proposed an animal–plant nitrogen cycle akin to the well-established carbon cycle.[46] Davy embellished the concept to involve the uric acid excrement of insects, and the 'xanthine oxide'[c] from spiders, writing from Barbados in 1946:

> In this tropical region, teeming with animal life, and equally so with vegetable, the quality of the urinary excrement of spiders as well as of insects, considering their composition … seems to be peculiarly in harmony with an adaptation of means to ends, and affording an example of that happy economy which is so often to be witnessed in the processes of nature. Both appear to be specially fitted to form a part of the food of plants. Both are only slightly soluble in water. Both in their unmixed state appear to be rejected by animals of every description when in search of food. Ants here, which may be considered the principal scavengers of the tropics, especially as regards putrefactive animal matter, leave untouched, as I have observed, the urinary excrement both of spiders and of insects. This exemption from destruction may be said to insure to the soil productive of vegetables a constant source of manure;

---

[c] i.e. guanine.

the vegetables in such a climate as this supporting innumerable insects, and the insects in their turn supporting in great numbers spiders and other animals – such as birds, lizards, batrachians – the excretions of which have similar qualities, and are well adapted to perform the same part. Ought not this to be a lesson to man to husband excrementitious matters generally, making no exception, and to bestow them on the soil as its peculiar and appropriate fertilizers?[47]

Guano started to be imported into Britain in 1840. Farmers found that it was vastly more effective than ordinary farmyard dung or Liebig's fertilisers or any of the other manufactured products that were starting to appear.[48] By the early 1850s, Britain was importing around 200,000 tons of guano per year, providing large amounts of nitrogen, phosphate and other nutrients to delighted farmers. Faced with serious homeland soil depletion through repeat cropping without replacement, the United States imported over three times more and became reliant on it to feed its rapidly expanding population. In his first State of the Union address in 1850, President Millard Fillmore specified that:

Peruvian guano has become so desirable an article to the agricultural interest of the United States that it is the duty of the Government to employ all the means properly in its power for the purpose of causing that article to be imported into the country at a reasonable price. Nothing will be omitted on my part toward accomplishing this desirable end.[49]

As the price of guano was set high by the Peruvian Government, American businessmen started looking elsewhere for similar natural deposits.[50] In 1856, the Federal Government duly passed the Guano Islands Act of 1856, legitimising in the nation's eyes the 'claiming' of uninhabited islands across the world and placing American feet firmly in imperialist waters. Eventually, around 200 such islands were so possessed by the US, but these did not fully live up to their promise, as the nitrogen had mostly been washed away by the rain. Nevertheless, the deposits on many islands were removed by the Pacific Guano Company for their phosphate and potassium content and mixed with fish corpses to add nitrogen to a manufactured fertiliser. One remote island annexed by the US for guano, Johnston Atoll, came in handy later for testing nuclear and biological weapons.

Peru's easy income from selling its natural resources led to the country sliding into social and political indolence.[51] Its dependence on the guano trade resulted in the 'Guano War' of 1864–1866, in which a Peruvian alliance with Chile terminated the Spanish occupation of the Chincha Islands. An 1853 report on Peruvian guano written for United States farmers by the Peruvian government agent in Baltimore was at pains to point out that supplies were inexhaustible.[52] However, Liebig considered the lucrative trade to be international plundering. He was correct, as, despite the enormous size of some of the deposits,[d] the guano mining took its toll. By the time the reserves were exhausted in the 1870s, Peru had exported around 12 million tons.[53] The American and European fallback then became the natural deposits of nitrates discovered in the Atacama Desert and in Antofagasta, again in South America, as well as relatively small amounts of ammonium sulphate being released in industrial countries as a by-product from converting coal to coke. How the South American nitrate deposits came to be there is not fully resolved but may have involved the disintegration of marine organisms and the precipitation of atmospheric nitrogen via lightening, with the extreme climactic dryness of the regions preventing nitrogen wash off. The export of nitrates from South America rose from 935 tons in 1830 to 2,478,000 tons in 1912, during which time the trade was fought over in the War of the Pacific (1879–1883), in which Chile annexed the resources from Peru and Bolivia.[54]

The grand nitrogen challenge

So, by the late nineteenth century, South American nitrates had allowed a major agricultural expansion, with ensuing European and American

---

[d] Some had a depth of 200 feet or more.

population explosions; however, the problem was that the food security was unsustainable and unstable since guano was running out and Chile controlled 80% of the world nitrogen supply.[55] It was William Crookes (1832–1919) (Figure 14.2(a)) who reminded everyone of the Malthusian jeopardy. Crookes is mostly remembered as the inventor of the Crookes tube. This was a major innovation, which, for example, enabled the discovery of X-rays by Wilhelm Röntgen in 1895 and was later the starting point for televisions. Crookes was a scientific giant of the Victorian era and was awarded the (Humphry) Davy medal of the Royal Society in 1888 'For his investigations on the behaviour of substances under the influences of the electric discharge in a high vacuum'. Ten years later, he was elected president

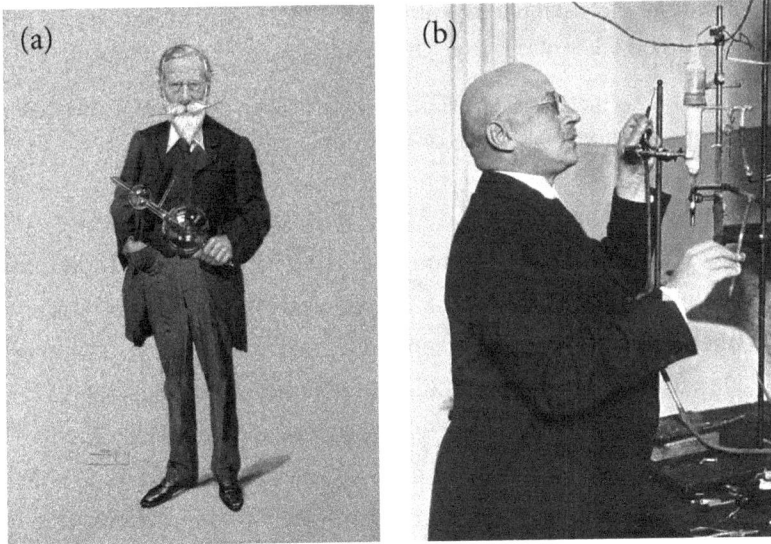

Figure 14.2.

(a) William Crookes in 1902, painted holding one of his glowing tubes by Leslie Ward (Spy). The painting had the caption '*ubi Crookes ibi lux*' ('where there is Crookes, there is light'). Three years earlier, Crookes had given his presidential address to the British Association for the Advancement of Science, in which he foresaw a global doomsday due to food shortages related to population growth. He laid down the scientific grand challenge of extracting atmospheric nitrogen from the air to provide plant fertiliser.

(b) Fritz Haber around 1914.

(*Continued*)

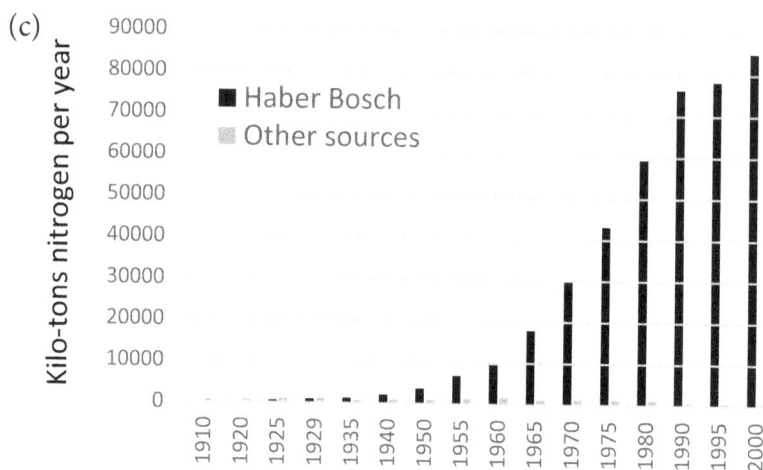

Figure 14.2. (*Continued*)

(c) Estimated global consumption of nitrogen fertilisers obtained through the Haber–Bosch process and other means (e.g. Chilean nitrates, ammonia from coke ovens).

Source: (a) Courtesy of the Wellcome Collection, public domain; (b) via Wikimedia Commons, public domain: (c) graph generated using data from Smil. Enriching the Earth, 2001, appendix L.

of the British Association for the Advancement of Science, and he divided his presidential address at the annual meeting in September 1898 into two parts. The first part of his address was an analysis predicting that Europe would not be able to obtain sufficient nitrogen for food security beyond the 1930s. He supported this with detailed statistics on wheat harvests in Britain and the rest of the world, together with the rates of population growth. Keen not to be perceived as a herald of doom, Crookes reminded the audience that 79% of atmospheric air is elemental nitrogen and that there are around 20 million tons of nitrogen over each square mile of the Earth's surface. He threw down the grand challenge of harnessing free nitrogen from the air to feed the world: 'It is the chemist that must come to the rescue of the threatened communities. It is through the laboratory that starvation may be turned into plenty'.[56] Atmospheric nitrogen (N_2) is very stable since the two nitrogen atoms are linked by a triple bond; however, as mentioned, it was known that the atoms could be separated by the immense energy of a lightning bolt, bringing nitrates down to earth in the rain. Crookes had conducted a presentation at a Royal Society soirée six years previously on the 'Flame of Burning Nitrogen', showing that nitrous and nitric oxide could form when passing a strong electric current through the air but realised that the energy needed to fix nitrogen using his technique on an industrial scale was currently prohibitive. He suggested that the hydro-electric potential of the Niagara Falls might be harnessed to do it at scale.[57]

The end of Crooke's presidential address dwelt on the paranormal, in which he had a longstanding interest, and indeed, he had been made president of the Society for Psychical Research the previous year.[58] Crooke was not alone in believing in spiritual phenomena, sharing this with Sherlock Holmes's author Arthur Conan Doyle (1859–1930) and the evolutionist Alfred Wallace, among many other eminent mid-late Victorians. In Crooke's case, his championing of psychic research was encouraged by the recent discoveries of radiation. His conjectures were mostly met with deep suspicion among his scientific peers, and the supposedly real phenomena that he believed in turned out to be frauds. His devoting part of his address to psychic research was no doubt appreciated by the imaginative section of the audience, but it created a scientific credibility gap that rather played into the hands of the many ears unsympathetic to his glum food forecasting.[59] The following day, *The Times* reported that there was still plenty of uncultivated land in Eastern Europe and Australia.[60] The paper then published a letter from the agricultural reformers John Lawes and Henry Gilbert arguing essentially that nitrogen supplies were less of a problem than poor farming practices.[61]

Despite the immediate hostile reaction from the agricultural establishment, Crookes's message was listened to both at home and abroad.[62] It was particularly heard in Germany, which had a rapidly growing urbanised population and imported 10 times more nitrate from Chile than Britain.[63] Land expansion or colonisation was one solution to more food, but that would mean war; war required explosives; and explosives at that time also required nitrogen. Bird excrement containing 'saltpetre' had been protected for this purpose by various English administrations over the years, long before any detailed understanding of the chemistry involved. For instance, the exhaustion of gunpowder supplies after the English Civil War became an emergency for the interregnum government and, in February 1645, led to a special bill giving saltpetre-men the authority to appropriate piles of droppings from pigeon houses.[64] Much later, Alfred Nobel made his fortune using nitrates imported from South America to manufacture dynamite.[65]

Various chemists took up Crookes' challenge and tried to fix nitrogen artificially from the air, for explosives, fertilisers or both. The process invented by Adolph Frank (1834–1916) and Nikodem Caro (1871–1935) converted calcium carbide and gaseous nitrogen to calcium cyanamide ('itrolime', $CaCN_2$) and carbon, and this was scaled up by industry to make inorganic nitrogen fertiliser. However, as with Crooke's technique, the process required too much electricity to be practicable at scale. The German chemist Fritz Haber (1868–1934) (see Figure 14.2(b)) then made the breakthrough in 1909, when he announced that he had succeeded in assimilating nitrogen into ammonia at high pressure and high temperature. The ammonia so generated could then relatively simply be oxidised to nitric acid for the generation of nitrates. The procedure was relatively energy efficient and suitable for large-scale production, which was duly developed by the industrialist Carl Bosch (1874–1940) – and henceforth came to be known as the 'Haber–Bosch process'.

As we all know, the European sabre rattling over continental and colonial resources led to World War I. Germany enacted the longstanding Schlieffen plan for rapidly overwhelming France on the west, followed by the equally rapid conquest of Russia on the east, thereby avoiding a war on two fronts. Once this failed, Germany found itself bogged down in trench warfare, and its supply of natural nitrates from Chile was cut off by the British Royal Navy, initially at the Battle of the Falkland Islands on 8 December 1914 and then by naval blockade. The Haber–Bosch process became critical for Germany continuing the prolonged and costly conflict, as it would not otherwise have had enough nitrogen for explosives to continue the war beyond 1915. By building a huge industrial complex that made available the nitrogen the military needed, Germany fought on for three further years of attrition.

Haber also contributed to the German war effort by his advocacy of gas warfare, starting with the use of chlorine gas at the second battle of Ypres in 1915.[66] After that, Haber's life began to unravel like a Greek tragedy. Within a week, his devastated pacifist wife Clara shot herself with his service revolver. Perpetuating the family tragedy, his son Herrmann committed suicide in 1946, and his daughter Claire followed on in 1949. She had been working as a chemist in the United States and made her fatal decision when she heard that her work on an antidote to chlorine gas had been superseded by work on the atom bomb. After the war, Haber went into mental decline.[67] The Treaty of Versailles required Germany to pay 50,000 tons of gold in reparations, and Haber tried in vain to develop a means to help his country by extracting gold from seawater. The technique worked, but there just wasn't enough gold in the water to make a difference. In 1933, he resigned his chair in chemistry at the Kaiser Wilhelm Institute in Berlin in protest at the sacking of Jewish colleagues by the Nazis. He moved briefly to England, where a fellowship was arranged by William Pope (1874–1940), a British counterpart in the development of WWI gases. Haber was appointed to a chair at the Daniel Sieff Institute in Palestine[e] but died from heart disease in the Hotel Euler in Basle on the way there.[68] Although he had converted to Christianity, Haber was Jewish by descent and was airbrushed out of Adolf Hitler's historical narrative.

Haber and Bosch received separate Nobel Prizes for Chemistry, Haber in 1918 and Bosch in 1931. Given the contribution to death and destruction, it seems odd that these should have come their way, and certainly many thought so at the time – particularly in Haber's case. Haber himself believed that killing the enemy with gas was justified, as it achieved the desired effect more rapidly than explosives. Be that as it may, Haber failed to mention either explosives or poison gas in his Nobel Prize acceptance lecture of June 1920, focusing instead on his research having

---

[e] Now, the Weizmann Institute of Science in Israel.

been driven by the impending crisis due to declining nitrogen reserves for food production and increasing food demand from an expanding industrialised population.

Nitrogen free from constraint

The Haber–Bosch process has enabled a massive expansion of nitrogen availability for agriculture, with 236 million metric tons of ammonia being snatched from the air across the world in 2021 alone (see Figure 14.2(c)).[69] It is for the impact on food production that the Haber–Bosch process has been described as the most important invention of all time, enabling more people to live and to live longer. This process has disconnected human populations from the constraints of the natural nitrogen cycle in which uric acid and other nitrogenous compounds released by animals play such a central role (see Figure 14.3) and has enabled the food needed for the world population to grow from 1.65 billion to 6 billion over the twentieth century, with a doubling since 1970. In the first six months of 2022, births around the world exceeded deaths by nearly 50 million. The world could now no longer feed itself without industrial nitrogen fixation to make fertiliser, as more land would be needed than exists without massive deforestation for equivalent yields from organic farming.[70] However, as Malthus pointed out, populations cannot expand forever, and the handle on agricultural productivity can only be turned so hard.[71] One major downside to the huge agro industrial effort that now supports much of the world's food production is the negative environmental impact of nitrogen fertilisers and food waste. These result in the release of nitrogen dioxide and stratospheric ozone-depleting nitrous oxide, the latter no longer Humphry Davy's laughing gas but now 7% of all greenhouse gases and one of the most damaging.[72] The huge successes achieved by humans stepping outside the natural balance between animals and plants are now offset by climate change and global ecological failure. This does not have the public's attention in nearly the same way as the 'carbon footprint'.[73]

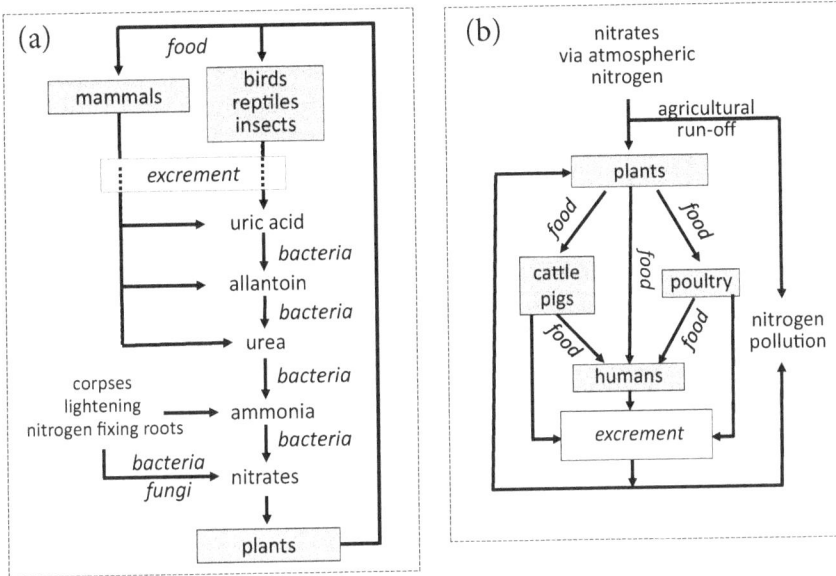

(a)
food
mammals
birds
reptiles
insects
excrement
uric acid
↓ bacteria
allantoin
↓ bacteria
urea
↓ bacteria
corpses
lightening
nitrogen fixing roots → ammonia
↓ bacteria
bacteria
fungi → nitrates
↓
plants

(b)
nitrates
via atmospheric
nitrogen
agricultural
run-off
plants
food / food
cattle
pigs
poultry
food
food
nitrogen
pollution
humans
food
food
excrement

Figure 14.3.

(a) The natural nitrogen cycle, in which nitrogen availability limits the ecosystem linking animal and plant populations. See Chapter 13 for more details.

(b) The ability to extract nitrogen from the air has bypassed the nitrogen cycle and allowed massively enhanced food supply and population growth. Limitations to indefinite growth include the accessibility of the energy needed for nitrogen extraction, water, agricultural space, climate change and, not least, political considerations.

The other major downside of industrial amounts of readily available nitrogen is commercial overproduction, historically encouraged in high-output nations by government subsidies. In the United States, for example, government farming subsidies for cash crops, such as corn (maize) at the expense of more diverse farm products have led to high energy sugars and vegetable fat being passed on to food manufacturers, as well as being fed to livestock for cheaper meat.[74] One consequence of this is the commercial trend towards marketing fattening low-profit/high-sales food and soft drinks high in sugars, salt and fats, to which those on low budgets naturally gravitate. Hence, the paradox that in both the US and Europe, obesity is closely related to poverty.[75] Agricultural surpluses attributable to government subsidies also result in the export of processed foods, or the commodities to make them, from high-income to middle- and low-income nations. Such processed foods are then priced to outcompete local produce and hence undermine local agriculture and contribute to rural migration to local cities and beyond. When James Parkinson wrote *Whilst the Honest Poor are Wanting Bread* in the wake of the French Revolution (see above), he could not have had in mind the offerings of today's multinational food and beverage industry, marketed not for health but for tastiness and profitability. Just as industrial agriculture has taken its major toll on the environment, the related food industry with which it is integrated is wreaking havoc on world health.

The Geography of Body Weight

Correlations exist at population levels across the world between increases in available food energy and increases in body weight.[76] The percentages of men and women globally who are overweight with a body mass index (BMI) of more than 25 have been estimated as increasing between 1980 and 2013 from 28.8% to 36.9% of men and from 29.8% to 38.0% of women.[77] Widespread obesity was first a modern problem in high-income countries, with, for example, a US Department of Health and Human Services survey of adults published in 2013 showing 1.8% underweight (BMI <18.5), 36.1% appropriate weight (BMI 18.5–25), 34.8% overweight (BMI 25–30) and 27.4% obese (BMI >30). Body weight in high-income countries is now settling at a high level; however, a ripple effect has spread obesity across the planet, aided and abetted by the commercial activities of multinational corporations encouraging the adoption of Westernised lifestyles and the purchase of Western foods and drinks.[78] Perhaps the most extreme example is the Micronesian island of Nauru, now stripped out by European companies of its valuable guano excrement and devoid of agricultural fertility. During its export heyday, the islanders became rich but, because of misadministration, now depend on income as a holding centre for refugees wishing to enter Australia.[79] The dietary transformation imposed by the need to import food, which is then compounded by poor nutritional choices and a lack of physical exercise, has led to Nauro being the most overweight country in the world, with an average BMI in both men and women of over 32 kg/m². In many middle- and low-income countries, there is now a double burden of malnutrition, with those who can afford relatively cheap imported high-energy food becoming obese and the very poor remaining undernourished and thin.[80]

Body weight and gout

A US population study found that a high body weight is the strongest predictor of a raised urate level, far exceeding the direct effects of specific lifestyle and environmental factors covered in Chapter 12.[81] Furthermore, the hyperuricaemia of obesity translates to an increased risk of gout.[82] One mechanism underlying this association is the shared direct effects of fructose on both uric acid and fat synthesis (see Chapter 12), but there is probably also another mechanism(s) by which a high body weight raises urate levels.[83] One suggestion is that fat tissue releases hypoxanthine, which is then converted to uric acid in the liver.[84]

Given all the knowledge we now have of causes and treatments, gout should now be an unusual disease. However, it is hardly surprising that the obesity pandemic is accompanied by an increasing prevalence of gout worldwide (see Figure 1.3), and what used to be a disease of the well-off has extended along with rising body weights to the poor. In the UK, the prevalence of gout has increased by 63.9% from 1997 to 2012, and in British Columbia, Canada, the age- and sex-standardised prevalence of gout increased by 59% from 2000 to 2012.[85] A similar increase has been seen by the United States National Health and Nutrition Examination Surveys of 2007–2008 and 2015–2016 when compared with the 1988–1994 interval.[86] As with obesity, there is global ripple, which will particularly affect genetically susceptible populations, such as in Oceania. In Nauru, for example, even in 1972, 63.6% of men had a high blood urate level (>0.42 mmol/l, or 7 mg/100 ml) and 6.9% suffered from clinical gout.[87] While detailed information on urate levels and gout in most middle- and low-income countries is lacking, these are likely to follow the obesity trend.[88]

Gout as a Sentinel of Non-Communicable Diseases

As is well known, obesity, and particularly abdominal obesity, is a major risk to health and longevity well beyond gout. It is a hub of non-communicable chronic diseases, including insulin resistance, type II diabetes, a high level of triglycerides in the blood and high blood pressure.[89] This constellation of symptoms is referred to as the 'metabolic syndrome', arguably a modern 'irregular Gout' (see Chapter 1). Each of the components is a separate risk factor for heart attacks and strokes, with their contributions summating.[90] Several studies have found that hyperuricaemia is associated with adverse cardiovascular outcomes, a good example being a prospective study of over 80,000 Austrian men in whom uric acid levels were significantly linked statistically to congestive heart failure and stroke.[91] Similarly, the urate level has been associated with the risk of death from coronary heart disease, congestive heart failure and stroke in post-menopausal women.[92] Having gout rather than just hyperuricaemia puts people at additional risk of cardiovascular disease, perhaps through the extra effects of inflammation.[93] For example, the release of inflammatory mediators from affected tissues may accelerate atherosclerosis, the chronic inflammatory process in the walls of arteries that results in heart attacks and strokes. In this, gout is no different from other inflammatory diseases, such as rheumatoid arthritis, inflammatory bowel disease and psoriasis.[94]

Thomas Sydenham may have had gout in mind when he famously said, 'A man is as old as his arteries'. It is certainly tempting to revive the old panic about uric acid (see Chapter 7) and put it at the centre of the metabolic syndrome, but unpicking cause and effect when there are so many possible interactions between the different components is fraught with difficulty in separating causation from correlation. The net influence of uric acid is complex, as, on the one hand, it may be a cardiovascular irritant and, on the other hand, it is an important protective antioxidant (see Chapter 13). Furthermore, the activity of xanthine oxidase, the enzyme that generates uric acid, may increase as a defensive strategy against stress, raising the possibility of 'reverse causation', whereby a raised urate level is a consequence rather than a cause of cardiovascular disease.[95] Current evidence is that uric acid does not itself actually cause disease other than gout. First, Mendelian randomisation studies (see Chapter 11) have mostly not shown that genetic variants that influence urate levels also directly impact cardiovascular disease risk.[96] Second, the results of clinical trials with the urate-lowering febuxostat have failed to show reductions in heart attacks and strokes, although there may be some benefit in preventing decline in kidney function.[97]

Final Reflections

As discussed at the start of this chapter, the food insecurity of the late eighteenth and early nineteenth centuries meant that the poor could not afford to have gout. This has all changed with the ready supply of food energy, enabled by the industrial extraction of nitrogen and the overriding of the ecological nitrogen cycle involving uric acid. Healthcare costs attributable to gout are considerable but obviously a tiny fraction of the total costs of the related non-communicable diseases.[98] These are taking up large parts of the national budgets of high-income countries, are politically weaponised to the point of swinging elections and are ultimately becoming unaffordable. Likewise, non-communicable chronic diseases now consume an increasing part of the budgets of middle- and low-income countries that can even less well afford to treat them. If there is one common denominator within this book, it is the failure to dissociate the fight against disease from business interests, be it those of the avaricious eighteenth-century physicians, the manufacturers of secret and pseudoscientific proprietary medicines, some modern pharmaceutical companies or industrial agriculture and food producers. The fact that these costs are maintained, and indeed continue to spiral, is to a large extent attributable to the financial interests of stakeholders in keeping them high. Power over world health has become concentrated in recent years in the hands of a relatively small number of giant transnational corporations with little interest in changing agricultural policies and providing high-quality, less-processed food and affordable pharmaceutical products, on the one hand, or in preventing rather than treating disease, on the other.[99] When linked to the difficulties of ageing populations, corporate commercial priorities with their grips on employment ecosystems and government policies present formidable challenges to global health.[100]

Glossary

Adenine: A *purine* and one of the four *nucleobases* that link up to form *nucleic acids*. Adenine is broken down in the body via *hypoxanthine* to *xanthine* and then to *uric acid*.

Afferent: Towards, as in a blood vessel taking blood towards a tissue. The opposite of *efferent*.

Alkaloid: A naturally occurring nitrogenous plant compound which has a *physiological* or *pharmacological* effect on animals.

Alkaptonuria: A rare genetic *inborn error of metabolism* with a *recessive inheritance*. The accumulation of homogentisic acid causes urine to turn brownish-black on standing.

Allantoin: A breakdown product resulting from the action of *uricase* on *uric acid*. It is so named after its discovery in the embryonic fluid of cows.

Allantoinase: The enzyme that digests *allantoin*. It is inactive in most mammals, in which the end-product of *purine* breakdown is therefore allantoin. Humans and hominid primates are exceptions among mammals, as the absence of *uricase* means they do not make allantoin, and they excrete its precursor *uric acid* instead.

Allele: A variant form of a specific *gene*. Mammals have a pair of alleles for each gene, one from each parent.

Note: Items in italics are explained in separate entries.

347

Allopurinol: A *purine* analogue that became the first drug to inhibit *xanthine oxidase* and hence reduce *uric acid* production.

Amino acids: Nitrogenous compounds that combine in sequence to form *proteins*. There are 22 amino acids encoded by *DNA*, with each amino acid derived from a unique *codon* of three *nucleobases*.

Ammonia: A simple organic molecule consisting of one nitrogen and three hydrogen atoms. It acts as the link in the *nitrogen cycle* between the breakdown of *nitrogenous* compounds in animal waste and their synthesis in plant tissues. Two molecules of ammonia derive from one of *urea*.

Amoeba: A single-cell lifeform with the capability to move and to engulf and ingest particulate matter for food.

Anion: An electrically negative-charged atom or molecule that can combine with a positively charged *cation*. An example is *urate*, which combines with positively charged hydrogen ions to form *uric acid*.

Anti-phospholipid antibodies: Autoantibodies that react with phospholipids in the body and which are linked to spontaneous miscarriages. They may occur on their own or be secondary to *systemic lupus erythematosus*.

Antioxidant: A compound that can inhibit *oxidation* and the generation of toxic *free radicals*. *Uric acid* is one of the most plentiful antioxidants in human blood.

Aqueous: Based on water.

Arthritis: Inflammation of a joint.

Atherosclerosis: A chronic inflammatory degeneration of large- and medium-sized arteries, characterised by the accumulation of oxidised lipids and other tissue debris. It is responsible for most heart attacks and strokes.

Autonomic nerves: The nerves that supply internal organs, glands and blood vessels.

Bacteria (singular: bacterium): A large domain of free-living single-cell organisms. Bacteria in soil are critical for processing *urea, uric acid* and other *nitrogenous* compounds for *nitrogen* uptake by plants. Some soil bacteria also fix nitrogen from the air and feed it into the *nitrogen cycle*. Bacteria form a major part of the mammalian intestinal *microbiome*. A minority of bacteria cause disease.

Beta radiation: A form of radioactivity of limited penetrance and danger, released, for example, by *tritium*.

Bone marrow: The central core within bones that makes red blood cells (erythrocytes) and most white blood cells (*leukocytes*).

Bowman's capsule: The outer casing surrounding the *capillary* tufts of kidney *glomeruli*. It drains into kidney *tubules*.

Bright's disease: A old term describing *protein* in the urine combined with *dropsy*. It was first described by Richard Bright (1789–1858), who realised that it signified kidney disease. Most of Bright's cases would have been due to *inflammation* in *kidney glomeruli* (glomerulonephritis).

Capillary: The smallest type of blood vessel, typically connecting small arteries (arterioles) with small veins (venules). The transfer of nutrients and oxygen from blood into the tissues predominantly takes place through the walls of capillaries. *Leukocytes* emigrate mostly downstream of capillaries through the walls of *post-capillary venules*.

Cartesian: Derived from the philosophy of René Descartes; for our purposes, it is indicative of a rational mathematical approach to understanding the body.

Cation: An electrically positive-charged atom or molecule that can combine with a negatively charged *anion*. Both hydrogen (H^+) and sodium (Na^+) are *cations* and can combine with urate, an organic *anion*.

Cell: The basic unit of life. During evolution, simple single-cell lifeforms developed into multi-cellular entities in which groups of cells perform both general functions and specialised functions related to the particular tissues in which they are situated. For example, the epithelial cells that line kidney *tubules* are specialised at transporting *urate* and other *anions* across the tubule wall, resulting in reabsorption or secretion out of or into urine depending on how *distal* the site on the tubule is from the *glomerulus*.

Cholesterol: A natural steroid-like substance that is needed for cell integrity. A high blood level of cholesterol is linked to *atherosclerosis*.

Chromosome: A long strand of *DNA*. Human cells have 46 chromosomes, of which 23 come from each parent.

Cloaca: A shared outlet for the urinary, intestinal and genital tracts found in birds and reptiles. It concentrates urinary *uric acid* prior to defaecation.

Clyster: An old term for an enema.

Codon: Three *nucleobases* within the *DNA* or messenger *RNA* sequence that encode a specific *amino acid* for *protein* synthesis.

Connective tissue: Fibrous material that provides structure to body tissues.

Consumption: An old term for chronic lung disease. Many cases of consumption would have been due to tuberculosis.

Corpuscle: A loosely defined old term that included blood *cells*.

Crystal: A homogeneous solid with a geometry particular to the specific substance.

Cutis: Skin.

Cyclodextrin: Compounds derived from the digestion of starch and widely used in chemical engineering.

Cyclooxygenase: An enzyme involved in the synthesis of *prostaglandins*.

Cytosine: A pyrimidine *nucleobase*.

Diploid: Having two sets of *chromosomes*, one from each parent.

Distal: Away from. Opposite of *proximal*.

Divalent: Able to combine with two other atoms. For example, *urate* is divalent and combines with two hydrogen atoms to form *uric acid* or with one hydrogen and one sodium atom to form *monosodium urate*.

DNA (deoxyribonucleic acid): A *nucleic acid*. The building blocks of DNA are the two purines *adenine* and *guanine* and the two pyrimidines *thymine* and *cytosine*. The order of their sequence in the DNA polymer provides the *genetic code* that becomes transcribed into messenger *RNA*, which in turn is translated into *protein*.

Dominant gene: In genetics, if the *allele* from one parent is dominant and the allele from the other parent is *recessive*, the trait encoded by the dominant allele will be expressed preferentially in the offspring.

Dropsy: An old term for *oedema*.

Efferent: Away from, as in a blood vessel taking blood away from a tissue. The opposite of *afferent*.

Empiric: An ambiguous term meaning either experimental or unorthodox.

Endogenous: Within the body.

Enzyme: A molecule that accelerates a chemical reaction. Most enzymes are *proteins*.

Epigenetic: An intracellular mechanism for varied heritability not involving differences in a *DNA* sequence.

Ester: A chemical compound produced by a reaction between an acid and an alcohol.

Excretion: Elimination from the body.

Febuxostat: A drug that inhibits *xanthine oxidase* and hence reduces *uric acid* production.

Fixed air: An old term for carbon dioxide.

Free radicals: Unstable atoms that can damage tissue. They are often a product of *oxidation* reactions.

Gene: The unit of inheritance. By and large, a gene encodes a *protein*.

Genetic code: The precise sequence of *nucleobases* in *DNA* or *RNA* that lead to the synthesis of the string of *amino acids* that make a specific *protein*. Each amino acid within a protein is encoded by a *codon* of three nucleobases within the DNA sequence.

Genetics: The science of heredity and its variability.

Genome: The entire set of *genes*.

Genome–wide association study (GWAS): A study linking genetic variability across the whole *genome* to a given characteristic.

Genotype: The two *alleles* of a *gene*.

Glomerulus (plural: glomeruli): A network or 'tuft' of *capillaries* in the *kidney* that filters water and some *solutes* from blood into kidney *tubules*.

Guanine: A *purine* compound and one of the four *nucleobases* that form *nucleic acids*, such as *DNA* and *RNA*.

Guano: A natural deposit formed from animal excrement and remains with high levels of nitrogen and other substances.

Haploid: Having one set of chromosomes.

Hypertension: High blood pressure.

Hyperuricaemia: A high level of monosodium urate in the blood.

Hypouricaemia: A low level of monosodium urate in the blood.

Hypoxanthine: A purine generated by the breakdown of *adenine*. In turn, it is converted to *xanthine* and then *uric acid*.

Inborn error of metabolism: A term introduced by Archibald Garrod (1857–1936) to describe an inherited metabolic abnormality caused by the variation of a single *gene*.

Inflammasome: A complex of proteins within cells that is responsible for the release of *interleukin-1 beta*.

Inflammation: A tissue response to injury. Classically, inflammation is demonstrated by swelling, redness, warmth and pain, as in an acute attack of gouty *arthritis*.

Innate immunology: The science of the workings of the immune system that are inherited and inbuilt and do not depend on sensitisation.

Interleukin-1 beta (IL-1β): A chemical signal that accelerates inflammation.

Ketone: An organic compound derived from the breakdown of fat.

Kidney: The organ that makes urine.

Kidney tubules: The tubes through which urine flows from the *glomeruli* to the *ureter*.

Laudanum: A tincture of opium in alcohol.

Leukocyte: A general term for white blood cells, including neutrophils, monocytes and lymphocytes.

Lithaemia: An old term for hyperuricaemia.

Lithia water: Water supposedly or actually containing lithium.

Lithiated soda: An old term for monosodium urate. Not to be confused with soda water with added lithium.

Lithic acid: An old term for uric acid.

Lithium: An element that amongst other things can combine with *urate* to form a compound with greater solubility than *monosodium urate*.

Macrophage: A *phagocyte* that may be resident in tissues or differentiate from a blood *monocyte*. There are various types of macrophages, which have different functions in *inflammation*. Some macrophages ingest *monosodium urate crystals* without perpetuating inflammation and may be important for the spontaneous resolution of an acute gout attack.

Major histocompatibility complex (MHC): A group of highly variable *genes* that make a major contribution to immune recognition and affect whether or not a tissue graft or an organ transplant from one individual to another is accepted. MHC variability also affects propensity to specific diseases and side-effects from drugs.

Malpighian body: The filtering apparatus of the kidney, being composed of a *glomerulus* surrounded by *Bownan's capsule*.

Manhattan plot: A way of presenting the results of a *genome-wide association study (GWAS)*. Genes are lined up horizontally on the *x*-axis, and the probability of each being linked to the object of the study (e.g. a disease or a laboratory variable) vertically on the *y*-axis. A horizontal bar is usually included to indicate whether the probability for a particular gene achieves statistical significance.

Microbiome: The mass of bacteria and other microorganisms that live internally within body cavities. The intestinal microbiome is the most studied and has recently been recognised to have a role in processing uric acid within the bowel.

Microtubule: A dynamic polymeric tubular structure composed of tubulin subunits.

Mitosis: A form of cell division involving chromosome duplication and resulting in two offspring cells which are identical to the parent cell.

Monocyte: A type of *leukocyte* that engulfs unwanted particles through *phagocytosis* and releases chemical signals that promote inflammation. The naked *monosodium urate crystal* is one such particle, and *interleukin-1 beta* is one such chemical signal.

Monogenic: A trait (or disease) governed by a single gene *allele*.

Monosodium urate: A urate *anion* combined with one hydrogen and one sodium *cation*. This is the form in which urate is found in solution in blood and other body fluids and is what crystallises in gout.

Neutrophil: The most numerous type of blood *leukocyte*. Interaction of neutrophils with *monosodium urate crystals* plays a major role in triggering acute gouty inflammation.

Nitrogen: An element required for the growth and function of biological tissues, either plant or animal.

Nitrogen cycle: The life cycle through which nitrogen passes from plants to animals and back to plants. Uric acid is a major component, taking nitrogen from birds, reptiles, insects and, to a lesser extent, mammals to soil bacteria, which digest it for uptake by plants.

Nitrogenase: An enzyme in soil *bacteria* that can 'fix' *nitrogen* in the air and convert it into organic compounds for plant growth.

Nitrogenous: Nitrogen-rich.

Nucleic acid: Polymers of *nucleobases* that carry *genetic code*. Nucleic acids are found in every self-sustaining lifeform.

Nucleobase: Nitrogen-rich compounds that act as the building blocks of *nucleic acids*. The nucleobases in *DNA* are *adenine, guanine, thymine* and *cytosine*. They are the same in RNA, except that uracil is used rather than *thymine*.

Oedema: Accumulation of fluid, commonly demonstrated by swollen ankles. It has a number of possible causes, including loss of protein through the kidneys and heart failure.

356 The Gout: A Medical Microcosm in a Changing World

Ornithine–urea cycle: A set of biochemical reactions that shunts *nitrogen* derived from *protein* degradation into soluble *urea*. It is an important means by which multicellular organisms avoid surplus nitrogen accumulating in toxic *ammonia*. In mammals, 95% of nitrogen in the urine is derived from the ornithine-urea cycle.

Osmosis: Movement of water towards a higher concentration. An example is water being pulled by urea into urine.

Oxidation: Addition of an oxygen atom to a molecule, as in the conversion of *xanthine* into *uric acid* by *xanthine oxidase*. Also used conventionally for the loss of a hydrogen atom, as in the conversion of *uric acid* into *allantoin* initiated by *uricase* (aka urate oxidase).

Oxypurinol: A metabolite derived from the action of *xanthine oxidase* on *allopurinol*. Oxypurinol then inhibits the ability of xanthine oxidase to generate *uric acid*.

Parkinson's disease: A neurodegenerative condition characterised by slow movement and a tremor.

Pathological: Induced by disease.

Peristalsis: The rhythmic contraction of the bowel that moves its contents along.

pH: An acid-alkali index. A pH of 7 is neutral. Reducing below 7 is increasingly acidic, and increasing above 7 is increasingly alkaline.

Phagocyte: A cell that can eat up an external particle or cell. Examples of cells that can phagocytose monosodium urate crystals are neutrophils, monocytes and macrophages.

Phagocytosis: The process of engulfment and internalisation of particulate material by a cell. One such particle is the monosodium urate crystal.

Pharmacological: Drug-induced.

Phenotype: The observable result of genetic combination. An offspring will have the phenotype determined by a dominant gene if both parents pass on a dominant variant or if one passes on a dominant and the other a recessive variant. Both parents need to pass on the recessive variant for the offspring to have the recessive phenotype.

Physiological: The normal function of the body.

Polygenic: The consequence of variations in more than one *gene*. The genetic contribution to *monosodium urate* levels in humans is polygenic.

Polyploid: Having more than the *diploid* quota of chromosomes.

Post-capillary venules: The small veins that capillaries pass blood into.

Probiotics: Live bacteria or yeasts that are taken to improve the microbiome.

Prodrug: A drug that needs to be converted into the active form once within the body. An example is azathioprine, which is inert until it is converted internally into the active 6-mercaptopurine.

Prostaglandins: A group of lipid compounds that have physiological hormone-like effects and which play a major role in the amplification of inflammation.

Protein: A nitrogen-rich macromolecule composed of one or more chains of *amino acids*. They perform multiple structural and functional roles in the body, including acting as *enzymes*.

Proximal: Near. Opposite of *distal*.

Pseudogene: Non-functional segments of DNA that have the appearance of genes. Many pseudogenes are the vestigial remnants of genes that ceased to be actively expressed at some point during species evolution. *Uricase* is a pseudogene in humans and hominid primates.

Purine: A theoretical nitrogen-rich entity that is the structural common denominator of a family of compounds, including *adenine*, *guanine*, *hypoxanthine, xanthine* and *uric acid*. Purine does not actually exist as such. *Caffeine* is also a purine.

Pus: The creamy fluid within an abscess composed in large part of dead *leukocytes*.

Recessive inheritance: In genetics, if the *allele* from one parent is recessive and the allele from the other parent is *dominant*, the trait encoded by the recessive allele will fail to be expressed in the offspring.

Rheumatic fever: The systemic illness due to a throat infection with a particular strain of streptococcal bacteria. It involves *Sydenham's chorea*, acute *arthritis* and injury to the heart, among other things.

Rheumatic gout: An old term for chronic arthritis, that would mostly be what we now call rheumatoid arthritis.

Rheumatism: A very general and largely old term to cover musculoskeletal maladies. Acute rheumatism would mainly have been what we now call *rheumatic fever*.

RNA (ribonucleic acid): A *nucleic acid* that performs various intermediary roles translating *DNA* into *protein*. The building blocks are the two *purines adenine* and *guanine* and the two pyrimidines *uracyl* (rather than *thymine* in DNA) and *cytosine*. Messenger RNA is one form of RNA, which serves to take the genetic code from DNA to the machinery in the cell that translates it into protein.

Serum: The fluid left after the solid matter is removed from a blood clot. Biochemical measurements on the blood (e.g. of monosodium urate) are commonly made on serum.

Solubility: A measure of the ability to be dissolved in a fluid, for example in water.

Solute: A substance or substances dissolved in a fluid.

Solute transporter channel: A large molecule inserted in a cell membrane that acts as a pathway for specific *solute* transportation into or out of the *cell*. *Monosodium urate* relies on a number of different solute transporter channels for passage into and out of different organs, and their genetic variation accounts for much of the heritable component of the blood urate level.

Spectroscopy: The identification of chemicals or the measurement of their concentrations by the wavelength or intensity of their colour or mass.

Spindles: The *microtubule* structures that pull duplicated *chromosomes* apart during *mitosis*.

Stable isotope: A non-radioactive variant of an atom that can be distinguished through mass spectrometry. Stable isotopes of *nitrogen* and carbon were incorporated into *amino acids* to track their fate in the body and to map the amino acid origin of the different atoms that make up *uric acid*.

Suppuration: *Pus* formation, as in an abscess.

Sydenham's chorea: The involuntary movements of the face and limbs occurring in rheumatic fever. Named after Thomas Sydenham.

Systemic lupus erythematosus (SLE): An autoimmune disease that causes widespread inflammation. It can cause a telltale 'butterfly' facial rash.

Tetraploid: Having four sets of *chromosomes*, two from each parent.

Theelin: An old term for oestrone, a female sex hormone.

Therapeutic index: Difference between the therapeutic and toxic doses of a drug. A low therapeutic index signifies a drug more likely to lead to side-effects.

Thymine: A pyrimidine *nucleobase*.

Tophus (plural: tophi): A white concretion of monosodium urate crystals deposited in tissues in chronic *hyperuricaemia*.

Transforming growth factor beta (TGFβ): A hormone-like compound with numerous functions. It is released by some macrophages in response to contact with monosodium urate crystals and acts to help suppress on-going inflammation.

Triploid: Having three sets of chromosomes, one from one parent and two from the other. Typically created by crossing diploid and tetraploid parents. Triploids are usually sterile.

Tritium: An isotope of hydrogen (^{3}H) and a *beta radiation* emitter. It is used in chemistry laboratories to label molecules and track their reaction products.

Tubules: See *kidney tubules*.

Tubulin: A protein that polymerises to form *microtubules*.

Urate: The *anion* component of uric acid and monosodium urate.

Urate of soda: *Monosodium urate*.

Urate oxidase: See *uricase*.

Urea: A *nitrogenous* compound that provides 95% of *nitrogen* excretion in mammalian urine, being the endpoint of *protein* breakdown within the body.

Urease: An enzyme that converts urea into ammonia, as in the processing of urea in mammalian urine by soil bacteria during the nitrogen cycle. Mammals and other land-living animals typically do not have urease.

Ureter: The tube that passes urine from the kidney to the bladder.

Uric acid: A purine created from *xanthine* by the action of *xanthine oxidase*. A uric acid molecule is formed by the combination of two hydrogen *cations* with one *urate anion*. Uric acid does not exist in blood and other body fluids, as one of the hydrogens is replaced by a sodium cation to form *monosodium urate*. Monosodium urate may convert to uric acid in urine if it is acidic, potentially resulting in uric acid crystallisation and the formation of uric acid stones.

Uricase: The first of three enzymes needed to convert *uric acid* into *allantoin*. Also known as urate oxidase.

Xanthine: A purine generated by the breakdown of *guanine* or *hypoxanthine*. In turn, it is converted by *xanthine oxidase* into *uric acid*.

Xanthine oxidase: The enzyme that converts *hypoxanthine* to *xanthine* and xanthine to *uric acid*. It is the molecular target of *allopurinol* and *febuxostat*. It is also known as xanthine oxidoreductase.

Endnotes

The endnotes for this book are available online as supplementary material. For more detail, please visit: https://www.worldscientific.com/worldscibooks/10.1142/q0486#t=suppl.

Index